Parent-Child Interaction Therapy with Toddlers

Emma I. Girard • Nancy M. Wallace
Jane R. Kohlhoff • Susan S. J. Morgan
Cheryl B. McNeil

Parent-Child Interaction Therapy with Toddlers

Improving Attachment and Emotion Regulation

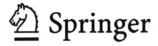 Springer

Emma I. Girard
School of Medicine
University of California, Riverside
Riverside, CA, USA

Nancy M. Wallace
Johns Hopkins School of Medicine
Kennedy Krieger Institute
Baltimore, MD, USA

Jane R. Kohlhoff
School of Psychiatry
University of New South Wales
Randwick, NSW, Australia

Susan S. J. Morgan
Karitane Toddler Clinic
Carramar, NSW, Australia

Karitane Toddler Clinic
Carramar, NSW, Australia

Cheryl B. McNeil
Department of Psychology
West Virginia University
Morgantown, WV, USA

ISBN 978-3-319-93250-7   ISBN 978-3-319-93251-4   (eBook)
https://doi.org/10.1007/978-3-319-93251-4

Library of Congress Control Number: 2018945224

This Springer imprint is published by the registered company Springer Nature Switzerland AG
The registered company address is: Gewerbestrasse 11, 6330 Cham, Switzerland

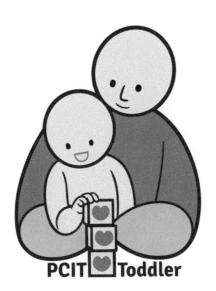

Emma:

Tony, my sincere gratitude for your profound love, support, and belief in me, ELE!

Holly, daughter of my heart, and Daniel, for inspiration to give entirely.

Thank you, Mom and Pop, for continuously leading by example.

Nancy, Jane, Sue, and Cheryl –

For the incredible discussions, weekend date nights, enthusiasm, and commitment.

Nancy:

I would like to thank my family and specifically, my parents, Bonnie and Richard, and brother, Christopher, for their ongoing support and encouragement of my professional endeavors. I would also like to thank Dr. Cheryl McNeil for her unwavering guidance as my advisor and beyond. Her vision for the future of children's mental health is inspiring and will continue to cause ripple effects in the field for years to come. Finally, I would like to thank my colleagues and patients at the Kennedy Krieger Institute for helping me to grow as a person and a professional.

Jane:
Thank you to Sue, who has walked this journey with me; Karitane, for all the opportunities you have provided; and most of all to Oscar, Reuben and my PK, who teach, support and inspire me every day.

Sue:
I would like to thank my family John, Tara, Claire, and Lianna for their continuing support and love with my passion in early intervention.

As well as the dedication of Jane Kohlhoff and the Karitane Toddler Clinic team.

Cheryl:
I am grateful for this amazing team of passionate and dedicated clinicians who worked long weekend and evening hours to share their successful therapy techniques with the world. I also want to acknowledge my mentor, Dr. Sheila Eyberg, who gifted all of us with PCIT and employed her impeccable science to fuel and refine the model. Thanks also to Dan, Danny, and Will who are eternally supportive of my efforts to expand the reach and effectiveness of PCIT.

Preface

Children are our most precious national resource; they are the living messages to a time we will not see, and new scientific advances are showing the crucial importance of the foundation years and especially the first 1001 days from conception until age 2 as a springboard for neuro-cognitive development, life-long health and well-being and socio-economic success.

National Scientific Council on the Developing Child, Harvard University. From AIMH website

Each and every human begins life biologically connected to its mother. Although such biological attachment is no longer present following birth, the trajectory of the human life continues to be intricately influenced by those who care for and raise babies into the adults that will go on to affect the world. The monumental responsibility afforded to parents and caregivers can be one of enormous joy and stress. When young children exhibit behavior difficulties, typical parenting stressors are exacerbated. Without support and intervention, such difficulties may negatively affect the parent-child attachment. Furthermore, such behavior concerns are likely to persist into the school-age years and contribute to social and emotional difficulties (Briggs-Gowan, Carter, Bosson-Heenan, Guyer, & Horwitz, 2006).

This book was written to guide mental health professionals in the practice of assisting parents in understanding and intervening in the earliest stages of toddlers' behavior difficulties through the implementation of a novel intervention entitled *Parent-Child Interaction Therapy with Toddlers: Improving Attachment and Emotion Regulation (PCIT-T)*. By helping parents connect with their toddlers and support their ongoing emotional development, the PCIT-T intervention is further expected to help prevent maladaptive behavioral trajectories and build the foundation for a strong, secure parent-child relationship.

Parent-Child Interaction Therapy with Toddlers is an early intervention program that involves coaching parents while they interact with their 12- to 24-month-old children. Adapting the play therapy and compliance training procedures of PCIT, parents are coded and coached in the use of therapeutic parenting practices proven to decrease problematic behaviors, improve children's language, and encourage young children to follow directions. Parents over-practice the "PRIDE" skills (praise, reflection, imitation, description, and enjoyment) until they display mastery. Numerous controlled studies have shown that these PRIDE skills improve children's behavior problems to within normal limits.

This PCIT-T book describes novel components for the special needs of toddlers, including specific procedures for promoting the attachment relationship and emotion regulation in both the caregivers and children. Central to the model is the understanding that difficult behaviors in toddlers are a sign of emotion dysregulation rather than deliberate defiance. It is with the assistance of a nurturing and sensitive caregiver that the child's capacity to manage emotion develops. The CARES model of PCIT-T involves coaching parents to come in, assist, reassure, validate emotions, and soothe when the toddlers experience the "big emotions" that are characteristic of this age range. Parents also are coached in their own set of adult CARES skills designed to promote relaxation and positive self-talk during stressful parenting situations. Finally, PCIT-T includes an adapted parent-directed interaction in which children learn to follow directions through a tell-show-try again-guide procedure and labeled praise for listening. Presenting referral concerns include the following:

- Tantrums
- Aggression (e.g., hitting, biting, pinching)
- Fussiness (e.g., screaming, whining, crying)
- Anger, frustration, head-banging
- Attachment difficulties (e.g., rejection of parent, difficult to comfort)
- Separation anxiety or withdrawal from parent
- Developmental concerns (e.g., autistic behaviors, language problems)
- Child abuse and neglect
- Parental stress (e.g., anxiety, dissatisfaction, difficulty coping, lack of confidence)

This book is divided into two major sections. The first section is comprised of ten chapters, each building upon the previous. In Chap. 1, a comprehensive overview of the theoretical underpinnings, empirical background, and program description are provided; thus, the rationale for PCIT-T is introduced in the context of an attachment and behavioral perspective. In Chap. 2, the core elements and primary treatment goals of PCIT-T are illustrated. In Chap. 3, the reader is guided through the background of and research support behind the development of PCIT. Chapter 4 illustrates the empirical evidence and application of PCIT to the toddler population prior to transitioning into the conceptualization of PCIT-T as an emotion regulation intervention for toddlers in Chap. 5. Chapter 6 discusses the use of behavior assessment throughout PCIT-T, while Chap. 7 includes details of toy selection and room set-up. Chapters 8 and 9 describe the skills used in the child-directed interaction (CDI-T) and parent-directed interaction (PDI-T) portions of PCIT-T, respectively. Lastly, concluding remarks and a summary of PCIT-T is presented along with necessary coaching considerations and training requirements reviewed in Chap. 10.

The second section provides therapists with a session-by-session guide complete with appendices of all materials necessary to implement PCIT-T with children and families. As such, it is recommended that consumers read the book in sequential order as section one provides clinicians with the information necessary to deliver PCIT-T with integrity and a thorough understanding of the background literature.

The PCIT-T model described in this book is based in large part on two initial research studies. The first, conducted by Kohlhoff and Morgan (2014) demonstrated initial support for an early version of the CDI phase of the PCIT-T model with evidence of decreased child behavior concerns. The second study was a waitlist-controlled trial and was nearing completion at the time of this book. Preliminary results of this study suggested notable improvements in child behavior concerns and parental emotional availability after just five weeks of intervention (Kohlhoff & Morgan, unpublished). In addition, 80% of children classified as having a disorganized attachment pattern prior to intervention shifted to an organized attachment pattern according to the Strange Situation Procedure (SSP; Ainsworth, Blehar, Waters, & Wall, 1978) when assessed 6 months later. Although these infant attachment results were demonstrated with a small group of 14 families and should be interpreted with caution, such findings remain promising, particularly given that few empirical studies of analogous interventions have resulted in similarly impressive outcomes. Currently, a randomized controlled trial is underway evaluating the relative effectiveness of PCIT-T in comparison to an established intervention (i.e. Circle of Security-Parenting) and waitlist control condition. Using a research-informed practice and practice-informed research model, results of ongoing clinical work and formal investigations will continue to influence the development of PCIT-T over time.

The five authors on this book are all applied, translational researchers who work directly with families in clinical practice. Fueled by our excitement about the encouraging outcomes obtained with treated families using the PCIT-T model, we wrote this book to make this approach widely accessible to early interventionists and policy makers. Outcomes of PCIT-T include enhancing parent-child attachment relationships, maximizing children's developmental outcomes, encouraging warmth and sensitivity in caregivers, improving emotion regulation for all family members, and decreasing children's behavior problems. We are inspired by the words from a PCIT-T parent who said, *"I came for help with my son's behavior. I didn't realize I would also develop a closer relationship with him."* It is our hope that PCIT-T provides therapists with helpful tools for improving children's behavior and family relationships, thereby creating bright futures for countless toddlers around the world.

Riverside, CA, USA   Emma I. Girard
Baltimore, MD, USA   Nancy M. Wallace
Randwick, NSW, Australia   Jane R. Kohlhoff
Carramar, NSW, Australia   Susan S. J. Morgan
Morgantown, WV, USA   Cheryl B. McNeil

Acknowledgments

The authors would like to acknowledge Sheila Eyberg, Ph.D., for her original creation of and pioneering work in the field of Parent-Child Interaction Therapy and Daniel M. Bagner, Ph.D. for his work in the field of behavioral parent training with infants. The authors would also like to highlight the visionary work of Anthony Urquiza, Ph.D.; Susan G. Timmer, Ph.D.; Jean McGrath, Ph.D.; Nancy Zebell, Ph. D.; Dawn Blacker, Ph.D.; and Stefan C. Dombrowski, Ph.D., for their creation of the Parent-Child Attunement Therapy adaptation. They also are grateful to Beth Troutman for her dedication to the integration of attachment theory and PCIT and Bryanne Barnett AM, an Australian pioneer in the field of attachment and early intervention and a personal mentor to many.

Additionally, the authors would like to thank Karen Willcocks for her assistance in creating the toddler emotion handout for this intervention, and Charlotte Hartle, graphic artist, for encapsulating the meaning of PCIT-Toddlers into a warm and heartfelt logo. Additionally, Charlotte Hartle designed the visual transition cards and graphic icons used with caregiver handouts presented in PCIT-T.

The authors would also like to thank Trista E. Vonada, LCSW, and the therapists at AWARE Inc. in Montana, for their thoughts and feedback in the early stages of protocol development, as well as the families, staff, and administration at the Karitane Toddler Clinic in Sydney, Australia, and the Preschool 0-5 Programs within the Riverside University Health System-Behavioral Health who have helped to inform the development of this model, especially P. Chris Home, LCSW, and Anna Loza, LCSW, for their leadership, advocacy, and emphasizing the importance of early intervention.

It is our hope that the creation of this book provides mental health experts with the tools and direction necessary to deliver effective treatment to children in their most formative developmental years while empowering caregivers to build a basis of connection, trust, consistency, and warmth that will profoundly shape children's lives and trajectories for years to come.

Contents

About the Authors

Emma I. Girard, PsyD is a Licensed Clinical Psychologist in private practice, Health Sciences Assistant Clinical Professor of Psychiatry with the University of California Riverside, School of Medicine and Senior Clinical Psychologist with Riverside University Health System-Behavioral Health: Preschool 0-5 Programs. As one of only twenty Master Trainers worldwide certified by Parent-Child Interaction Therapy, International (PCIT-I), she disseminates PCIT to 16 treatment labs throughout Riverside County California. Additionally, she has trained over 200 clinicians while simultaneously serving as a Training Partner with the University of California Davis PCIT Training Center. Dr. Girard also disseminates Teacher-Child Interaction Training (TCIT), an adaptation PCIT for school educators. She and her team in Riverside received the "Bright Idea Award" from the Ash Center for Democratic Governance and Innovation at Harvard Kennedy in 2015 for their Mobile Prevention and Early Intervention (MPEI) program. Dr. Girard is an international and avid presenter in PCIT disseminating information to locations including Australia, Japan, Portugal, Itlay, Germany, and throughout the United States. Her passion to bring clinical experience from community-based organizations to inform research has produced significant collaborations with the Clinical Child Program at West Virginia University and the University of California Davis PCIT Training Center. These aforementioned collaborations have examined the impact of barriers to treatment, outcomes of emotion regulation on the caregiver and child, homework completion rates and use of incentives as a clinical motivator, as well as testing a PCIT clinician training model. When not at the office, Dr. Girard loves travel, dance, and a glowing campfire outdoors.

Jane R. Kohlhoff, Phd is a Clinical Psychologist and Senior Lecturer in the School of Psychiatry, University of New South Wales, Australia. Dr. Kohlhoff works in collaboration with a leading Australian parenting organization, Karitane, to conduct clinically oriented and translational research in the areas of perinatal, infant, and early childhood mental health. She has particular interest in attachment theory and clinical applications, disruptive behaviors in early childhood, early interventions to improve outcomes for vulnerable and marginalized families, and the roles of early environmental and biological factors in the intergenerational transmission of poor parenting and psychological outcomes. She has a strong commitment to attachment-based research and clinical work and is an accredited Strange Situation Procedure and Adult Attachment Interviewer coder. Dr. Kohlhoff is currently leading programs of research evaluating the efficacy of the PCIT-Toddlers intervention. She has published widely, presented at numerous international conferences, and received a number of awards including the 2017 Ingham Institute Early Career Researcher Award and a prestigious 2017 Australian Research Council Discovery Early Career Award.

Cheryl B. McNeil, Phd is a Professor of Psychology in the Clinical Child program at West Virginia University. Her clinical and research interests are focused on program development and evaluation, specifically with regard to abusive parenting practices and managing the disruptive behaviors of young children in both the home and school settings. Dr. McNeil has co-authored several books (e.g., *Parent-Child Interaction Therapy: Second Edition, Short-Term Play Therapy for Disruptive Children, Handbook of PCIT for Children with ASD*), a continuing education package (*Working with Oppositional Defiant Disorder in Children*), a classroom management program (*The Tough Class Discipline Kit*), and a Psychotherapy DVD for the American Psychological Association (*Parent-Child Interaction Therapy*). She has a line of research studies examining the efficacy of Parent-Child Interaction Therapy and Teacher-Child Interaction Training across a variety of settings and populations, including over 100 research articles and chapters related to the importance of intervening early with young children displaying disruptive behaviors. Dr. McNeil is a master trainer for PCIT International and has disseminated PCIT to agencies and therapists in many states and countries, including Norway, New Zealand, Australia, Taiwan, Hong Kong, and South Korea.

Susan S. J. Morgan, MMH is a Registered Nurse/Midwife who graduated in 1977 and supplemented her qualifications with a Masters in Perinatal Infant Mental Health in 2010. She has worked extensively with parents, infants, and toddlers for over 30 years and has a strong dedication to working within an attachment-based framework. She currently manages the Karitane Toddler Clinic in Sydney, Australia's only community-based PCIT clinic. Susan is a Level II Trainer with PCIT International and passionate supporter of the model. Susan's clinical and research interests have focused on early intervention and work with children under the age of 2 years. As the primary clinician and trainer on the initial studies of PCIT-Toddler, she served as the key informant for the methods in this book. Susan has published a number of peer-reviewed journal articles and has presented at international forums. Her aspiration is for all families to have the opportunity to learn how to care for their children in a safe and sensitive way so the children can reach their full potential.

Nancy M. Wallace, Phd is a postdoctoral fellow at the Kennedy Krieger Institute, Johns Hopkins School of Medicine. She recently completed her doctoral studies in clinical child psychology at West Virginia University under the mentorship of Dr. Cheryl McNeil. Her primary research interests include the dissemination and implementation of evidence-based parent-training approaches used to treat children with disruptive behavior difficulties. Specifically, Dr. Wallace is committed to the research and clinical practice of Parent-Child Interaction Therapy (PCIT). She has co-authored over three dozen publications, book chapters, encyclopedia articles, manuals, and professional presentations related to PCIT including a dissertation examining the implementation of a PCIT-based program in a community-based wraparound system. Clinically, Dr. Wallace holds certification as a Level I trainer for PCIT International and is especially passionate about the practice and adaptation of PCIT for populations including toddlers, children with selective mutism, and in-home community-based wraparound services. For her commitment to research and community service, Dr. Wallace has won numerous awards including the 2015 Dr. Stephen Boggs Graduate Student PCIT Research Excellence Award by PCIT International and a grant by the Community Engagement Grant Program at West Virginia University to support her dissertation work.

Part I
Parent-Child Interaction Therapy with Toddlers: Theoretical Underpinnings, Empirical Background and Program Description

Chapter 1
An Introduction to PCIT-T: Integrating Attachment and Behavioral Principles

"Jack," aged 19 months, was referred to the PCIT-T clinic by his pediatrician for assistance with tantrums and aggressive behaviors. Strategies implemented by the pediatrician had not led to any change in his behavior.

Jack attended the initial assessment session with his mother, "Rachel," and his father, "Tim." On assessment, Rachel and Tim said that Jack had been displaying difficult behaviors on a daily basis including biting, hitting, hair pulling, head banging, and tantrums (screaming, flopping to the floor, and swinging his head back and forth during the tantrum). His anger and frustration appeared to be primarily directed at his mother and older brothers. Rachel and Tim did not know the origin of the challenging behaviors and found it difficult to identify any specific triggers or precipitants for Jack's aggression and tantrums.

Rachel expressed significant distress at being unable to manage Jack's behavior and said that she did not feel emotionally connected to him. She said that she often became overwhelmed and struggled to control Jack's behavior, especially in public places. Rachel and Tim had both spanked Jack in the past and had also tried to ignore his behaviors, but they had not found these techniques to be effective. Discouraged and frustrated, the parents reached out for help and were referred for PCIT-T.

© Springer Nature Switzerland AG 2018
E. I. Girard et al., *Parent-Child Interaction Therapy with Toddlers*,
https://doi.org/10.1007/978-3-319-93251-4_1

PCIT-T Overview

PCIT-T is an adaptation of PCIT that aims to meet the unique developmental needs of toddlers aged 12–24 months presenting with behavioral concerns. The original PCIT program, developed by Dr. Sheila Eyberg, is a well-established intervention for 2–7-year-old children referred for a range of behavioral and emotional problems. PCIT is unique in that it uses in vivo coding and coaching techniques (typically conducted from behind a one-way mirror using a Bluetooth device) to help parents reach mastery on a set of play therapy and discipline skills proven to increase child compliance, decrease aggression, and improve the parent-child relationship. Coaching behind the one-way mirror is ideal to allow the parent-toddler dyad to be the sole focus within the treatment room and to provide to the toddler the experience that all interaction is coming directly from their parent without the distraction of the clinician in the room. From a research perspective, PCIT has demonstrated some of the largest effect sizes in the realm of children's mental health (e.g., $d = 1.65$; Ward, Theule, & Cheung, 2016) and is considered a best practice for the treatment of trauma associated with child maltreatment, defiance, aggression, hyperactivity, and anxiety in preschoolers (McNeil & Hembree-Kigin, 2010).

PCIT-T incorporates the basic structure of PCIT, including coding, coaching, mastery criteria, play therapy techniques, and compliance training, while adapting the program to fit the developmental needs of younger children between 12 and 24 months of age. Like the original PCIT program, PCIT-T has theoretical underpinnings in attachment and social learning theories. A distinguishing feature of PCIT-T, however, is the strong emphasis on recognizing and supporting the toddler's emotional and physical needs. The PCIT-T model stands in direct contrast to the concept that it is possible to "spoil a baby," a notion that may have contributed to some parents' apprehension about meeting young children's needs out of fear of doing damage. Rather, the PCIT-T model assumes that the parent's (or caregiver's) role is to meet the needs of the infant or toddler and in doing so to help the child develop the skills and capacities that will optimize social-emotional functioning across the life span (Tronick & Beeghly, 2011).

Emotion regulation, defined as "the processes by which individuals influence which emotions they have, when they have them, and how they experience and express these emotions" (Gross, 1998, p. 275), is a foundational component of the developmental process. Therefore, the three key assumptions of PCIT-T are (i) that disruptive behaviors in children aged less than 2 years are signs of emotional dysregulation rather than deliberate, intentional attention-seeking acts or as components of a coercive parent-child interaction cycle (as is typically the case with older children referred for treatment of behavior problems) (Patterson, 1982), (ii) that the early parent-child attachment relationship is the vehicle through which capacities for emotion and behavior regulation emerge and are consolidated (Sroufe, 1995), and (iii) that toddlers have the capacity to learn how to listen to instructions and that parents can play a key role in helping this skill to develop (McNeil & Hembree-Kigin, 2010). The emphasis of PCIT-T is therefore on improving the quality of the parent-child relationship with a particular focus on improving the parent's sensitivity to the child's needs and his/her capacity to support the child's emotion regulation. In this context, parental sensitivity is defined as the ability to correctly recognize and identify the child's emotional needs and then to respond appropriately and in a timely way. Withdrawing attention and implementing negative consequences for inappropriate behavior are included but adapted to better fit the developmental needs of the young population. Importantly, rather than selectively ignoring or using the standard PCIT parent-directed interaction time-out sequence, in PCIT-T the parent is coached to interpret disruptive child behavior as a sign that the child is experiencing a "big" emotion and that they need the parent's support to be able to manage it.

Young children typically cannot verbalize emotional states, and it can be difficult for an onlooker to ascertain when a "big emotion" is present for a child. Our operational definition for a big emotion is a change in the child's behavior, often associated with crying, whining, or yelling, that appears to indicate an overwhelming emotional reaction that is difficult to control. The big emotion often includes anger and frustration. It grows in intensity and involves either a strong need for immediate access to the parent or a blatant rejection of the parent (e.g., pushing away the parent). Big emotions involve a change of facial expression and vocalizations beyond simple crying, whining, or yelling and may include physical aggression, destruction of property, flailing, arching the back, falling to the floor, and even unusual behaviors such as turning to the corner, freezing, withdrawing from the parent, or self-injury.

Through repeated experiences with a sensitive and responsive parent who is able to successfully support the toddler's emotion regulation, the child gradually requires less "scaffolding" and develops the ability to regulate emotions independently. Many parents have poor emotion regulation skills themselves and struggle to be sensitive and responsive to the child when he/she is emotionally dysregulated. An important part of the PCIT-T intervention is therefore the parallel processes, whereby the therapist provides a "secure base" for the parent – recognizing and validating the parent's feelings and then coaching them in real time to remain calm and develop their own emotion regulation skills – while at the same time teaching the parent to do the same for his or her child. Thereby, the toddler is taught to follow directions and accept parental guidance and limits.

PCIT-T differs from traditional PCIT with respect to limit setting. A guided compliance approach, as used in applied behavior analysis, is included instead of time-out for repeated noncompliance to a direct command. Commands appropriate for children in this developmental range are specified in this manual. To accommodate the attention span of toddlers, session time is shorter than typical PCIT with older children. Finally, the Eyberg Child Behavior Inventory (ECBI; Eyberg & Pincus, 1999) is not used as a measure of behavior change due to its lack of validity for children below 2 years of age. Additionally, the ECBI provides information related to conduct problems without information related to a child's social and emotional health. Therefore, the Devereux Early Childhood Assessment (DECA; LeBuffe & Naglieri, 2003; LeBuffe & Naglieri, 2009; Mackrain, LeBuffe, & Powell, 2007) or the Brief Infant Toddler Social Emotional Assessment (BITSEA; Briggs-Gowan, Carter, Bosson-Heenan, Guyer, & Horwitz, 2006) and supplemental measures such as the Parenting Stress Index – Short Form (PSI-SF; Abidin, 1995) are used to monitor change at specific points throughout treatment.

Enhancements to the typical PCIT procedure are included in an effort to tailor the intervention to a toddler's unique developmental needs. Such enhancements include a specified protocol for transition between the therapist's waiting room and the therapy room; the use of a soft, calming tone of voice during interaction; as well as increased awareness and use of physical touch (e.g., back rubs). The importance of enjoyment in the caregiver-child interaction is enhanced by the use of caregiver's animated expressions of delight including clapping, positive facial expressions characteristic of an upbeat affect, and gleeful noises during play. Finally, a particular focus is placed on the use of developmentally appropriate toys, the therapy room layout, and the need for routine. In an effort to account for the developmental needs of toddlers, handouts meant to provide psychoeducational information on sleep, nutrition, developmental milestones, teething, and the influence of illness on toddler behavior are provided. Given the level of intervention, the estimated length of treatment ranges from 12 to 18 sessions. It is recommended that caregivers attend sessions with their toddler twice per week to assist with experiential learning due to the short recall cycle for toddlers and their need for consistent frequent exposure to assist in learning. There is also a wide variation seen in the number of sessions needed based on the child's developmental needs and acquisition of skills of the caregiver and consistency of attendance. Due to the age of the toddler, missing one session creates great delays, and illness in not uncommon in this age group. Therefore, it is important to make up missed sessions as soon as possible. We hope that this book may help to fulfill a previously existing gap in the clinical literature while also aiding clinicians in the effective treatment of this complex, yet highly rewarding, group of young children and their families.

The Incorporation of an Attachment Perspective

In contrast to a purely behavioral approach, PCIT-T incorporates an attachment perspective, critical for effective work with very young children and their caregivers. A purely behavioral conceptualization indicates that the parent-child relationship is strengthened with increasing levels of positive reinforcement within the relationship. An attachment perspective, in contrast, suggests that the relationship is strengthened as the parent becomes increasingly self-reflective and attuned to the child's needs and subsequently able to respond to the child's needs sensitively, thereby decreasing conflict and increasing flow and mutual reciprocity within the dyadic interaction (Troutman, 2015). As suggested by Stern (1995), the parent-child relationship is an interdependent "system," and so changes in any one element of the system (e.g., parental behavior, parental representations of the child) invariably lead to changes in other elements (e.g., child behavior, the child's representations of the parent). As both the parent and child begin to experience mutual enjoyment, each learns tolerance and patience, and the parent's working model of the child begins to shift to a more positive understanding (Troutman, 2015). As a result of these changes within the parent, the child's working model of the parent also changes, and the child comes to expect sensitive responsiveness, safety, and nurturance. Although quantitative skill mastery, critical to the success of PCIT, is retained within PCIT-T, attachment-focused aspects of the program are not as clearly defined and measured. Instead, attachment-based skills are developed throughout the course of the program and may change as the child grows. Ultimately, it is hypothesized that attachment-based skills will help the caregiver and therapy team to become intricately in tune with the child's cues, emotions, and behaviors, critical to a healthy parent-child relationship and therapeutic success. Such work falls in line with the theoretical and empirical basis of attachment-focused work. Therefore, it is critical that PCIT-T therapists are familiar with terms and concepts foundational to the attachment literature.

Empirical conceptualization of attachment theory formally originated with the work of John Bowlby (1951; 1958; 1969; 1973; 1980; 1988) who, after initially studying the impact of maternal withdrawal on personality development, went on to develop the "Ethological Theory of Attachment." Bowlby argued for the existence of the attachment behavioral system, suggesting that attachment behaviors are fundamental to human survival as they increase the likelihood of an infant gaining proximity to their caregiver and, in turn, the chances of infant's needs being met. Bowlby's pioneering work informed Mary Ainsworth's original conceptualization of the three primary attachment styles derived from her observations of infant-mother interactions in Uganda (Ainsworth, 1967) and Baltimore, Maryland (Ainsworth, Blehar, Waters, & Wall, 1978). From such observations, Ainsworth developed a structured observation paradigm, entitled the Strange Situation Procedure (SSP; Ainsworth et al., 1978), whereby a 12-month-old infant is systematically separated from and reunified with his or her caregiver. In Ainsworth's original SSP coding system, infants were classified as having one of three patterns of behavioral organization, namely, secure, avoidant, and resistant/ambivalent. A securely attached infant typically demonstrates distress or other cues indicative of yearning for his or her parent on separation, and is likely to seek comfort, often in the form of physical contact with the parent prior to returning to play on reunification. It has been observed that parents of securely attached children are typically sensitive and responsive and provide support to the child's cues and emotions (Fearon & Belsky, 2016). In contrast, an infant with an avoidant style of attachment is unlikely to show distress following separation (despite feeling distressed) and tends to avoid engagement with the parent upon reunification. Infants with this attachment pattern are likely to have experienced a withdrawn or disengaged caregiver. Finally, an infant with a resistant/ambivalent style of attachment may appear upset with the parent and inconsistently indicate a need for contact with and distance from the parent, or they may show helpless, passive behavior. Upon reunification, the infant may exhibit signs of distress while maintaining attention on the parent. These children have often experienced inconsistent parenting whereby the parent may have demonstrated intense and intrusive behavior followed by disengagement (Fearon & Belsky, 2016). In 1986, Main and Solomon recognized the need for a fourth category, which they labeled "disorganized/disoriented." A disorganized/disoriented attachment pattern is characterized by odd, disorganized behaviors that are frequently presented in contrast to one another in the presence of the parent (Main & Solomon, 1986). An infant with a disorganized attachment style may, for example, clearly seek contact with the parent but then show indications of fear or disengagement such as freezing. Most often, the disorganized attachment patterns have been found to occur with infants who have experienced interactions with a parent who was either frightening or seemingly frightened (Main & Hesse, 1990).

The infant attachment patterns described by Ainsworth et al. (1978) and Main and Solomon (1986) have been replicated across a wide range of samples (Fearon & Belsky, 2016). The clinical applicability and relevance of attachment theory and the SSP have been seen in evidence from meta-analytic and longitudinal studies showing infant attachment security to be predicted by higher levels of caregiver sensitivity (Fearon & Belsky, 2016), particularly when in combination with increased parental capacity for "reflective functioning," that is, the caregiver's capacity to understand themselves and others in terms of mental states such as feelings, wishes, and beliefs – a capacity that enables the parent to think about the inner world of the child and to understand and respond contingently and sensitively to his/her emotional and physical needs (Fonagy & Target, 1997; Slade, 2005). Further support and clinical relevance come from the large body of evidence showing insecure and disorganized infant attachment patterns to be associated with significantly higher risk of externalizing disorders in childhood (Fearon, Bakermans-Kranenburg, Van IJzendoorn, Lapsley, & Roisman, 2010) and psychopathology across the life span (Sroufe, 2005).

The goal of PCIT-T is to teach parents the skills that optimize secure attachment patterns in children. An attachment-based conceptualization of parent-child relationships and child behavior problems will also influence the PCIT-T therapist's understanding of the child's behaviors and needs. Many of the behaviors that a parent may view at the start of treatment as "problematic" or "difficult" may indeed be better understood as outward expressions of an underlying insecure or disorganized attachment pattern. For example, a toddler who in coaching sessions is frequently upset or angry with the parent, but who also indicates a need for contact (e.g., displays clingy, whining behavior), may have an ambivalent attachment style. As outlined in Table 1.1, this child may have experienced parenting characterized by a mix of intrusiveness and disengagement, and so coaching should focus on helping the parent to be consistently emotionally and physically available for the child. This way, the child will come to learn that the parent is a secure base and source of comfort and support when needed. Alternatively, a toddler with an avoidant attachment style may seem self-sufficient and unaffected by the parent's engagement or disengagement during play sessions but may regularly tantrum when challenges arise with toys or when he doesn't get his own way. This toddler would benefit from parental coaching focused on enhancing the parent's ability to actively and sensitively support the child's emotion regulation rather than avoiding or withdrawing when the child is upset. Finally, parents of children with disorganized attachment styles may benefit from coaching that challenges their feelings of helplessness and disapproval of, and disconnection from, the child.

Table 1.1 Attachment styles, notable features of the child, and associated parenting characteristics

Child attachment style	Notable features of the child	Associated parenting characteristics
Secure	Distress upon separation; Cues indicate yearning for parent, upon separation; Seek comfort (e.g., physical contact) with the parent prior to returning to play upon reunification	Sensitive, responsive style; Provides appropriate support in response to the child's cues and emotions
Avoidant	Fails to demonstrate negative emotion following separation; Continues to apathetically avoid engagement by failing to interact with the parent throughout interactions	Withdrawn or disengaged throughout interaction with the child; Discourages interaction with the child
Resistant/ ambivalent	Appears upset with the parent or help-lessly passive; Inconsistently indicates a need for contact with and distance from parent; May exhibit signs of distress while maintaining attention on the parent during reunification	Inconsistent parenting style; Parent may have demonstrated intense and intrusive behavior followed by disengagement
Disorganized	Seeks contact with the parent followed by indications of fear or disengagement with odd behaviors such as freezing; Behaviors are contradictory to one another and may occur in quick succession	Most often occurs with infants who have experienced frightening or frightened parenting

It is important to remember that parents also bring their own relationship and attachment histories to the parent-child relationship. In addition to attending to the toddler's attachment pattern and the impact of these on behavior, the PCIT-T therapist must therefore also be aware and sensitive to the attachment characteristics and needs of the parent. The Adult Attachment Interview (AAI; Hesse, 2008) is a semi-structured interview designed to assess an adult's state of mind regarding past and current attachment relationships. The interview identifies four categories of adult attachment state of mind, secure-autonomous, insecure-preoccupied, insecure-dismissing, and disorganized/disoriented, categories that are useful to be mindful of when working with parents within an attachment-based framework. Detailed discussions about the characteristic features of the AAI classifications (Hesse, 2008), their impact on engagement in parenting and other therapeutic programs (Heinicke et al., 2006; Teti et al., 2008), and the intergenerational transmission of attachment insecurity as measured using the AAI and SSP can be found elsewhere (Van IJzendoorn, 1995). But in relation to PCIT and PCIT-T, as alluded to by Troutman (2015), parents with an insecure attachment style may struggle to manage their own emotions in the face of the child's difficult emotions. They may be less eager or indeed able to incorporate the therapist's suggestions or have difficulty accepting critical feedback. Behavioral skills coaching in PCIT-T therefore functions as a primary mechanism of behavior change, but it also must be adapted to the suit the unique combination of the toddler's attachment characteristics as well as that of their parents.

PCIT-T coaches are therefore tasked with helping parents to increase their reflective functioning capacities so that they can correctly identify, interpret, and respond sensitively to their children's emotional and attachment needs. The PCIT-T therapist must view the parent-child dyad through an attachment-focused lens, considering and being sensitive to the parent's own attachment characteristics and associated interpretations of the child's emotions and behavior. Through a parallel process, the PCIT-T therapist provides emotional support and scaffolding for the parent, as he or she learns to do this for the child.

Following from such attachment-based conceptualization, behavioral skills coaching in PCIT-T functions not only as a primary mechanism of behavior change but must also adapt to the unique combinations of toddler's attachment characteristics as well as that of their parents. As coaches, therapists are tasked with helping parents respond appropriately to their children while also understanding the parent's interpretation of such emotions and behavior through an attachment-focused lens (Troutman, 2015).

Attachment and Behaviorally Based Components of PCIT-T

Intervention targeting a toddler-aged population fosters a unique opportunity to integrate attachment and behavioral theory. The current treatment approach is grounded in evidence-based treatment and previous research in the fields of child development, attachment, and behaviorism. Therefore, components of both models are combined in an effort to best serve the developmental needs of toddlers and their parents. Table 1.2 details the core elements of PCIT-T within both the attachment and behavioral perspectives.

"Getting in Early": PCIT-T as an Early Intervention Program

Disruptive behaviors commencing in early childhood, if left untreated, can be the start of a trajectory toward poor outcomes across the life span including social-emotional concerns, academic problems, and conduct disorders in middle childhood and adolescence (Campbell, 1995; Campbell, Spieker, Burchinal, Poe, & Network, 2006), as well as psychopathology and antisocial behavior in adulthood (Campbell, 1995; Campbell, Shaw, & Gilliom, 2000; Kim-Cohen et al., 2003). Given the significant personal and societal costs associated with disruptive behaviors in early childhood, the urgency of providing effective intervention is clear. Encouragingly, research

Table 1.2 Core elements of PCIT-T within the attachment and behavioral perspectives

Attachment components	Behavioral components

• Parallel process (coach as secure base for parent so parent is secure base for child)
• Coach as an external source of emotion regulation for parents – scaffolding emotion regulation skills until they have the capacity to independently implement such skills
• Reflection, understanding and recognition of the impact of the parent's emotions and behavior on the child's emotions and behavior
• The CARES model (implementation for the child by the parent and parent use of self-CARES)
   o Emotion dysregulation, rather than negative attention-seeking, perspective of difficult behavior
   o Emphasis on meeting toddler's emotional and behavioral needs rather than correcting misbehavior
   o Emphasis on coaching the parent to correctly identify the child's needs and cues and to respond sensitively
• Setup of the room to promote positive and harmonious interaction and promote exploration and parent as secure base
• Focus on psychoeducation about the child's developmental stage including emotional needs and the importance of the parent-child relationship in child's emotional and behavioral regulation
	• PRIDE skills as primary positive reinforcement schedule
	• Learning-based immediate coaching, feedback, coding throughout intervention
	• Parent-directed interaction-toddler (PDI-T)-guided compliance procedure – a scaffolding technique to facilitate learning
	• Repetitive use of the PDI-T listening language to assist with and reinforce language formation and retention
	• Under-reaction technique as a minor limit-setting procedure – withdrawal of attention
	• Use of physical cues and pointing in PDI-T
	   Aggression consequence procedure – limit setting
	• Constant assessment – Dyadic Parent-Child Interaction Coding System (DPICS) observation, coding of CARES, coding of emotion labels, graphing, mastery criteria
	• Emphasis on modeling/imitation
	• Homework practice to reinforce skill acquisition

suggests that by effectively intervening in the very early years of life, trajectories toward poor outcomes can be altered before coercive parent-child behaviors and interactions become entrenched. Converging evidence indicates that treatments should be provided as early as possible, i.e., in infancy and the toddler years, to provide the best opportunity for success (All Party Parliamentary Group for Conception to Age 2 - First 1001 Days, 2015). The known plasticity of neurobiological systems during the infancy and toddler periods highlights this period as a key time for intervention and prevention (Fox & Hane, 2008; National Scientific Council on the Developing Child, 2007; Schore, 2001).

Meta-analytic evidence suggests that interventions that are brief, have a behavioral component, and enhance parental sensitivity are most likely to bring about lasting improvements in children's attachment security and thus capacity for learning, as well as positive improvements in behavioral and emotion regulation (Bakermans-Kranenburg, Van Ijzendoorn, & Juffer, 2003). Such interventions are also likely to buffer the effects of early-life adversity on brain functioning (Glaser, 2000; Gunnar, 1998).

It is well known that prenatal, birth, medical status, and early-life experiences have a striking influence on toddlers given their young developmental age. Limited expressive and receptive language abilities, developing cognitive understanding, and strong biological needs (e.g., sleep, hunger, health, attention, comfort) powerfully influence a toddler's ability to regulate his or her emotions. Therefore, a caregiver's consistent and predictable responses to a toddler's behavioral and emotional cues powerfully shape the toddler's attachment to his or her caregiver(s). In turn, such responses inform a toddler's understanding of the world as a safe or unsafe environment.

In addition, decades of landmark child development research has clearly demonstrated the need for and potential impact of parent-focused programs in the lives of their young children. Notably, in 1995, researchers Betty Hart and Todd Risley published a book entitled, "Meaningful Differences in the Everyday Experiences of Young American Children." The text described work conducted over the course of 2.5 years in which the language-based home environments of 42 children from welfare, working class, and professional backgrounds were intricately examined. Research began when the children were just 7 months old. After transcribing 1300 h of adult conversation spoken in front of the child, results were staggering. By the age of 4, the children from welfare backgrounds had heard 13 million words, while children from professional families had heard 45 million words, a difference of 32 million words. The types of words that children from each group heard also differed. Children from welfare backgrounds heard more negatively framed speech and were more likely to hear the same words repeated over and over as compared to professional children who were more likely to be exposed to a larger variety of words. As the children entered school, the significant differences in the language-based quality of their home environments became pronounced in their academic abilities – their vocabularies and reading abilities in particular (Hart & Risley, 1995; Leffel & Suskind, 2013). For the over 13.2 million children living in poverty in America in 2016, the impact of early language handicap upon children's futures is profound. As time continues, such disparities are likely to widen, placing children from low SES homes at further risk of academic impairment and, ultimately, financial difficulty (Leffel & Suskind, 2013). Despite the unfortunate picture painted by such statistics, parent-focused interventions in the early lives of such children hold the potential for effective, sustainable, positive change that may effactually counter the effects of such environmental deficits while helping to position children on a more secure developmental path. The speech and language literature has utilized parent-based approaches with young children suffering from early language delays through interventions such as Hanen Centre's "It Takes Two to Talk" (The Hanen Centre, 2018). The 6–8-h group-based approach is led by a speech-language pathologist with the primary goal of helping parents to become more responsive to their child's language and behavior. Therefore, techniques include skills in each of the three following categories: child-oriented behaviors, interaction-promoting strategies, and language modeling.

More recently, Hart and Risley's findings inspired the creation of Project ASPIRE (ASPIRE, 2013) and the Thirty Million Words Project (Center for Early Learning and Public Health, 2018) aimed at enhancing the language-based environments of young children from low socioeconomic environments, specifically, those with hearing loss and typically developing children, respectively (Leffel & Suskind, 2013). The parent-focused interventions focus on increasing parental skills, knowledge, and sense of efficacy while positioning parents as the primary change agent via Dyadic Parent-Child Interactions. The belief that parents have a profound opportunity to positively impact children's brain development is infused throughout both interventions. Additionally, therapists provide parents with qualitative feedback on videotaped interactions in verbal discussion. Skills focus on teaching parents skills to increase the quality and quantity of their communication with their child. Aptly named "the three Ts," such skills include tuning in, talking more, and taking turns (Dubner, 2015). Specifically, "tuning in" teaches parents to allow children to lead the interaction and speak to them in an upbeat, enthusiastic voice. "Talking more" focuses on using a wide variety of vocabulary words while speaking often and about topics that are relevant to the parent and child's actions in the moment. Finally, "taking turns" prompts parents to respond to children's sounds and verbalizations. Quantitative feedback is provided via an electronic device (Language Environment Analysis (LENA)) designed to quantify spoken words as well as the quality of the language environment (e.g., television versus spoken language). Using such technology, the parent and therapist are able to set language-based goals and track progress.

Results of a randomized research trial examining the effects of the Thirty Million Words Project showed that the intervention significantly increased parents' understanding of their impact on children's language development as well as the frequency and variability of language spoken to the child. Additionally, results indicated that the frequency of children's speech also increased following intervention, lending evidence to the enrichment of the early language environment. Unfortunately, the effects of such change were not maintained post-intervention, speaking to the need for additional supports and structures to enhance the sustainability of intervention efforts (Leffel & Suskind, 2013). PCIT-T includes several skills aimed at enhancing the language environment of the toddler, such as reflections (which promote active listening) and behavioral descriptions (which increase parental talk), with the hope of decreasing language disparities in at-risk families (Tempel, Wagner, & McNeil, 2009).

A critical need for effective, evidence-based, and parent-focused programs aimed at improving children's long-term developmental and mental health outcomes clearly exists. Implementation of the PCIT-T treatment package has the potential to have a sustained and widespread impact on children via two primary avenues: (1) PCIT-T may be used as an early intervention tool with children already experiencing behavior difficulties (e.g., hyperactivity, aggression, tantrums, difficulty settling), language delays, problematic attachment styles, separation anxiety, autistic behaviors, and/or trauma histories (e.g., child maltreatment, witnessing family violence), and (2) PCIT-T may also be used as a *prevention* tool applied to children at risk for such issues in an effort to minimize or thwart their ongoing effects.

References

Abidin, R. R. (1995). *Parenting stress index: Professional manual* (3rd ed.). Lutz, FL: Psychological Assessment Resources, Inc.

Ainsworth, M., Blehar, M. C., Waters, E., & Wall, S. N. (1978). *Patterns of attachment: assessed in the strange situation and at home*. Hillsdale, NJ: Erlbaum.

Ainsworth, M. D. S. (1967). *Infancy in Uganda: Infant care and the growth of love*. Baltimore, MD: Johns Hopkins University Press.

All Party Parliamentary Group for Conception to Age 2 - First 1001 Days. (2015). *Building Great Britons*. Retrieved from www.1001criticaldays.co.uk:

ASPIRE, P. (2013). *The power of parent talk*. Retrieved from project-aspire.org

Bakermans-Kranenburg, M. J., Van Ijzendoorn, M. H., & Juffer, F. (2003). Less is more: Meta-analyses of sensitivity and attachment interventions in early childhood. *Psychological Bulletin, 129*(2), 195.

Briggs-Gowan, M. J., Carter, A. S., Bosson-Heenan, J., Guyer, A. E., & Horwitz, S. M. (2006). Are infant-toddler social-emotional and behavioral problems transient? *Journal of the American Academy of Child and Adolescent Psychiatry, 45*, 849–858.

Campbell, S. B. (1995). Behavior problems in preschool children: A review of recent research. *Journal of Child Psychology and Psychiatry, 36*(1), 113–149.

Campbell, S. B., Shaw, D. S., & Gilliom, M. (2000). Early externalizing behavior problems: Toddlers and preschoolers at risk for later maladjustment. *Development and Psychopathology, 12*, 467–488.

Campbell, S. B., Spieker, S., Burchinal, M., Poe, M. D., & Network, T. N. E. C. C. R. (2006). Trajectories of aggression from toddlerhood to age 9 predict academic and social functioning through age 12. *Journal of Child Psychology and Psychiatry, 47*(8), 791–800.

Center for Early Learning and Public Health. (2018). Retrieved from http://tmwcenter.uchicago.edu

Dubner, S. J. (Producer). (2015). *Does "Early Education" come way too late? a new Freakonomics radio podcast*. Retrieved from http://freakonomics.com/podcast/does-early-education-come-way-too-late-a-new-freakonomics-radio-podcast/

Eyberg, S., & Pincus, D. (1999). *Eyberg child behavior inventory and Sutter-Eyberg student behavior inventory*. Lutz, FL: Psychological Assessment Resources.

Fearon, R., Bakermans-Kranenburg, M. J., Van IJzendoorn, M. H., Lapsley, A. M., & Roisman, G. I. (2010). The significance of insecure attachment and disorganization in the development of children's externalizing behavior: a meta-analytic study. *Child Development, 81*(2), 435–456.

Fearon, R. M. P., & Belsky, J. (2016). Precursors of attachment security. In J. Cassidy & P. R. Shaver (Eds.), *Handbook of attachment: Theory, research, and clinical applications* (3rd ed., pp. 291–313). New York, NY: The Guilford Press.

Fonagy, P., & Target, M. (1997). Attachment and reflective function: Their role in self-organization. *Development and Psychopathology, 9*, 679–700.

Fox, N. A., & Hane, A. A. (2008). Studying the biology of human attachment. In J. Cassidy & P. R. Shaver (Eds.), *Handbook of attachment: Theory, research, and clinical applications* (pp. 217–240). New York, NY: The Guilford Press.

Glaser, D. (2000). Child abuse and neglect and the brain - a review. *Journal of Child Psychology and Psychiatry, 41*(1), 97–116.

Gross, J. J. (1998). The emerging field of emotion regulation: an integrative review. *Review of General Psychology, 2*(3), 271–299.

Gunnar, M. R. (1998). Quality of early care and buffering of neuroendocrine stress reactions: Potential effects on the developing human brain. *Preventative Medicine, 27*, 208–211.

Hart, B., & Risley, T. R. (1995). *Meaningful differences in the everyday experience of young American children*. Baltimore, MD: Brookes.

Heinicke, C. M., Goorsky, M., Levine, M., Ponce, V., Ruth, G., Silverman, M., & Sotelo, C. (2006). Pre- and postnatal antecedents of a home-visiting intervention and family developmental outcome. *Infant Mental Health Journal, 27*(1), 91–119.

Hesse, E. (2008). The adult attachment interview: Protocol, method of analysis, and empirical studies. In J. Cassidy & P. R. Shaver (Eds.), *Handbook of attachment: Theory, research, and clinical*. New York, NY: Guilford Press.

Kim-Cohen, J., Caspi, A., Moffitt, T. E., Harrington, H., Milne, B. J., & Poulton, R. (2003). Prior juvenile diagnoses in adults with mental disorder. *Archives of General Psychiatry, 60*, 709–717.

LeBuffe, P. A., & Naglieri, J. A. (2003). *The Devereux Early Childhood Assessment Clinical Form (DECA-C): A measure of behaviors related to risk and resilience in preschool children*. Lewisville, NC: Kaplan Press.

LeBuffe, P. A., & Naglieri, J. A. (2009). The Devereux Early Childhood Assessment (DECA): A measure of within-child protective factors in preschool children. *NHSA Dialog, 3*(1), 75–80.

Leffel, K., & Suskind, D. (2013). Parent-directed approaches to enrich the early language environments of children living in poverty. *Seminars in Speech and Language, 43*(4), 267–278.

Mackrain, M., LeBuffe, P., & Powell, G. (2007). *Devereux early childhood assessment infants and Toddlers*. Lewisville, NC: Kaplan Early Learning Company.

Main, M., & Hesse, E. (1990). Parents' unresolved traumatic experiences are related to infant disorganized attachment status: Is frightened and/or frightening parental behavior the linking mechanism? In M. Greenberg, D. Cicchetti, & E. M. Cummings (Eds.), *Attachment in the preschool years: Theory, research and intervention* (pp. 161–184). Chicago, IL: University of Chicago Press.

Main, M., & Solomon, J. (1986). Discovery of an insecure-disorganized/disoriented attachment pattern. In T. B. Brazelton & M. W. Yogman (Eds.), *Affective development in infancy* (pp. 95–124). Westport, CT: Ablex Publishing.

McNeil, C. B., & Hembree-Kigin, T. (2010). *Parent-child interaction therapy*. New York, NY: Springer.

National Scientific Council on the Developing Child. (2007). *The timing and quality of early experiences combine to shape brain architecture* (Working Paper #5). Retrieved from http://developingchild.harvard.edu/resources/reports_and_working_papers/working_papers/wp5/

Patterson, G. R. (1982). *Coercive family process*. Eugene, OR: Castalia.

Schore, A. (2001). Effects of a secure attachment relationship on right brain development, affect regulation, and infant mental health. *Infant Mental Health Journal, 22*(1-2), 7–66.

Slade, A. (2005). Parental reflective functioning: An introduction. *Attachment & Human Development, 7*(3), 269–281.

Sroufe, L. A. (1995). *Emotional development. The organization of emotional life in the early years*. Cambridge, UK: Cambridge University Press.

Sroufe, L. A. (2005). Attachment and development: A prospective, longitudinal study from birth to adulthood. *Attachment & Human Development, 7*(4), 349–367.

Stern, D. N. (1995). *The motherhood constellation: A unified view of parent-infant psychotherapy*. London, UK: Karnac books.

Tempel, A. B., Wagner, S. M., & McNeil, C. B. (2009). Parent-child interaction therapy and language facilitation: The role of parent-training on language development. *The Journal of Speech and Language Pathology – Applied Behavior Analysis, 3*(2-3), 216–232.

Teti, D. M., Killeen, L. A., Candelaria, M., Miller, W., Reiner Hess, C., & O'Connell, M. (2008). Adult attachment, parental commitment to early intervention, and developmental outcomes in an African American sample. In H. Steele & M. Steele (Eds.), *Clinical applications of the adult attachment interview* (pp. 126–153). New York, NY: The Guilford Press.

The Hanen Centre. (2018). *It takes two to talk: The Hanen program for parents*. Retrieved from http://www.hanen.org/helpful-info/research-summaries/it-takes-two-to-talk-research-summary.aspx

Tronick, E., & Beeghly, M. (2011). Infants' meaning-making and the development of mental health problems. *The American Psychologist, 66*(2), 107–119.

Troutman, B. (2015). *Integrating behaviorism and attachment theory in parent coaching*. New York, NY: Springer.

Van IJzendoorn, M. H. (1995). Adult attachment representations, parental responsiveness, and infant attachment: a meta-analysis on the predictive validity of the Adult Attachment Interview. *Psychological Bulletin, 117*(3), 387–403.

Ward, M. A., Theule, J., & Cheung, K. (2016). Parent–Child interaction therapy for child disruptive behaviour disorders: A meta-analysis. *Child & Youth Care Forum, 45*(5), 675–690.

Chapter 2
Core Elements and Treatment Goals of PCIT-T

Introduction

PCIT-T retains many of the core components of PCIT (outlined in Chap. 3) including in vivo coaching during parent-child play sessions and utilization of the child-directed interaction (CDI) phase in which parents are coached to increase the use of positive verbalizations and decrease the use of negative verbalizations during dyadic interactions with their child. However, the CDI phase in the current intervention will be entitled CDI-toddler (CDI-T) to differentiate it from standard CDI in PCIT. The PCIT-T intervention also comprises a number of unique features to meet the specific developmental needs of toddlers including increased emphasis on assessment and emotion regulation, ongoing consideration of child development, provision of parental education about typical toddler development, and parental coaching around implementation of an age-adapted parent-directed interaction-toddler (PDI-T) phase that focuses on teaching listening skills rather than implementing negative consequences for noncompliance. It should be noted that although the current program is intended for children between the ages of 12 and 24 chronological months of age, it may be applied to children slightly older (e.g., 26 months) or slightly younger (e.g., 11 months) based on the child's developmental level and corresponding need. If it is determined that a child has developmentally passed the PCIT-T range and behavior concerns perpetuate, standard PCIT may be considered.

Philosophy of Coaching in PCIT-T

Scientifically, the unique provision of live, moment-to-moment feedback during ongoing parent-child interactions is perhaps the most powerful element in PCIT, contributing to the large effect sizes often discussed in PCIT literature (Kaminski, Valle, Filene, & Boyle, 2008). As in standard PCIT, PCIT-T coaching occurs via a

© Springer Nature Switzerland AG 2018
E. I. Girard et al., *Parent-Child Interaction Therapy with Toddlers*,
https://doi.org/10.1007/978-3-319-93251-4_2

bug-in-the-ear Bluetooth or walkie-talkie device, while the therapist speaks to the parent from behind a one-way mirror. The setup is meant to simulate a realistic dyadic environment, whereby the parent and child may interact without the presence of the therapist. Furthermore, the technique enables parents to implement and practice skills learned in didactic discussion while experiencing their effects upon the child during real-time interactions. When emotional and behavioral difficulties arise, coaching provides the framework from which learning, and ultimately successful, resolution occurs. Apart from the scientific, technique-driven perspective of coaching as a critical change element of high-fidelity treatment implementation, effective coaching is a complex, carefully delivered therapeutic art. At its heart, coaching must remain positive and focused on building upon the strengths of the parent-child dyad while remaining focused on the central goal of skill acquisition.

Parents of toddlers are often particularly sensitive to remarks about and any perceived judgment of themselves as parents. Unlike parents of preschoolers, parents of toddlers have had less than 2 years to develop their identity as parents with their current child and to understand the temperment and needs of this child. During this time, parents of toddlers undergoing PCIT-T are likely to have experienced personal, child-focused, or dyadic disruptions that, in turn, may have contributed to the child's behavior, parents' sense of competence, and fragility of the current parent-child relationship. Such difficulties may include parent and/or child medical trauma (e.g., a complicated and/or especially painful birth experience), postnatal depression and/or anxiety, marital discord, child developmental delays, and a multitude of other potential individual factors. Given the child's young age, the effect of such events may still bring about raw emotion for the parent. Furthermore, the parent's own relationship with his or her parents and the effect of their parents' parenting style are likely to have a powerful impact upon themselves as a parent. The experience of having their own child may cause strong emotions regarding parenting beliefs and practices based on their past experiences and perceptions as a child. In addition, unlike preschoolers, toddlers' spoken language abilities are often limited, if not nonexistent. Such lack of communication can contribute to feelings of confusion, frustration, and fear particularly during moments in which big emotions are being expressed and the parent is unsure of the child's needs or how to properly attend to them. Therefore, a primary goal of each PCIT-T session is to help parents feel more confident and competent in their role as parents.

Given the emotional fragility of the parent-toddler dyad, coaches must use their intuition and empathetic, therapeutic nature to guide the parent toward or away from specific skills or behaviors during dyadic interactions. Recognition of the parent and child's mood is critical as the coach must balance the needs of the dyad with the intensity of the scheduled session. For example, the therapist may determine that the child is in need of a snack prior to the start of the session. In other circumstances, the therapist may decide not to awaken a sleeping toddler in order to discuss important information with the parent. The coach must model calm, confident, warm leadership in the midst of parental and child distress. It is likely that such traits will be internalized and transferred from therapist to parent to child through the parallel attachment process. Given the powerful impact of coaching on children and their parents, coaches must thoughtfully choose their words and tone of voice during coaching so as to only model language and display a demeanor that they wish parents to replicate. Specifically, as is central to the spirit of PCIT-T, only positive language should be utilized. When corrections must be made, they should be phrased as constructive suggestions, without the words no, don't, stop, quit, or not. To avoid negative feedback, one of the most common techniques during coaching is the use of tactical ignoring. In this technique, the coach (1) ignores a parent mistake (e.g., asking a question, giving, a command, or using negative talk), (2) waits for the first time a parent engages in a behavior that is the exact opposite of the mistake, and (3) provides a labeled praise for the opposite behavior (e.g., "nice job saying that as a statement that time," "I like how you are following her lead now," "great job using your positive words now"). Furthermore, for each correction or command, a coach should provide the parent with five positive remarks or praise statements to compensate for the potential negative emotional impact of such statements.

The novel observation and coaching modality may cause parents to feel initially uncomfortable and/or anxious. If therapists sense parental anxiety regarding the coaching format, brief discussion should occur whereby therapists provide empathy while also explaining the purpose behind the modality. The therapist may also elicit the parents' fears behind the approach. In many cases, the supportive, strengths-based feedback is likely to quell such fears and disconfirm cognitive distortions related to the model.

Similarly, new coaches may also experience anxiety prior to implementation of the novel approach. Over time, ongoing practice and observation of clear therapeutic benefit is likely to diffuse such fears. Additionally, core coaching skills such as providing feedback to parents after each verbalization help to create rhythm within the coaching sequence. Such frequent feedback should be brief and telegraphic in nature, often limited to 3–7 words so as not to interrupt the momentum of the interaction. Basic coaching entails praising parents' use of PCIT-T skills just following their implementation. Higher-order coaching statements extend such skill-based praise to include psychoeducational knowledge of the effect of the statement upon the child (e.g., "That reflection helps his speech." "Those behavioral descriptions keep her on task.") or observations of the effect of skills on the child or the dyadic interaction ("He is sharing more because of your imitation." "She put another one away because you praised her for cleaning up." "Your hug makes him happy."). Longer explanations and discussions may occur following the session or over the phone in between sessions. When interactions are going well, coaching remains highly positive, gentle, and skill-focused. When difficult circumstances arise or parents begin to engage in negative interactions, coaching may become more directive in an effort to re-engage the dyad in calm, effective skill implementation (e.g., "Pick up that toy and start pushing the buttons. Nice redirection."). The concept of scaffolding or challenging an individual to achieve just above their expected level is used throughout PCIT-T coaching, particularly given the likely novelty of many parenting techniques to this population. Although the most powerful learning comes as a result of repeated experience and exposure to a variety of clinical situations, additional coaching guidance and information are provided as a reference in Appendix A at the conclusion of this book.

The PRIDE Skills

Similar to PCIT, the PRIDE (praise, reflect, imitate, describe, enjoy) skills are taught and coached to mastery within the child-directed interaction-toddler (CDI-T) phase of the intervention. This stage of the intervention encourages caregivers to have a 5-min daily therapuetic play session with their child in which they use the PRIDE skills at a high level, as would be seen in a clinic-based professional play therapy session, to work on the parent-child relationship. The PRIDE skills serve as the foundational mechanism whereby parents develop a strong, positive relationship with the child while learning to manage a wide variety of child behaviors using positive attention. The PRIDE skills are based on Eyberg and Funderburk (2011).

Labeled Praise

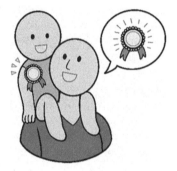

Perhaps the hallmark of such skills is the "P," otherwise known as labeled praise. Unlike unlabeled praise, labeled praise specifically indicates the behavior or attribute to which the parent attributes the positive evaluation. For example, a parent may indicate, "thank you for sitting on your bottom." Such praise is likely to result in a myriad of positive effects including an increased chance that the behavior will be repeated, enhancing the child's self-esteem, and improving the positivity of the parent-child interaction.

Reflection

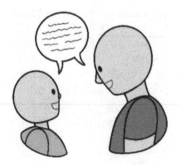

The "R" stands for reflection or the verbal repetition or restatement of the child's speech. Given the critical period of language development that occurs during the toddler years, verbal reflections serve as a vital tool whereby parents reinforce, scaffold, and model appropriate language skills. Additionally, verbal sounds, a vital component to toddler's speech and learning, are also reflected as they serve as an approximation to speech.

Imitation

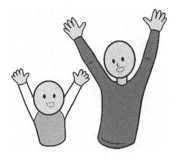

Next, the "I" signifies behavioral imitation. Although the skill is not quantified, a qualitative evaluation of the parent's ability to mimic the child's play is provided after each dyadic sequence. Imitation serves as a primary tool whereby children learn foundational skills such as cause and effect, and appropriate behavior may be modeled and reinforced.

Description

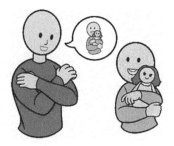

Description, or the "D" stands for behavior description in which a running commentary on the child's actions is provided. Such high-quality language reinforces appropriate behavior while also pairing verbal descriptions of the child's actions to the child's immediately completed behaviors. Each word, therefore, is meaningful to the child as it is linked to his or her interests and activities. In addition to verbal benefits, behavior descriptions also serve a vital role in helping to maintain a child's attention to task and thereby enhance learning within a single activity.

Enjoyment

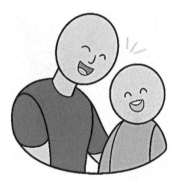

Finally, the "E" stands for enjoyment. Although the skill serves to increase the reinforcing value of the interaction for a child of any age, the enthusiastic quality of the parent's voice and facial expressions is emphasized further in PCIT-T. Enthusiastic expression of language serves to engage toddlers in play and contributes to the enhanced bond created between the parent and child. For more information on the PRIDE skills, including examples and detailed descriptions, see Chap. 6.

Mastery Criteria

Like PCIT, parents are held to mastery standards whereby they must provide the child with ten labeled praise statements, ten verbal reflection statements, and ten behavior description statements with three or fewer questions, commands, and critical statements in a 5-min coded sequence at the beginning of the session. Given that many children in this age range may not speak ten times during the 5-min coding segment, the mastery criterion for parents in this situation is considered achieved when 75% of all child verbalizations receive an appropriate reflection statement by the parent. In turn, such standards cause parents to become intricately aware of the type and quality of their speech during interactions with the child.

The CARES Model

A vital and unique component of PCIT-T is its focus on assisting young children in learning to regulate their emotions. Broader lifespan development research examining predictors of life satisfaction clearly position childhood emotional health and child conduct far above intellectual development (Layard, Clark, Cornaglia, Powdthavee, & Vornoit, 2014). Such work provides compelling evidence for an increased focus on factors likely to have a positive effect on emotional health such as the parent-child relationship, self-control, and emotion regulation (Banyard, Hamby, & Grych, 2017; Brauner & Stephens, 2006; Moffitt et al., 2011; White, Moffitt, Earls, Robins, & Silva, 1990). Rather than viewing negative emotions and behaviors as problematic or attention-seeking in nature, such emotions and behaviors are viewed as opportunities for the parent to teach the child to better regulate his or her emotions. Such behaviors and emotions are viewed through a developmental lens in which biological needs (e.g., hunger, thirst, sleep, toileting) are considered.

The CARES model therefore serves as a concrete set of steps to be used when guiding parents of toddlers through the child's expression of intense emotions and behaviors. The basic premise of such steps serves to support the child's feeling through expressions of warmth and understanding, rather than punishment. Parents, therefore, help to teach their young children coping skills in order to guide them through emotions, rather than blame them and provide consequences for their occurrence. Given the stressful and often overwhelming nature of helping very young children cope with their emotions, the CARES steps are to be simultaneously applied to the parent via therapist coaching. The application of such skills to the parent serves to model the techniques while also strengthening his or her emotional ability to then apply such skills to the child. Through this process, parents learn to anticipate and predict their child's emotional cues, as, in turn, the therapist does for the parent. Parents are thereby able to understand and quickly intervene with their young child's difficult emotions prior to escalation, a hallmark feature of a strong parent-child bond.

Similar to the PRIDE skills, each letter of the CARES model stands for a behavioral step to be applied within the dyadic interaction (Table 2.1). In some cases, only a single step of the CARES model may be necessary, where in others, all steps may be used. Although the steps may be used in any order depending on the nature of the particular situation, the steps will be described in the sequential order of the model below. For examples and a more detailed explanation of the model, refer to Chap. 8, Child-Directed Interaction-Toddler.

Table 2.1 Labeling the CARES model acronym

The CARES model	
"C"	Come in
"A"	Assist child
"R"	Reassure child
"E"	Emotional validation
"S"	Soothe

Come In

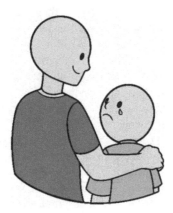

The "C" in CARES stands for "come in." Physical proximity to young children is vital to the rewarding nature of interactions. When managing difficult emotions and behaviors, such proximity communicates responsivity, availability, warmth, as well as a message of support and understanding. Additionally, such closeness allows parents to utilize and children to benefit from other CARES skills, thereby making the step foundational to the model's use.

Assist Child

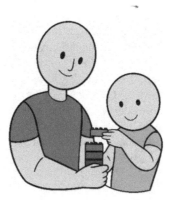

The "A" stands for "assist," whereby parents are coached to help the child rectify the particular issue they have encountered. Scaffolding should guide such assistance as parents use the opportunity to support, rather than completely resolve, the difficulty. Should such scaffolded guidance fail to result in the child's emotional de-escalation and resolution, the parent may complete the task for the child. However, the therapist should be mindful of the percentage of instances in which complete resolution by the parent is necessary, and if necessary, consider decreasing the developmental difficulty of provided toys to allow the child's increased independence.

Reassure Child

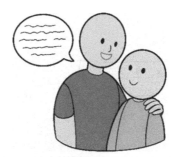

Unlike previous steps in which physical movement is central to implementation, verbal consolation or "reassurance" constitutes the foundation of the "R." While the content of such words should clearly convey a message of care and nurturance, the tone and quality of these verbalizations as soothing, warm, and calm are of even greater importance. The therapist's role in using this skill to support the parent's emotion regulation is vital to the parent's ability to appropriately implement the skill with the child. In sum, the "R" is primarily focused on conveying a message of care and emotional presence.

Emotional Validation

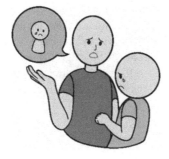

The "E" stands for "emotional validation" and is used to label the child's emotion. Such verbal classification serves to authenticate the child's emotion by ascribing a vocabulary word to its experience, a core component of emotional intelligence.

While common emotions such as happy, sad, and mad are likely to be experienced, noticed, and labeled, the step supports the expansion of the child's vocabulary through the use of more complex emotions such as frustrated, excited, and disappointed.

Soothe

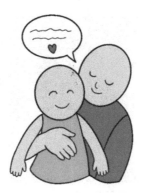

Finally, the "S" stands for "soothe" and is likely to permeate each of the other CARES steps. Through this step, parents use a comforting verbal tone, voice, and physical touch during interactions with the child. The foundational CARES skills provide the child with emotional comfort and support while communicating a premise of care, love, and nurturance – a natural bonding agent within any dyadic interaction.

In order for parents to effectively implement the CARES model with their children, they must also feel supported in their ability to apply the model to themselves, particularly during moments of child distress. Therapists play a vital role in this parallel process as they coach parents to translate and implement the CARES skills to themselves. The adult CARES approach is used to assist the caregiver in learning to acknowledge and regulate their own emotions to model and facilitate the toddler's ability to manage big emotions. Among other skills, CARES for parents involves self-soothing through breathing and relaxation techniques. The specific use of emotion regulation skills for parents is described in Chap. 8.

Under-Reaction and Redirection

The use of selective attention, or the strategic provision of attention for appropriate behavior and immediate removal of such attention upon the occurrence of misbehavior, is a core behavior management skill in standard PCIT. However, implementation of the skill assumes a level of negative attention-seeking intentionality, often learned from a history of behavioral escalation in the coercive cycle. Within this context, the skill may be appropriately applied to older children within instances in which a strong, negative emotion is present (e.g., a classic tantrum). Given the developmental considerations of emerging emotion regulation abilities in the toddler population, the classic implementation of selective attention is not applied, and instead the CARES model is used. However, it is likely that older toddlers, in particular, may attempt to engage parents in cause and effect-based activities in an effort to elicit a parental response. Such instances are not likely to include a strong negative emotional component. Instead, the child is likely to remain emotionally calm and happy, perhaps smiling and making bids for the parent's attention in a game-like manner. In such circumstances, a reaction from the parent (whether positive or negative) is likely to result in perpetuation of the child's behavior, and so a quiet "under-reaction and redirection" response is warranted. During the implementation of such a response, the parent should refrain from acknowledging the child's action and instead verbally engage in an alternative activity. A specific praise for the positive opposite of the child's negative behavior can be provided. If the under-reaction response is implemented immediately, the child's behavior should quickly cease. Should behavioral or emotional escalation occur, CARES should be applied. For a more detailed explanation of the under-reaction and redirection skill as it applies to the motivations behind toddlers' behavior, please refer to Chap. 8.

Management of Aggressive and Destructive Behaviors

Although the expression of difficult emotions in young children may occur in the form of aggressive and destructive behavior, the potential perpetuation of such behaviors is highly problematic and potentially dangerous. The implementation of high-level consequences (e.g., time-out in a chair) in response to such behaviors, as is done with older children in standard PCIT, would be developmentally inappropriate for children in the toddler age group. In PCIT-T, therefore, a mild, developmentally appropriate consequence procedure is applied following aggressive (e.g., hitting, kicking, pushing, biting) and destructive (e.g., breaking a toy) behaviors in an effort to decrease the chances that such behaviors occur again. The procedure is intentionally brief. Verbiage stated within the procedure is meant to be conveyed in a clear but firm tone, in direct contrast to the upbeat, enthusiastic demeanor emphasized in the remainder of the program. Specifically, steps consist of covering and holding the child's hands, providing him or her with direct eye contact, firmly stating

"No hurting," and looking away from the child for 3 seconds. A second phrase, "No hurting. Gentle hands," is then provided. The child's hands are then released, and the child is physically rotated toward another toy. Redirection is used to re-engage the child in appropriate play using the PRIDE skills. Finally, the CARES model may be utilized as necessary. The procedure is repeated upon the recurrence of aggression. Emphasis is placed upon such redirection and use of the CARES steps as young children may be likely to experience ongoing emotion regulation difficulties following the presence of aggression. Similarly, attempting to prevent aggression using high levels of praise for "safe hands and feet," appropriately playing with toys, and remaining calm during upsetting situations are critical to the child's ability to learn to regulate his or her emotions and behaviors. Additionally, the parent and therapist's ability to recognize the child's cues prior to the expression of aggressive and destructive behaviors will help to prevent the occurrence of such high-level behaviors. Further examples and explanation of the procedure can be found in Chap. 8 under the heading "Dangerous and Destructive Behaviors."

Parent-Directed Interaction-Toddler

The parent-directed interaction-toddler (PDI-T) portion of PCIT-T diverges most widely from procedures used during standard PCIT. Conceptually, it is emphasized that young children must be taught how to follow directions, a skill found to be fundamental to educational success. Early intervention research supports the critical importance of self-control, attention, and compliance within emotion regulation. For example, in 2015, economists Fryer, Levitt, and List created a preschool in a poor area of Chicago with the primary goal of testing the effects of a traditional, academically focused curriculum and a curriculum focused on nonacademic skills such as sitting calmly, working memory, and executive functioning abilities (Fryer, Levitt, & List, 2015). In addition, a simultaneous parent academy was created whereby parents could earn monetary incentives for attending parent sessions, as well as when their children turned in homework or their children displayed improved test performance. The Woodcock-Johnson test was used to measure cognitive abilities, while the Blair and Willoughby Measures of Executive Function and the Preschool Self-Regulation Assessment assessed nonacademic skills. Results of the study indicated that children with below-average difficulties on nonacademic skills did not reap any gains from the program, regardless of their cognitive abilities at pretreatment. Conversely, children with pretreatment test scores of above average difficulties of non-cognitive abilities amassed notable gains from the program, thereby speaking to the foundational nature of such abilities to children's academic potential.

For toddlers, it is critical to recognize that noncompliance does not occur from intentional defiance as is found in preschool-aged children but rather from insufficient learning and behavioral practice. Therefore, the PDI-T procedure consists of concrete, graduated steps in which scaffolding is used to teach young children listening skills, instead of the implementation of punishment-based consequences for noncompliance. The rules of effective commands are taught, as included in standard PCIT: commands are stated directly, rather than indirectly, given one at a time, specific, and provided in a neutral tone of voice with brief explanations either prior to the command or following compliance. Additionally, parents should remain mindful of the number of commands provided throughout the day and, specifically, the proportion of commands to positive statements (e.g., PRIDE skills). Unlike standard PCIT, emphasis is placed on pairing a positive touch with the delivery of the command in order to assist in orienting the child to the expected action. Additionally, the proximity between the parent and child is included as a second critical area of emphasis. Such proximity assists in gaining and maintaining the child's attention to the stimulus. Such proximity also positions each command as a dyadic, teaching opportunity in which the parent is actively supporting the child's learning process. Finally, the PCIT-T PDI-T protocol diverges from standard PCIT in the types of commands that may be delivered. In standard PCIT, any developmentally appropriate command may be implemented. In the PCIT-T PDI-T procedure, however, only a few, concrete, predetermined commands thought to be vital to toddlers' understanding and developmental level may be delivered. Additionally, parents are asked to rank such commands in order of progressive difficulty for the child. During this process, parents may reference the likelihood and consistency with which the child may have been previously exposed to the command. Following such rank ordering, young children are then guided through a listening procedure to learn such commands until mastery of each successive command is achieved.

Known in applied behavior analysis as guided compliance, the procedure consists of concrete steps labeled as "tell," "show," "try again," and "guide." The procedure includes a combination of verbal and visual cues to appeal to and assist toddlers with varying developmental strengths and abilities. Each successive step is initiated when listening has not occurred during a previous step. Upon compliance, a specific, enthusiastically delivered labeled praise paired with a positive touch is provided. Such touch is emphasized in the current population due to its importance in enhancing the value of the praise and warmth of the relationship. Additionally, particularly younger toddlers may have difficulty comprehending spoken words and, therefore, may derive greater reinforcement from the enthusiastic quality of the parent's voice and the physical touch paired with labeled praise statement. The PDI-T procedure is meant to serve a foundational role in teaching young children basic listening skills in an effort to prevent later compliance difficulties. This compliance training phase also fosters an early pattern of consistency, predictability, and follow-through within the parent-child relationship.

As part of PDI-T, the therapist works with parents to help them appreciate that gaining independence is an important developmental process in this age range. As such, teaching listening skills must be balanced with supporting the child's natural need to assert independence and develop a sense of control in the world. During daily living, parents are encouraged to use indirect commands and provide choices whenever possible to foster toddler independence. PDI-T procedures are used in ways that set the child up for success. As such, the 5 min PDI-T practice sessions are conducted only when the child is in a positive mood, and listening practice is structured as an upbeat teaching tool to celebrate the child's emerging ability to follow directions. The PDI-T procedure is purposefully limited and practiced at a maximum of three times a day.

Intervention Goals

The specific goals of PCIT-T focus on three primary categories: (1) caregiver skills, (2) child behavior, and (3) the quality of the caregiver-child relationship. Regarding caregiver skills, PCIT-T aims to (1) improve the positivity of caregiver speech by increasing positive child-directed vocalizations and decreasing negative child-directed vocalizations, (2) decrease caregiver distress and overall stress levels, (3) increase caregiver understanding of the toddler's developmental needs based on appropriate developmental expectations, (4) improve caregiver ability to assist the child in regulating his or her emotions, and (5) improve caregiver ability to regulate his or her own emotions. Regarding children's behaviors, PCIT-T aims to improve toddler social-emotional functioning, positive social skills, and emotion regulation ability. Finally, PCIT-T aims to improve the quality of the caregiver-child relationship by (1) enhancing the caregiver and child's reciprocal enjoyment by assisting the dyad in developing mutually rewarding experiences, and (2) decreasing the caregiver's negative perceptions of the toddler and his or her behavior by enhancing understanding of the child's need for assistance with emotional regulation (see Table 2.2).

In alignment with such goals and considering the unique developmental needs of toddlers, a number of key components differentiate PCIT-T from standard PCIT. Given the premise that a toddler's negative behavior typically relates to an expression of need and the developmental challenge of regulating emotion, PCIT-T assists parents in providing nurturance and support to the distressed toddler and assisting the child with emotion regulation. An intensifying approach meant to manage higher-level disruptive behavior (e.g., physical aggression, self-injurious behavior) in a developmentally appropriate, yet theoretically grounded, manner is therefore applied. A key component of such work is a focus on helping parents recognize and appropriately respond to toddlers' indications of emotion dysregulation in an effort to foster warm, responsive parenting skills while scaffolding young children's appropriate behaviors (e.g., verbalizations, pointing). Whenever possible, antecedent management (e.g., preventative praising of opposite behaviors, responding to early cues of child distress) is used to prevent the occurrence of disruptive behaviors (e.g., aggression, toy throwing). However, when such behaviors do occur, techniques such as under-reaction, distraction, and a brief consequence procedure are used to teach toddlers emotion regulation skills.

Given the importance of children's emotion regulation, developmentally appropriate redirection and transition techniques are emphasized and over-practiced to the point of mastery (i.e., positive parental response becomes automatic). While the therapist typically coaches the caregiver from behind a one-way mirror using a

Table 2.2 PCIT-T intervention goals and methods of measurement

PCIT-T intervention goals	Methods of measurement for PCIT-T intervention goals
Improve the positivity of caregiver speech by increasing positive child-directed vocalizations and decreasing negative child-directed vocalizations	Mastery criteria obtained in PRIDE skills and Avoid Skills
Decrease caregiver distress and stress levels	Improved scores on the Parenting Stress Index measure and Edinburgh Postnatal Depression Scale over the course of treatment
Increase caregiver understanding of toddler needs based on appropriate developmental expectations	Satisfactory implementation of Toddler CARES model
Provide caregiver with clearly defined tools to support the toddler's ability to regulate emotions	Satisfactory implementation of Toddler CARES model
Improve caregiver ability to regulate their own emotions	Satisfactory implementation of Adult CARES model
Improve toddler social-emotional functioning	Improved scores on the DECA or BITSEA over the course of treatment
Improve toddler positive social skills	Improved scores on the DECA or BITSEA over the course of treatment
Improve toddler emotion regulation abilities	Improved scores on the DECA or BITSEA over the course of treatment
Enhance caregiver and toddler reciprocal enjoyment by assisting the dyads in developing mutually rewarding experiences	Mastery criteria obtained in PRIDE skills and Avoid Skills; Satisfactory implementation of "Other Positive Skills"
Decrease caregiver negative interpretations of child behavior by enhancing understanding of the child's need for assistance with emotion regulation	Satisfactory implementation of Toddler CARES model

Bluetooth device, the therapist may come into the treatment room at times to assist the caregiver, particularly should any of the following three high-risk situations arise: (1) the child is displaying high levels of aggressive behavior, (2) the therapist feels that there is potential risk for maltreatment, or (3) the caregiver appears emotionally overwhelmed and is unable to assist the child in regulating his or her behavior. Following such situations, the therapist may provide the in-person comfort and support needed by the parent and child to resume, rather than end, the play.

References

Banyard, V., Hamby, S., & Grych, J. (2017). Health effects of adverse childhood events: Identifying promising protective factors at the intersection of mental and physical well-being. *Child Abuse & Neglect, 68*, 88–98.

Brauner, C. B., & Stephens, C. B. (2006). Estimating the prevalence of early childhood serious emotional/behavioral disorders: challenges and recommendations. *Public Health Reports, 121* (3), 303–310.

Eyberg, S., & Funderburk, B. W. (2011). Parent-child interaction therapy protocol. Gainesville, FL: PCIT International.

Fryer, R. G. J., Levitt, S. D., & List, J. A. (2015). *Parental incentives and early childhood achievement: A field experiment in Chicago heights.* Retrieved from http://www.nber.org/papers/w21477

Kaminski, J. W., Valle, L. A., Filene, J. H., & Boyle, C. L. (2008). A meta-analytic review of components associated with parent training program effectiveness. *Journal of Abnormal Child Psychology, 36*(4), 567–589.

Layard, R., Clark, A., Cornaglia, F., Powdthavee, N., & Vornoit, J. (2014). What predicts a successful life? a life-course model of well-being. *The Economic Journal, 124*(580), F720–F738.

Moffitt, T. E., Arseneault, L., Belsky, D., Dickson, N., Hancox, R. J., Harrington, H., ... Caspi, A. (2011). A gradient of childhood self-control predicts health, wealth, and public safety. *PNAS, 108*(7), 2693–2698.

White, J. A., Moffitt, T. E., Earls, F., Robins, L., & Silva, P. A. (1990). How early can we tell?: Predictors of childhood conduct disorder and adolescent delinquency. *Criminology, 28*(4), 507.

Chapter 3
Setting the Empirical Stage: An Overview of Standard PCIT

Parent-Child Interaction Therapy: Overview

Parent-Child Interaction Therapy (PCIT) is backed by a strong, extensive empirical research base that has demonstrated its efficacy across a range of children presenting with a variety of behavioral and emotional concerns (Eyberg & Funderburk, 2011). Developed in the 1980s by Dr. Sheila Eyberg at the Oregon Health Sciences University, the treatment was originally developed to treat children between 2 and 7 years of age with primary disruptive behavior concerns (e.g., tantrums, noncompliance, aggression). Rooted in a strong theoretical base of operant conditioning, social learning, and attachment theories, the intervention incorporates seminal contributions by pioneering clinicians and researchers in the field of parenting and the parent-child relationship (Eyberg, 1988; McNeil & Hembree-Kigin, 2010). Diana Baumrind's authoritative parenting style frames the context of the intervention as a balance between positive, warm, sensitive caregiving and the importance of limits, consequences, and control. Gerald Patterson's coercive cycle (1982) contributes to our understanding of the escalating pattern of parent-child interactions that has previously reinforced negative child behavior by allowing children to delay and escape from parental demands that lead to noncompliance (McNeil & Hembree-Kigin, 2010). The balance of such concepts is reflected in the intervention's two-stage treatment model, originally developed and clinically implemented by Eyberg's early mentor, Dr. Constance Hanf (Reitman & McMahon, 2013).

In the first stage of the intervention, child-directed interaction (CDI), parents are taught and coached using an in vivo format to reach mastery levels of positive attention skills including specific praise ("Thank you for sitting so nicely"), verbal reflection of appropriate child speech (child, "I like to build houses"; parent, "You do like to build houses"), and behavioral description ([child is stacking blocks], parent: "You are stacking the red block on top of the green block"). Qualitative skills such as imitation of appropriate behavior and reciprocal enjoyment are a primary focus of the phase. Additionally, parents learn to minimize their use of questions ("What do

© Springer Nature Switzerland AG 2018
E. I. Girard et al., *Parent-Child Interaction Therapy with Toddlers*,
https://doi.org/10.1007/978-3-319-93251-4_3

you want to do now?"), commands ("Sit down"), and critical statements ("I don't like how you are behaving") that serve to take the lead away from the child and provide attention toward negative, inappropriate behavior (Eyberg & Boggs, 1998). These PRIDE skills (praise, reflection, imitation, description, and enjoyment) are based in part on techniques used in traditional play therapy to establish rapport quickly with young children. Selective attention skills are taught and practiced in the CDI phase as the primary form of behavior management. Such high levels of positive attention for appropriate child behavior and minimal attention for negative attention-seeking misbehavior function to reinforce acceptable behavior and improve the warmth and quality of the parent-child relationship while decreasing the occurrence of negative behaviors. Additionally, the implementation of such skills increases the quality of the parent-child relationship in an effort to build positivity, trust, and the foundation of a warm relationship. In the second phase of the intervention, parent-directed interaction (PDI), parents gradually incorporate the use of effective commands provided in a clear, direct, positive, age-appropriate manner. The use of such commands begins with simple play-based commands ("Please hand me the red block") before progressing to larger, real-life commands ("Please take off your shoes"). Initiation of compliance is expected within 5 s of the original command or the subsequent warning statement before parents enter into a step-by-step time-out procedure designed to prevent escape and minimize attention toward negative behavior. The final steps of the treatment include the application of skills to enhance selected real-life situations (e.g., diaper changing, nap time) (Eyberg & Bussing, 2010).

In addition to the strong evidence base behind the use of such specific skills, the methods behind the instruction, delivery, and transfer of skills from therapist to parent to child are foundational to treatment success within the parent-training literature (Kaminski, Valle, Filene, & Boyle, 2008). Such methods include the provision of live, active coaching, coding, and real-time feedback. The aforementioned techniques allow parents to acquire and implement novel skills with their child while receiving active guidance. With practice, such skills are likely to be incorporated into the parent's natural repertoire and occur habitually across a variety of real-life settings (e.g., home, public places) thereby allowing the benefits of focused therapy and Home Therapy Practice sessions to occur across the child's day. However, it should be noted that although generalization of intensely practiced skills is likely to occur, it is unrealistic to expect parents to implement therapeutic parenting techniques in response to their young children's behavior on a minute-to-minute basis throughout the day. The concept of "good enough parenting," originally developed by pediatrician and psychoanalyst, Dr. Donald Winnicott (1953), has been framed as a realistic conceptualization of the balance between parenting perfection and reality. Therefore, therapists should emphasize the importance of daily, intensive practice of skills as it is built into the model while empathizing with perfectionistic parents surrounding the realities of attempting to consistently apply therapeutic parenting techniques to their temperamentally challenging toddlers. Examples and further discussion regarding the implementation of such complex concepts will occur throughout the PCIT-T protocol as described later in the session-by-session guide.

Parent-Child Interaction Therapy: Evidence Base

A strong base of meta-analytic reviews clearly demonstrates the impact of PCIT on decreasing disruptive behavior concerns in young children as evidenced by particularly large effect sizes from pre- to post-treatment (e.g., $d = 1.65$; Ward, Theule, & Cheung, 2016), even surpassing that of other evidence-based parenting programs (e.g., Triple P) (Costello, Chengappa, Stokes, Tempel, & McNeil, 2011; Eyberg & Bussing, 2010; Eyberg & Funderburk, 2011; Eyberg, Nelson, & Boggs, 2008; Thomas & Zimmer-Gembeck, 2007; Ward et al., 2016). A number of efficacy (Eyberg et al., 2008; Hood & Eyberg, 2003; Nixon, Sweeney, Erickson, & Touyz, 2003) and effectiveness studies (Abrahamse, Junger, & Lindauer, 2012; Lanier, Kohl, Benz, Swinger, & Drake, 2014; Pearl et al., 2011) contribute to the strong research base that qualifies PCIT as an efficacious treatment using standards set by Chambless and Hollon (1998). The positive effects of the robust treatment have been demonstrated across a wide variety of populations including maltreated children (Chaffin, Funderburk, Bard, Valle, & Gurwitch, 2011) and children exposed to domestic violence (Timmer, Ware, Urquiza, & Zebell, 2010). Such work had led to the national recognition of PCIT by the National Child Traumatic Stress Network (NCTSN) as one of six evidence-based treatments for children that have experienced trauma. Additionally, PCIT has been shown to effectively decrease negative child behaviors and improve parent-child interactions in vulnerable populations such as low-income, single mothers (Naik-Polan & Budd, 2008) and foster parents (Mersky, Topitzes, Janczewski, & McNeil, 2015). For a more comprehensive understanding of the PCIT research literature, see Lieneman, Brabson, Highlander, Wallace, and McNeil (2017).

Parent-Child Interaction Therapy: Treatment Settings

Typically, PCIT delivery occurs in the context of a university-based or outpatient community clinic. A one-way mirror is used to allow the therapist to separate him or herself from the adult-child dyad playing on the opposite side of the mirror. Bug-in-the-ear or walkie-talkie and microphone systems are used to enable communication between the dyad and therapist during live coaching of the parent-child interaction throughout the session. In addition to adaptations of the PCIT model, modifications to the treatment location, outside of the typical university or outpatient setting, have also been implemented and tested. Namely, Teacher-Child Interaction Training (TCIT), a comprehensive adaptation for the implementation of PCIT in the school system, has been applied to preschool and kindergarten classrooms with impressive outcomes. Results have indicated improved teacher skills and teacher-student interactions across classrooms as well as increased rates of student compliance and high teacher satisfaction with the treatment program (Fernandez, Gold, Hirsch, & Miller, 2015; Lyon et al., 2009; Stokes, Tempel, Costello, & McNeil, 2010). Finally, improved rates of child negative behaviors have also been reported in the home environment of student receiving TCIT (Campbell, 2011). Although many PCIT skills remain the same in the TCIT model, teachers are coached to reduce questions and commands. Additionally, teachers use behavior descriptions and labeled praise statements to provide attention to students displaying positive behavior while selectively ignoring students displaying inappropriate behavior. Finally, the traditional PDI time-out procedure is often replaced by a classroom-specific consequence that serves to decrease attention toward the behavior while also complying with school-based policies and procedures.

PCIT adaptations in the home environment have led to improved rates of positive child behavior as well as increased use of positive parenting skills in the home environment (Ware, McNeil, Masse, & Stevens, 2008). Particular strengths of the home-based adaptation have been noted including increased validity of PCIT procedures (e.g., time-out) to the individual context of the home environment as well as decreased attrition rates (Fowles et al., 2017; Masse & McNeil, 2008). Drawbacks of the in-home model include the lack of control over the real-life environment, the use of the in-room coaching environment, and potential costs associated with therapist travel to and from the family's home (Masse & McNeil, 2008). Since this research, the in-home coaching adaption has been disseminated across an entire state with careful attention paid to the scientific implementation of the powerful model (Beveridge et al., 2015; Fowles et al., 2017).

Parent-Child Interaction Therapy: Treatment Populations

In an effort to better meet the needs of the variety of populations to which PCIT has been applied, researchers have developed and implemented adaptations to the PCIT model. Early on, McNeil and Hembree-Kigin (2010) described an adaptation for older children, ages 7–8 years, whose developmental level would otherwise fall outside of the typical PCIT age range. Although the same behavioral principles (e.g., positive reinforcement, selective attention, limit setting) remain consistent, the adaptation accounts for school-age children's physical size and advanced cognitive abilities. Specifically, the adaptation recommends that caregivers use reduced levels of child-directed skills while making such verbalizations more complex and varied in structure (Stokes, Tempel, Costello, & McNeil, 2017). Additionally, individual therapy time is added to sessions to increase rapport between the therapist and child client. Finally, the parent-directed interaction phase of PCIT is divided into stages in which effective commands are taught and implemented prior to the implementation of a modified time-out procedure with an added token economy incentive system.

Emotion regulation has been studied using standard PCIT for 2- to 8-year-old children with disruptive behavior (Lieneman, Girard, Quetsch, & McNeil, 2018). Both caregiver and child emotion regulation were evaluated in a sample of 66 primarily Hispanic and low-income families receiving treatment at a community mental health center. Caregivers completed the Difficulties in Emotion Regulation Scale

(DERS; Gratz & Roemer, 2004), a self-report measure of adult emotion dysregulation. Parents also completed the Emotion Regulation Checklist (ERC; Shields & Cicchetti, 1997) regarding their children's emotion regulation. The ERC yields two subscales: adaptive regulation and lability/negativity. Pre- and posttesting revealed that caregivers reported significant improvements in their own emotion regulation following PCIT (*Cohen's d* = 0.78). Similarly, parents reported that their children displayed large improvements in their abilities to regulate their emotions after PCIT (*Cohen's d* for lability/negativity = 1.93). Emotion regulation improvements in caregivers and children occurred during both the CDI and the PDI phases of treatment, demonstrating a largely linear improvement over time. The authors considered the caregiver improvements in emotion regulation to be attributable to the PCIT skills of ignoring disruptive child behavior, learning to stay in the moment and focus on the caregiver-child relationship, becoming more in tune with their own emotions and the emotions of their child, responding in a neutral and scripted fashion to child disruptive behavior, and learning to calmly underreact to stressful interactions with the child. The large improvements in child emotion regulation paralleled the positive changes in child disruptive behavior. The Lieneman et al. (2018) study adds significantly to the PCIT literature in that it is the first study to demonstrate changes in both parent and child emotion regulation following PCIT. The reductions in children's emotional dysregulation in the areas of lability and negativity have important implications for future mental health. Research has repeatedly demonstrated that emotion regulation in childhood is linked to social/emotional functioning, academic success, and overall well-being later in life (Lieneman et al., 2018). The emotion regulation changes seen in this study suggest that PCIT is more than just a behavior modification program. It also addresses the overall emotional functioning of the family unit.

The concept of emotion regulation also has been addressed using PCIT with children displaying internalizing disorders. Given the behavioral manifestation of early childhood depression and anxiety as well as the critical influence of the environment on the development and treatment of such symptoms, researchers have explored PCIT's effects on internalizing difficulties. Namely, Lenze, Pautsch, and Luby (2011) developed an adaptation for PCIT for depressed preschool children. Specifically, child-directed and adult-directed module components are limited to six sessions, regardless of mastery levels. A unique Emotional Development (ED) module was added to increase children's emotional awareness and emotion regulation abilities. During the module, parents are taught to help children regulate their emotions using techniques such as labeling the emotion and prompting the child to use relaxation skills. Research outcomes of the adaptation indicated clinically significant decreases in children's levels of depressive symptoms as well as increases in prosocial behaviors and emotional coping. Later, Comer et al. (2012) tested the implementation of the Coaching Approach behavior and Leading by Modeling (CALM) Program, an adaptation of PCIT for anxious preschoolers including those diagnosed with separation anxiety, social anxiety, generalized anxiety, and/or specific phobias. Rather than focusing on discipline procedures to target noncompliance, parent skills are used to coach parents as they gradually expose their child to the feared stimulus, thereby promoting brave behaviors and decreasing anxious reactions. Research outcomes indicated diagnostic and functional improvements such that most participants did not meet criteria for an anxiety disorder at post-treatment.

Given the well-known prevalence of attention-deficit hyperactivity disorder (ADHD) and its symptomatic presentation in young children, an adaptation of PCIT has also been developed to target emotion regulation in preschoolers with ADHD. Adapted from the PCIT-ED program for the treatment of preschool depression, the PCIT emotion coaching protocol enables caregivers to react to their child's emotion by following a decision sequence in which they label and reflect children's positive and negative emotions provided the disruptive behavior is absent (Chronis-Tuscano et al., 2016). Results of such adaptations indicated reduced impairment in child symptoms and improved childhood emotion regulation skills at the post-treatment time point.

Approximately one dozen studies have shown that PCIT improves disruptive behavior in children on the autism spectrum (see McNeil, Quetsch, and Anderson (In Press) for details about these investigations). As an example, Zlomke, Jeter, and Murphy (2017) studied 17 children on the autism spectrum and found results in PCIT similar to those obtained with children displaying typical development. Scores on the Eyberg Child Behavior Inventory improved from outside of normal limits to within normal limits (Cohen's d effect size of 2.45), and compliance rates improved from 41% to 87%. An adaptation of PCIT for children with an autism spectrum disorder has also been developed (Lesack, Bearss, Celano, & Sharp, 2014). Adaptations to the child-directed phase of PCIT for children with an autism spectrum disorder included reflecting only functional communication and the provision of toys to minimize the likelihood of perseverative or stereotypic play. Adaptations to the parent-directed interaction phase of PCIT included the use of the child's name prior to the command, a hand-over-hand guided compliance sequence to teach a specific command, reduced time-out duration, and the use of a holding chair procedure following escape from time-out. Case study results utilizing such adaptations resulted in decreased child disruptive behaviors as well as increased use of positive parent verbalizations and decreased negative parent verbalizations.

Finally, the robust effects of PCIT have been adapted to a variety of cultures around the world with positive outcomes including Latino/Latina populations (McCabe, Yeh, Garland, Lau, & Chavez, 2005), the indigenous people of New Zealand (Capous, Wallace, McNeil, & Cargo, 2016; McNeil & Hembree-Kigin, 2010), European (Abrahamse et al., 2012), and Asian groups (Leung, Tsang, Heung, & Yiu, 2009). Each cultural adaptation maintains the core tenets of PCIT while simultaneously modifying and incorporating key aspects of the individual culture's values. See Capous et al. (2016) for a complete review of PCIT across cultures.

References

Abrahamse, M. E., Junger, M., & Lindauer, R. J. (2012). The effectiveness of parent-child interaction therapy in the Netherlands: Preliminary results of a randomized controlled trial. *Neuropsychiatriede l'enfance et de l'adolesence, 60*, S88–S88.

Beveridge, R. M., Fowles, T. R., Masse, J. J., Parrish, B. P., Smith, M. S., Circo, G., & Widdoes, N. S. (2015). The dissemination and implementation of parent-child interaction therapy (PCIT): Lessons learned from a state-wide system of care. *Children and Youth Services Review, 48*, 38–48.

Campbell, C. (2011). *Bringing PCIT to the classroom: The adaptation and effectiveness of the teacher-child interaction training-preschool program.* Paper presented at the Biennial Parent-Child Interaction Therapy International Convention, Gainesville, FL.

Capous, D. E., Wallace, N. M., McNeil, D. J., & Cargo, T. A. (2016). Best Practices for Parent Child Interaction Therapy across Diverse Cultural Groups. In *Parent-child interactions and relationships: Perceptions, practices and developmental outcomes.* New York, NY: Nova Science Publishers.

Chaffin, M., Funderbunk, B., Bard, D., Valle, L. A., & Gurwitch, R. (2011). A combined motivation and parent-child interaction therapy package reduces child welfare recidivism in a randomized dismantling field trial. *Journal of Consulting and Clinical Psychology, 79*, 84–95.

Chambless, D. L., & Hollon, S. D. (1998). Defining empirically supported therapies. *Journal of Consulting and Clinical Psychology, 66*(1), 7–18.

Chronis-Tuscano, A., Lewis-Morrarty, E., Woods, K. E., O'Brien, K. A., Mazursky-Horowitz, H., & Thomas, S. R. (2016). Parent–child interaction therapy with emotion coaching for Preschoolers with attention-deficit/hyperactivity disorder. *Cognitive and Behavioral Practice, 23*(1), 62–78.

Comer, J. S., Puliafico, A. C., Aschenbrand, S. G., McKnight, K., Robin, J. A., Goldfine, M. E., & Albano, A. M. (2012). A pilot feasibility evaluation of the CALM program for anxiety disorders in early childhood. *Journal of Anxiety Disorders, 26*(1), 40–49. https://doi.org/10.1016/j.janxdis.2011.08.011

Costello, A. H., Chengappa, K., Stokes, J. O., Tempel, A. B., & McNeil, C. B. (2011). Parent-child interaction therapy for oppositional behavior in children: Integration of child-directed play therapy and behavior management training for parents. In A. A. Drewes, S. C. Bratton, & C. E. Schaefer (Eds.), *Integrative play therapy.* Hoboken, NJ: Wiley.

Eyberg, S. (1988). Parent-child interaction therapy: Integration of traditional and behavioral concerns. *Child & Family Behavior Therapy, 10*(1), 33–46.

Eyberg, S., & Funderburk, B. W. (2011). Parent-child interaction therapy protocol. Gainesville, FL: PCIT International.

Eyberg, S. M., & Boggs, S. R. (1998). Parent-child interaction therapy for oppositional preschoolers. In C. E. Schaefer & J. M. Briesmeister (Eds.), *Handbook of parent training: Parents as cotherapists for children's behavior problems* (2nd ed., pp. 61–97). New York, NY: Wiley.

Eyberg, S. M., & Bussing, R. (2010). Parent-child interaction therapy for preschool children with conduct problems. In R. C. Murrihy, A. D. Kidman, & T. H. Ollendick (Eds.), *Clinical handbook of assessing and treating conduct problems in youth* (pp. 132–162). New York, NY: Springer.

Eyberg, S. M., Nelson, M., & Boggs, S. R. (2008). Evidence-based psychosocial treatments for children and adolescents with disruptive behavior. *Journal of Clinical Child and Adolescent Psychology, 37*(1), 215–237.

Fernandez, M. A., Gold, D. C., Hirsch, E., & Miller, S. (2015). From the clinics to the classrooms: A review of teacher-child interaction training in primary, secondary, and tertiary prevention settings. *Cognitive and Behavioral Practice, 22*, 217–229.

Fowles, T. R., Masse, J. J., McGoron, L., Beveridge, R. M., Williamson, A. A., Smith, M., & Parrish, B. P. (2017). Home-based vs. clinic-based parent–child interaction therapy:

Comparative effectiveness in the context of dissemination and implementation. *Journal of Child and Family Studies*, 1–15. https://doi.org/10.1007/s10826-017-0958-3

Hood, K. K., & Eyberg, S. M. (2003). Outcomes of parent-child interaction therapy: Mothers' reports of maintenance three to six years after treatment. *The Family Journal: Counseling and Therapy for Couples and Families, 8*, 180–186.

Kaminski, J. W., Valle, L. A., Filene, J. H., & Boyle, C. L. (2008). A meta-analytic review of components associated with parent training program effectiveness. *Journal of Abnormal Child Psychology, 36*(4), 567–589.

Lanier, P., Kohl, P. L., Benz, J., Swinger, D., & Drake, B. (2014). Preventing maltreatment with a community-based implementation of parent-child interaction therapy. *Journal of Child and Family Studies, 23*(2), 449–460.

Lenze, S., Pautsch, J., & Luby, J. (2011). Parent-child interaction therapy emotion development: A novel treatment for depression in preschool children. *Depression and Anxiety, 28*, 153–159.

Lesack, R., Bearss, K., Celano, M., & Sharp, W. G. (2014). Parent–child interaction therapy and autism spectrum disorder: Adaptations with a child with severe developmental delays. *Clinical Practice in Pediatric Psychology, 2*(1), 68–82.

Leung, C., Tsang, S., Heung, K., & Yiu, I. (2009). Effectiveness of parent-child interaction therapy (PCIT) among Chinese families. *Research on Social Work Practice, 19*, 304–313.

Lieneman, C. C., Brabson, L. A., Highlander, A., Wallace, N. M., & McNeil, C. B. (2017). Parent–child interaction therapy: Current perspectives. *Psychology Research and Behavior Management, 10*, 239–256.

Lieneman, C. C., Girard, E. I., Quetsch, L. B., & McNeil, C. B. (2018). Emotion regulation and attrition in parent-child interaction therapy. *Manuscript submitted for publication.*

Lyon, A., Gershenson, R., Farahmand, F., Thaxter, P., Behling, S., & Budd, K. (2009). Effectiveness of teacher-child interaction training (TCIT) in a preschool setting. *Behavior Modification, 33*(6), 855–884.

Masse, J. J., & McNeil, C. B. (2008). In-home parent-child interaction therapy: Clinical considerations. *Child & Family Behavior Therapy, 30*(2), 127–135.

McCabe, K. M., Yeh, M., Garland, A. F., Lau, A. S., & Chavez, G. (2005). The GANA program: A tailoring approach to adapting parent child interaction therapy for Mexican Americans. *Education & Treatment of Children, 28*(2), 111.

McNeil, C. B., & Hembree-Kigin, T. (2010). *Parent-child interaction therapy.* New York, NY: Springer.

McNeil, C. B., Quetsch, L. B., & Anderson, C. M. (In Press). *Handbook of parent-child interaction therapy with children on the Autism Spectrum.* New York, NY: Springer.

Mersky, J. P., Topitzes, J., Janczewski, C. E., & McNeil, C. B. (2015). Enhancing foster parent training with parent-child interaction therapy: Evidence from a randomized field experiment. *Journal of the Society for Social Work and Research, 6*(4), 591–616.

Naik-Polan, A. T., & Budd, K. S. (2008). Stimulus generalization of parenting skills during parent-child interaction therapy. *Journal of Early and Intensive Behavior Intervention, 5*(3), 1–92.

Nixon, R. D. V., Sweeney, L., Erickson, D. B., & Touyz, S. W. (2003). Parent-child interaction therapy: A comparison of standard and abbreviated treatments for oppositional defiant preschoolers. *Journal of Consulting and Clinical Psychology, 71*, 251–260.

Patterson, G. R. (1982). *Coercive family process.* Eugene, OR: Castalia.

Pearl, E., Thieken, L., Olafson, E., Boat, B., Connelly, L., Barnes, J., & Putnam, F. (2011). Effectiveness of community dissemination of parent-child interaction therapy. *Psychological Trauma: Theory, Research, Practice, and Policy, 4*(2), 204–213.

Reitman, D., & McMahon, R. J. (2013). Constance "Connie" Hanf (1917-2002): The mentor and the model. *Cognitive and Behavioral Practice, 20*, 106–116.

Stokes, J. O., Tempel, A. B., Costello, A. H., & McNeil, C. B. (2010). *Parent-child interaction therapy with an 8-year-old child: A case study.* Paper presented at the Association for Behavioral and Cognitive Therapies 44th Annual Conference, San Francisco, CA.

Stokes, J. O., Tempel, A. B., Costello, A. H., & McNeil, C. B. (2017). Parent-child interaction therapy with an eight-year-old child: A case study. *Evidence-Based Practice in Child and Adolescent Mental Health, 2*(1), 1–11.

Thomas, R., & Zimmer-Gembeck, M. J. (2007). Behavioral outcomes of parent-child interaction therapy and triple P-positive parenting program: A review and meta-analysis. *Journal of Abnormal Child Psychology, 35*(3), 475–495.

Timmer, S. G., Ware, L., Urquiza, A., & Zebell, N. M. (2010). The effectiveness of parent-child interaction therapy for victims of interparental violence. *Violence & Victims, 25*, 486–503.

Ward, M. A., Theule, J., & Cheung, K. (2016). Parent–child interaction therapy for child disruptive behaviour disorders: A meta-analysis. *Child & Youth Care Forum, 45*(5), 675–690.

Ware, L. M., McNeil, C. B., Masse, J., & Stevens, S. (2008). Efficacy of in-home parent-child interaction therapy. *Child & Family Behavior Therapy, 30*(2), 99–126.

Winnicott, D. (1953). Transitional objects and transitional phenomena. *International Journal of Psychoanalysis, 34*, 89–97.

Zlomke, K. R., Jeter, K., & Murphy, J. (2017). Open-trial pilot of parent-child interaction therapy for children with Autism Spectrum Disorder. *Child and Family Behavior Therapy, 39*(1), 1–18.

Gratz, K. L., & Roemer, L. (2004). Multidimensional assessment of emotion regulation and dysregulation: Development, factor structure, and initial validation of the Difficulties in Emotion Regulation Scale. *Journal of Psychopathology and Behavioral Assessment, 26*(1), 41–54. https://doi.org/10.1023/B:JOBA.0000007455.08539.94.

Shields, A., & Cicchetti, D. (1997). Emotion regulation among school-age children: The development and validation of a new criterion Q-sort scale. *Developmental Psychology, 33*(6), 906–916. https://doi.org/10.1037/0012-1649.33.6.906.

Chapter 4
The Application of PCIT to the Toddler Age Group

The strong framework embedded within the PCIT approach has enabled its implementation and empirical success with children aged less than 2 years across a wide variety of treatment settings, populations, and diagnoses. While the nuances of each PCIT adaptation differ, common to all is an emphasis on improving the quality of the parent-child relationship in bringing about positive child behavior change and an acknowledgment that the unique developmental capacities and needs of toddlers aged 12–24 months prohibit the application of classic PCIT procedures. PCIT-T shares features with a number of other attachment-based intervention approaches targeting high-risk infants/toddlers and caregivers including attachment and biobehavioral catchup (Yarger, Hoye, & Dozier, 2016) and child-parent psychotherapy (Lieberman, Silverman, & Pawl, 2005). An additional intervention, the family checkup (FCU), uses a brief consultation model (rather than a parent coaching model) focused on motivational interviewing-based techniques. Longitudinal outcomes of this intervention have included improved child behavior and language abilities (Lunkenheimer et al., 2008). Despite the differences between attachment-based and behaviorally based intervention approaches, additional literature has emerged illustrating the bidirectional benefits of a combined approach. Dombrowski, Timmer, Blacker, and Urquiza (2005) were among the first to adapt and apply the PCIT evidence based to toddlers, specifically those that had experienced maltreatment. Named Parent-Child Attunement Therapy (PCAT) , the intervention focused on toddlers aged 12–30 months. Despite many similarities to traditional PCIT (e.g., technology, mastery attainment, PRIDE skills, selective attention for negative behaviors), adaptations such as the use of less complex language, decreased session time, increased enthusiasm, the absence of time-out, and increased use of touch are used. Results of an original case study indicate improved positivity and quality of the dyadic interaction.

PCIT tailored to the unique developmental needs of children aged 12–24 months has been found to increase verbalizations in samples of young children currently experiencing, or at risk for experiencing, language-based developmental delays (Bagner, Garcia, & Hill, 2016; Blizzard, Barroso, Ramos, Graziano, & Bagner,

© Springer Nature Switzerland AG 2018
E. I. Girard et al., *Parent-Child Interaction Therapy with Toddlers*,
https://doi.org/10.1007/978-3-319-93251-4_4

2017). Bagner et al. (2016) applied the Infant Behavior Program (IBP), a home-based, child-directed interaction-focused intervention to groups of ethnically diverse, at-risk infants with scores above the 75th percentile on the Brief Infant-Toddler Social and Emotional Assessment (Briggs-Gowan, Carter, Bosson-Heenan, Guyer, & Horwitz, 2006), a standardized measure of infant behavior difficulties. Throughout each coaching session, caregivers were guided to increase their use of PRIDE skills while applying selective inattention to negative behaviors, including aggression. Adaptations such as clapping and repeating verbal sounds were also encouraged. Finally, caregivers were asked to practice such skills during 5 min of dedicated Homework Practice each day. Following a maximum of seven sessions, results across both studies indicated that higher levels of PRIDE skills were related to higher attachment-based caregiving skills such as levels of parental warmth, parental sensitivity, and responsivity at the post-intervention time point (Blizzard et al., 2017). Traditional parent-training outcomes such as increased child compliance, decreased physical aggression, and decreased internalizing behaviors were also observed, which the authors noted as surprising given the lack of standard compliance-focused consequences for childhood noncompliance (Blizzard et al., 2017). Finally, increases in parental positive skills and decreases in parental negative skills were also found (Bagner, Garcia, et al, 2016).

Recently, members of our own team have begun to test the limits of this robust treatment by empirically elucidating its powerful intervention effects with clinic-based infant and toddler samples. Specifically, our adaptations for the toddler population have centered upon improving toddlers emotion regulation while using positive parenting techniques to limit the occurrence of negative behavior. Kohlhoff and Morgan (2014) first described and implemented a preliminary version of Parent-Child Interaction Therapy-Toddler (PCIT-T) with a group of 29 families with a child less than 2 years of age. These researchers outlined a number of noteworthy adaptations designed specifically to meet the developmental needs of the population. First, unlike PCIT sessions that typically occur over the course of a 45–60-min session, PCIT-T sessions lasted 30–45 min. Additionally, less emphasis was placed on discipline as typically conducted in PDI (e.g., simple commands). Instead, some PDI ideas were infused into the CDI phase. Redirection was used as a primary form of behavior management, and parent-focused psychoeducation of developmentally appropriate expectations was infused throughout the treatment. Finally, PCIT-T also

attempted to help parents prevent problem behavior prior to its occurrence by increasing their focus on creating a safe, developmentally appropriate environment and intervene quickly upon early signs of emotion dysregulation. Although the behavioral parent-training lens primarily used in PCIT remained at the core of many PCIT-T skills, an attachment-based emphasis on meeting the emotional and developmental needs of toddlers remained a key focus of the treatment. Although the authors noted a number of limitations that necessitated further research, results demonstrated promising treatment outcomes indicating decreased problem behavior, improved parenting skills, and high treatment satisfaction.

To expand on this work, Kohlhoff and colleagues are currently evaluating outcomes of the PCIT-T intervention with toddlers aged 15 to 24 months in a larger waitlist controlled study. Although this research is currently still in progress, preliminary data clearly points to the efficacy of the PCIT-T model (Kohlhoff, Morgan, & Mares, 2017). Of the first 27 parent-toddler dyads that completed the trial (14 allocated to the PCIT-T treatment condition and 13 allocated to the waitlist control condition), the toddlers who received PCIT-T group showed significantly larger decreases in externalizing and internalizing behaviors as assessed using the Child Behavior Checklist (CBCL; (Achenbach & Rescorla, 2000)[CBCL externalizing subscale, $F(1,23) = 10.26$, $p < 0.05$, $\eta_p^2 = 0.23$, i.e., large effect size; CBCL internalizing subscale, $F(1,22) = 15.01$, $p < 0.05$, $\eta_p^2 = 0.24$, i.e., large effect size]. Parental use of positive parenting skills such as labeled praise, behavioral descriptions, and reflections increased dramatically more in the PCIT-T group compared to the waitlist group [DPICS "do skills," $F(1,11) = 33.60$, $p < 0.001$, $\eta_p^2 = 0.75$, i.e., large effect size), and use of negative parenting skills such as criticisms, commands, and questions decreased significantly [DPICS "don't skills," $F(1,11) = 5.68$, $p < 0.05$, $\eta_p^2 = 0.32$, i.e., large effect size). Significantly, preliminary results of this study show trends toward statistical significance in terms of increases in parental emotional availability. Specifically, compared to parents in the waitlist condition, parents in the PCIT-T intervention group were rated using the Emotional Availability Scales (Biringen, Robinson, & Emde, 2000) as having shown greater increases in parental sensitivity and greater ability to structure the interaction for the toddler at the posttreatment/waitlist assessment ($ps < .08$). Trends for decreased parental intrusiveness and decreased parental hostility were also seen ($ps < 0.14$). Finally, in an attempt to elucidate the impact of the PCIT-T intervention on infant attachment pattern, the toddlers in this study are also being assessed using the SSP (Ainsworth, Blehar, Waters, & Wall, 1978) at baseline and then again 6 months later (i.e., around 4–5 months after completing PCIT-T intervention). While this part of the research study is an open trial and data collection/coding is still in process (at the time that this book was published, pre-post attachment data is available for fourteen toddlers), preliminary outcomes are extremely promising with five out of the six children classified as having a "disorganized" attachment pattern prior to the intervention having shifted to an "organized" attachment pattern at follow-up. Although these results are based on a small sample size and so should be interpreted with caution, they are noteworthy given that few empirical studies of analogous interventions have resulted in similarly impressive outcomes. Taken together, preliminary results from Kohlhoff and Morgan's work suggest that this early version of PCIT-T – which comprises the core components and the same basic underlying assumptions of the PCIT-T intervention described in the current book – is associated with positive gains not only in terms of parent and child behavior but also in the emotional quality of the parent-child interaction and the infant attachment pattern. When completed, Kohlhoff and Morgan's study will provide more definitive results. Future studies examining the latest iteration of the PCIT-T model (described in the current book) will also be undertaken in due course to confirm these findings.

In sum, it can be noted that adaptations of PCIT designed and delivered to children under 2 years have shown positive results including improved child behaviors such as increased compliance, decreased aggression, defiance, and internalizing difficulties. Increases in positive and decreases in negative parent behaviors have also been observed, and improvements in the quality of the parent-child relationship and emotional availability have been shown. Finally, such effects have been achieved after seven or fewer coaching sessions regardless of parent mastery (Bagner, Coxe, et al., 2016; Bagner, Rodríguez, Blake, & Rosa-Olivares, 2013; Kohlhoff & Morgan, 2014). The age of this population and positive impact of this adaptation have powerful implications for efforts to not only intervene but also prevent behavior problems in young children while helping to position them on positive, developmental trajectories (Dombrowski et al., 2005). Together, such studies elucidate the critical importance of combining both behavioral and attachment-based interventions and outcome measures during treatment with infants and early toddlers.

References

Achenbach, T. M., & Rescorla, L. A. (2000). *Manual for the ASEBA Preschool forms and profiles*. Burlington, V.T: University of Vermont, Research Center for Children, Youth & Families.

Ainsworth, M., Blehar, M. C., Waters, E., & Wall, S. N. (1978). *Patterns of attachment: Assessed in the strange situation and at home*. Hillsdale, NJ: Erlbaum.

Bagner, D. M., Coxe, S., Hungerford, G. M., Garcia, D., Barroso, N. E., Hernandez, J., & Rosa-Olivares, J. (2016). Behavioral parent training in infancy: A window of opportunity for high-risk families. *Journal of Abnormal Child Psychology, 44*(5), 901–912.

Bagner, D. M., Garcia, D., & Hill, R. M. (2016). Direct and indirect effects of behavioral parent training on infant language production. *Behavior Therapy, 47*, 184–197.

Bagner, D. M., Rodríguez, G. M., Blake, C. A., & Rosa-Olivares, J. (2013). Home-based preventive parenting intervention for at-risk infants and their families: An open trial. *Cognitive and Behavioral Practice, 20*(3), 334–348.

Biringen, Z., Robinson, J. L., & Emde, R. N. (2000). Appendix B: The emotional availability scales (; an abridged infancy/early childhood version). *Attachment and Human Development, 2*(2), 256–270.

Blizzard, A. M., Barroso, N. E., Ramos, F. G., Graziano, P. A., & Bagner, D. M. (2017). Behavioral parent training in infancy: What about the parent–infant relationship? *Journal of Clinical Child and Adolescent Psychology*, 1–13.

Briggs-Gowan, M. J., Carter, A. S., Bosson-Heenan, J., Guyer, A. E., & Horwitz, S. M. (2006). Are infant-toddler social-emotional and behavioral problems transient? *Journal of the American Academy of Child and Adolescent Psychiatry, 45*, 849–858.

Dombrowski, S. C., Timmer, S. G., Blacker, D. M., & Urquiza, A. J. (2005). A positive behavioural intervention for toddlers: Parent attunement therapy. *Child Abuse Review, 14*, 132–151.

Kohlhoff, J., & Morgan, S. (2014). Parent child interaction therapy for toddlers: A pilot study. *Child and Family Behavior Therapy, 36*(2), 121–139.

Kohlhoff, J., Morgan, S., & Mares, S. (2017). *Parent-Child Interaction Therapy for young Toddlers (PCIT-T): Changing experience as well as behaviour*. Paper presented at the International Attachment Conference, London, June 2017.

Lieberman, A. F., Silverman, R., & Pawl, J. H. T. (2005). Infant–parent psychotherapy: Core concepts and current approaches. In C. H. Zeanah (Ed.), *Handbook of infant mental health*. Guilford. New York.

Lunkenheimer, E. S., Shaw, D. S., Gardner, F., Dishioin, T. J., Connell, A. M., Wilson, M. N., & Skuban, E. M. (2008). Collateral benefits of the family check-up on early childhood school readiness: Indirect effects of parents' positive behavior support. *Developmental Psychology, 44*(6), 1737–1752.

Yarger, H. A., Hoye, J. R., & Dozier, M. (2016). Trajectories of change in attachment and biobehavioral catch-up among high-risk mothers: A randomized clinical trial. *Infant Mental Health Journal, 37*(5), 525–536.

Chapter 5
Conceptualizing PCIT-T as an Emotion Regulation Treatment for Toddlers

A critical difference between the current treatment and standard PCIT as it is applied to older children is rooted in the core conceptualization of emotion regulation. Older children are cognitively capable of intentionally engaging in negative behaviors for the primary purpose of gaining attention. Therefore, the implementation of selective attention serves to minimize such behaviors by decreasing their rewarding value while motivating children to build and utilize the emotion regulation skills that they are developmentally capable of utilizing independently. Toddlers, however, do not yet possess the cognitive or emotional skills necessary to independently manage and control such emotions. Furthermore, the developing parent-child bond remains in its most formative stages. Therefore, the influence of the parent's ability to recognize and regulate his or her emotions has a profound impact upon the toddler's ability to control his or her own feelings. Such emotion regulation skills may be transmitted via parent modeling as well as directly taught via the parent's ability to support the child's emotional development in a calm, consistent, and predictable manner. However, this principle assumes that parents have the skills and emotional capability of appropriately modeling and transmitting such developmentally informed emotion regulation skills to their child. PCIT-T serves as an interactive process whereby each member of the therapy team (e.g., therapist, parent, child) models, reinforces, and supports each other during the live application of such skills with one another. Specifically, the coach provides a secure emotional base for the parent, who is in turn able to provide the same support to the child in a sequence often referred to as the parallel process. One key, yet complex, element within the effective implementation of the parallel process lies in the coach's and parent's ability to accurately read, interpret, and respond to the underlying function behind a child's dysregulated behavior (e.g., screaming, physical aggression, toy throwing). Variation between motivations is likely to occur within a given session. Misinterpretation of the function of a given behavior may result in inappropriate responding, unnecessary emotional escalation, and a missed opportunity for parents and children to learn appropriate emotion regulation strategies. Table 5.1 summarizes the emotions that may motivate toddlers' behavior. Tables 5.2 and 5.3 are the respective handouts

Table 5.1 Possible motivation related to toddler's behavior and example PCIT-T coaching statements to guide parental response

Situation	Emotion/motivation	Child's need	Example coaching statement	Parental response
Situation: Child tries to independently pull a toy apart, and it won't come apart. Child begins to cry. Child throws the toy, stomps feet, and flings arms	Frustration/anger	Sensitive engagement and support in regulating emotions	"He needs your help. Go closer. Pick him up"	CARES steps are implemented. Parent moves in close [CARES STEP: COME IN], says, "I know you're upset. Mommy is here to help you" [CARES STEPS: EMOTIONAL VALIDATION and REASSURE CHILD and SOOTHE with tone of voice]. Parent partially pulls apart toy, thereby scaffolding the child's ability to complete the task independently [CARES STEP: ASSIST CHILD]
Situation: After some time in the same room, child begins walking and searching around the space, failing to engage with an activity. Child begins to whine/flail arms	Boredom	Stimulation, engagement, and support to get back into a productive play	"Looks like he might be getting a bit bored. Grab a new toy, and get excited about what you're doing. Make it fun." [Child joins the parent and begins to play] "Looks like you've got her back on task. I think she's getting tired. [if the session has gone long]. I think we'll end pretty soon"	Parent provides a new toy or activity change. High levels of enthusiasm are used to assist in engaging child. Assess the level of child fatigue, and consider a concluding session.
Situation: Child picks up a small piece of string found on the floor. Parent removes string from child's hand. Child hits parent	Anger at parent	Limit setting for choking hazard, sensitive engagement, and support in regulating emotions	Move in close to him, and hold his hands out in front of him. Firmly say, "No hurting," and look away for 3 s. Repeat, "No hurting," and look away for 3 s. Finally, say	Parent moves close to the child [CARES STEP: COME IN] and interrupts the physical aggression and begins to rub the child's back [CARES

Note: When an item must be taken away from the toddler, the item should be placed out of sight. Developmentally, toddlers are more likely to forget about the object if it is no longer in sight			"Gentle hands." Now say, "I know you're upset." Rub his back a bit. Grab another toy, and enthusiastically describe how you're playing with it	STEP: SOOTHE with gentle touch]. Parent says, "I know you're upset. Mommy is here." [CARES STEPS: EMOTIONAL VALIDATION and REASSURE CHILD]. Parent then picks up a new light-up toy nearby and begins to play with it. When child reaches for the toy, parent hands child the toy and says, "Good job playing!" [PRIDE SKILL: LABELED PRAISE]
Situation: After playing with a new, singing, light-up toy, child begins repeatedly spinning in circles and falling to the ground	Overstimulation	Redirection, change in environment, sensitive engagement, and support in regulating emotions	"Seems like he might be getting a little overexcited by the new toy. He might need a change of activity. Pick him up, rock him for a moment, and move him around the room. Describe what you see around the room"	Parent picks child up [CARES STEP: COME IN], rocks him [CARES STEP: SOOTHE], and says, "I can tell that you are excited. [CARES STEP: EMOTIONAL VALIDATION], I see the dump truck and some blocks! There are dinosaurs next to the blocks. I want to make a big, tall tower." [POSITIVE SKILL: DISTRACTION]
Situation: Child has not eaten in an extended period of time. Provision of multiple toys has not seemed to calm the child	Unmet physical need (e.g., hunger, thirst, toileting, sleep)	Food, physical comfort, sensitive engagement, and support in regulating emotions	"It doesn't look like new toys are helping him to calm down. I wonder if he might be hungry. Do you think he might need a bit of his drink and snack?"	Parent retrieves child's drink and a snack from diaper bag and says, "I know you're upset [CARES SKILL: EMOTIONAL

(continued)

Table 5.1 (continued)

Situation	Emotion/motivation	Child's need	Example coaching statement	Parental response
				VALIDATION]. I think you're hungry. Mommy's here with some milk for you [CARES SKILLS: REASSURE CHILD & ASSIST CHILD]." Parent hands child a drink.
Situation: Child attempts to pull the door handle to leave the room while looking at the parent and smiling	Attention-seeking game	Attention	"It looks like this might be turning into a little game. Let's try to redirect her attention. Grab a new toy, and enthusiastically start to play with it"	Parent quietly and calmly directs attention toward a novel light-up toy. Says, "Wow, I can make the animals spin around and around! [avoid commands, e.g., "Stay here" and negative talk, e.g., "Don't open the door."] [BEHAVIOR MANAGEMENT SKILL: UNDER-REACTION AND REDIRECTION]

Table 5.2 CARES emotion regulation skills for toddlers

 PCIT-T: Emotion Regulation for Toddlers

CARES

Steps provided in any order and often simultaneously

Picture Icon		Skill	How and why use this skill?
	C	**Come in**	• Move your body physically close to child • Make movements calm and slow • By moving closer, child sees you are present and available to them • Increases child sense of reliability with the caregiver
	A	**Assist child**	• Help child problem-solve current issue • Establishes early teaching experiences • Perform with child versus doing for child Example: (child) starts to fuss when unable to sort toy (parent) slowly turns toy while child remains holding toy to show placement in toy sort
	R	**Reassure child**	• Creates opportunity for increased trust • Verbal statement child will be taken care of by caregiver Example: (parent) "It's ok, Mommy/Daddy is here." (parent) "I've got you, you're alright."
	E	**Emotional validation**	• Label child's feeling being expressed • Creates sense of understanding and support • Helps to build emotional vocabulary Example (parent) "I know it's sad/frustrating when…" (parent) "You're proud/happy because…"
	S	**Soothe (voice/touch)**	• Provides sense of safety and security • Gives physical cues everything is okay • Model for child relaxed and calm demeanor Example (parent) Give cuddle to child or soft caress (parent) Use quiet, lulling tone of voice

Provide **REDIRECTION** after CARES

Use toys with sounds for distraction   Move to a different area/location
Note if child is tired, hungry, and wet   Increase facial and verbal animation

Table 5.3 CARES emotion regulation skills for adults

PCIT-T: Emotion Regulation for Adults
CARES

Picture Icon		Skill	How and why use this skill?
	C	**Check cognitions, clue into yourself**	• Before beginning special time with your toddler, recognize: ○ Your thoughts/reason why you are spending time together ○ The feelings you bring into a play ○ How your body language demonstrates your current style of engagement
	A	**Assist self**	• If not emotionally ready for play, implement relaxation techniques to help refocus energy: ○ Deep breathing ○ Quick shower ○ Progressive muscle relaxation ○ Call to supportive system
	R	**Reassure self**	• Parenting presents challenges, and no one technique works for all children therefore use: ○ Positive self-talk ○ Remind yourself of tender moments ○ Foresee future events that will take place with your child bringing joy
	E	**Emotional awareness**	• Toddlers and babies are remarkably good at sensing emotions. They seem to track and respond to stress • Special time allows for fun and connection to be experienced when we engage in a play with positive thoughts and emotions
	S	**Sensitive and soothing**	• Similar to using a soothing voice with your toddler, be kind and sensitive to yourself in how you reassure yourself and the tone of your own self-talk. Remind yourself learning is a process of trial and error, plotting and adjusting courses as you go

Steps provided in any order and often simultaneously

> The more **EMOTION REGULATION** we can create in ourselves, the greater the benefit to our children.

provided to parents to explain emotion regulation skills to implement with toddlers and how parent can implement emotion regulation skills for themselves, respectively. Examples are provided to guide therapists in coaching an appropriate parent response and should be used to apply the CARES model to each individual child. The CARES model is discussed in further detail in Chap. 8.

As noted in the examples provided above, PCIT-T does not focus on discipline techniques, given the working assumption that there is no coercive cycle in place. PCIT-T strives to improve relationship enhancement between the parent and toddler, as well as develop sensitive parenting practices by the caregiver. It is a model that emphasizes learning a toddler's cues and how to tune into a toddler's needs, rather than changing a toddler's behavior. PCIT-T, through the emotion regulation technique of CARES, provides the essential scaffolding to build trust between the parent and toddler, to teach skills to self-soothe for both the parent and toddler, and to quickly redirect a behavior as a method to move a child away from distress. In order to effectively redirect a toddler, the toddler must first be calm. The parent is also taught to manage their own feelings in order to sit with their toddler when they express emotions that can be difficult for the parent to experience such as frustration, fearfulness, and anger. During PCIT-T the parent does not deny their child the experience of difficult emotions, as this is a new educational experience for the toddler. Additionally, the child is never left alone, and understanding is provided through emotion coaching to the toddler by the parent (see "Emotion Labeling and Emotion Coaching" section in Chap. 8).

Chapter 6
Behavioral Assessment in PCIT-T

Similar to PCIT, PCIT-T is a data-driven treatment approach. The ongoing collection of clinical data is necessary to inform ongoing treatment. Given the two primary treatment targets of (1) decreasing toddlers' behavior difficulties and (2) improving parenting skills, either the Devereux Early Childhood Assessment (DECA; LeBuffe & Naglieri, 2003, 2009; Mackrain, LeBuffe, & Powell, 2007) or the Brief Infant-Toddler Social and Emotional Assessment (BITSEA; Briggs-Gowan, Carter, Bosson-Heenan, Guyer, & Horwitz, 2006) must be administered to measure changes in children's behavioral and emotional outcomes. In addition, the Dyadic Parent-Child Interaction Coding System (DPICS; Eyberg, Nelson, Duke, & Boggs, 2010) must be used to measure parents' skill acquisition. Outside these measures, it is recognized that clinical practices have varying needs, considerations, and limitations with regard to clinical assessment. Therefore, practitioners and agencies may determine which additional assessments will be administered at the baseline, mid-treatment, and posttreatment assessment points.

In addition to child assessments, the practitioner should be aware of adult mental health concerns that may affect the child's functioning and the parent-child relationship. PCIT-T therapists should particularly be cognizant of the high rates of anxiety and depression in parents of young children. One possible referral question for PCIT-T is whether postpartum depression (current or in remission) has resulted in residual attachment and child behavioral problems. If a caregiver presents with active symptoms of postpartum depression, or another mental health disorder, a referral for a comprehensive evaluation would be appropriate in order to ensure that appropriate medical/psychiatric treatment and other relevant referrals can be secured. Other mental health issues that might be present in caregivers include marital discord, substance abuse, and trauma histories. A thorough intake interview should be undertaken that evaluates the overall psychological functioning of the child's caregivers. If concerns are noted, the practitioner can supplement the battery with adult assessment devices, such as measures of anxiety and depression. A list of optional measures for both child and adult evaluation is provided below to assist practitioners in obtaining assessment data that may be used to more thoroughly inform clinical treatment.

© Springer Nature Switzerland AG 2018   55
E. I. Girard et al., *Parent-Child Interaction Therapy with Toddlers*,
https://doi.org/10.1007/978-3-319-93251-4_6

Required Assessment Measures

The Devereux Early Childhood Assessment (DECA)

1. The DECA (LeBuffe & Naglieri, 2003, 2009; Mackrain et al., 2007) is designed to assess emotional, social, and behavioral concerns commonly present in early childhood. Two versions of the DECA are available: the DECA-Infant (DECA-I) is designed for children aged 1–18 months, while the DECA-Toddler (DECA-T) is designed for children aged 18–36 months. The self-report measure typically takes 15 minutes to complete. Critical areas of developmental growth including adaptive skills, communication, motor skills, play, and pre-academic/cognitive abilities are also assessed. The DECA-I, a strength-based measure captures areas of children's growth in two protective factor scales: initiative, and attachment/realtionships and provides a score for total protective factors. The DECA-T measure captures areas of children's growth in three protective factor scales: initiative, attachment/relationships and self-regulation and also provides a score for total protective factors. Assessment results provide clinicians with t-scores and percentile ranks with which pre-post intervention changes may be measured.

OR

Brief Infant-Toddler Social Emotional Assessment (BITSEA)

2. The BITSEA (Briggs-Gowan et al., 2006) is a parent-report screening questionnaire used to assess social and emotional difficulties in children 12–36 months of age. The instrument includes 42 items, and results are categorized according to two subscales including a problem score and competence score. Psychometric evaluation demonstrated high rates of overlap between the BITSEA and the well-known Child Behavior Checklist (CBCL; Achenbach and Rescorla, 2000) as well as the longer version entitled the Infant Toddler Social Emotional Assessment (Carter, 2013; Carter, Briggs-Gowan, Jones, & Little, 2003).

AND

Dyadic Parent-Child Interaction Coding System (DPICS)

3. The DPICS (Eyberg et al., 2010) is a standardized coding system designed to assess the quality of a parent-child relationship. Each parent verbalization during a play-based parent-child interaction is broken down and categorized according to a system of coding rules. Aptly described as "do" skills, certain categories have been found to enhance the quality of the parent-child interaction. Such categories include labeled praise, (verbal) reflection, and behavior description. However,

other categories have been found to diminish the quality of the parent-child interaction. Such categories include questions, commands, and critical talk statements. Psychometric research has found the DPICS to be highly valid and reliable across coders trained in the system.

Supplementary Assessment List

Ages and Stages Questionnaire (ASQ)

1. The ASQ (Squires & Bricker, 2009) is a 30-item self-report questionnaire completed by parents and caregivers to assess children aged 1 month to 5.6 years on a range of developmental areas. Such areas include communication, gross motor skills, fine motor skills, problem-solving, and personal-social development. The assessment typically takes approximately 10–15 minutes to complete. Psychometric research has demonstrated high levels of reliability, validity, sensitivity (0.86), and specificity (0.85). Results of the assessment provide information to determine if a child's development is considered typical; and whether monitoring may be necessary or if further assessment is needed.

Parenting Stress Index-Short Form (PSI-SF)

2. The PSI-SF (Abidin, 1995) is a 36-question self-report measure used to assess stress related to parenting within the context of the parent-child dyad. Questions are designed to simultaneously assess both parent and child domain, which combine into a total stress scale score. Three subscales including the parental distress, parent-child dysfunctional interaction, and difficult child are included. An additional validity scale (defensive responding) also indicates if a parent is responding to items from a defense perspective. The scale can be completed in less than 10 minutes and used with families of children younger than 12 years. Psychometric research indicates that indices of reliability and validity are high. See Abidin (1995) for more information.

Edinburgh Postnatal Depression Scale (EPDS)

3. The EPDS (Cox, Holden, & Sagovsky, 1987) is a 10-item self-report scale originally designed to screen postnatal women for depressive symptoms. The brief measure can also be used to assess depressive symptoms in the antenatal population, in mothers of children up to age 4 years, and in fathers. Participants should be asked to reference the past 7 days when responding to questions. Total scores at or above 13 in an English speaking population are considered clinically significant and may indicate a need for additional services.

Child Behavior Checklist (CBCL)

4. The CBCL (Achenbach & Rescorla, 2000) is a 99-item self-report measure used to assess behavior difficulties in children aged 18 months and older. An internalizing and externalizing subscale combines to form a total scale score from which respective t-scale and percentile ranks can be calculated. The well-standardized measure demonstrates strong psychometric properties including high reliability and validity.

The Modified Checklist for Autism in Toddlers, Revised with Follow-Up (M-CHAT-R/F)

5. The Modified Checklist for Autism in Toddlers, Revised (M-CHAT-R/F; Robins et al., 2014) is a free parent-report screening tool used to assess for risk of autism spectrum disorder in children aged 16–24 months. The M-CHAT-R/F comprises two sections: (1) initial 20-item parent-report questionnaire and (2) follow-up questionnaire administered by a professional (e.g., nurse, general practitioner). The initial questionnaire requires parents to answer questions regarding their child's current skill levels using a yes/no format and takes approximately 5 minutes to complete. If children screen positive on the initial questionnaire (score > 3), parents are then asked structured follow-up questions in order for the assessor to obtain additional information (Robins, Fein, & Barton, 2009). In the follow-up, which takes between 5 and 10 minutes to complete, scores of >2 indicate that further diagnostic evaluation is needed. The test authors also suggest that if the initial screener is >8, the follow-up can be bypassed, and instead the child can be referred immediately for further diagnostic assessment.

Initial Behavioral Assessment

Following completion of the standardized assessment measures, the therapist will conduct a behavioral assessment of the caregiver's and child's level of baseline skill. Specifically, an assessment of the baseline quality of the caregiver and child interaction will be conducted and coded using the Dyadic Parent-Child Interaction Coding System (DPICS). The three assessment scenarios will last 5 minutes each and will attempt to simulate three common caregiver-child interaction situations. The coding sheet used to code caregiver verbalizations during each of the three situations can be found in Section 2 under Pretreatment Interview and Assessment Session. At the conclusion of the assessment, the therapist should also determine the caregiver's use of the positive skills (e.g., imitation, enjoyment, affection), redirection, and affective skills (e.g., mutual eye contact, animated tone of voice, facial expression, developmentally appropriate play style) in addition to the caregiver's use of the CARES steps in response to the child's emotion dysregulation.

Prior to the initiation of the assessment, the clinician should refer to the "toy selection and room setup" portion of this book to ensure that the space is well suited to the assessment and the child's developmental needs.

Child-Directed Interaction-Toddler (CDI-T): This situation is designed to assess the quality of the caregiver-child interaction when few demands are placed on the child. Instead, the caregiver is told to allow the child to choose the toys and activity in which to play and follow the child's lead.

> "In this situation, tell [child's name] that he/she may play with whatever he/she chooses. Let him/her choose any activity he/she wishes. You just follow his/her lead and play along with him/her" (Eyberg & Funderburk, 2011, p.13).

Allow parent and child to "warm-up" for 5 minutes prior to coding. After the warm-up period, begin to time, and code using the DPICS for the 5-minute situation.

Parent-Directed Interaction-Toddler (PDI-T): This situation is designed to assess the quality of the caregiver-child interaction when the caregiver must direct the child according to his or her wishes. Therefore, the desired toys may be restricted, non-preferred demands may be placed on the child, and disruptive behavior may occur. After reading the instructions below, begin the timer, and code DPICS for the 5-minute situation.

> "That was fine. Now we'll switch to the second activity. Redirect [child's name] to play with a different toy in the room that you have chosen and see if you can get [child's name] to play with you" (Eyberg & Funderburk, 2011; p.13).

Cleanup (CU): This final situation is designed to assess the quality of the caregiver-child interaction when the caregiver must direct the child to perform a typically undesirable task. Given the young age of this population, caregivers should assist the children in cleaning up the toys. After reading the instructions below, begin timer, and code DPICS for the 5-minute situation.

> "That was fine. Now please tell [child's name] that it is time to clean up the toys (Eyberg & Funderburk, 2011; p.13). Help him/her put all the toys in their containers and all the containers in the toy box [or designate location]."

Ongoing Behavioral Assessment

Given the high need for supervision and attention toward children in the toddler stage of development, the provision of a frequent, time-intensive assessment in PCIT-T will instead occur upon a more limited basis as compared to typical PCIT, where an Eyberg Child-Behavior Inventory (ECBI; Eyberg & Pincus, 1999) measure is provided at the initiation of each appointment. Instead, caregivers will be asked to complete the Devereux Early Childhood Assessment (DECA) or the Brief Infant-Toddler Social Emotional Assessment (BITSEA) and any additional measures as required by their agency at pre/mid/post-treatment points which often include the intake appointment, during the parent-directed interaction teach session, and at the conclusion of treatment, just prior to the graduation session. Feedback from such measures should be provided during the session following their provision (i.e., CDI teach session, PDI coach Session #1, and graduation session, respectively). Due to the age of this population and their developmental needs some children may graduate from treatment after the CDI-T phase and therefore measures obtained would be limited to pre/post time-points.

Upon the initiation of each session after completing a check-in with the parent, clinicians code the caregiver during interactions with the child in a 5-minute behavioral assessment using the Dyadic Parent-Child Interaction Coding System (DPICS). To conduct PCIT-T with fidelity, therapists should receive training in the DPICS, which is typically conducted in a live workshop with a PCIT International certified trainer. Basic training requires studying the DPICS-IV Clinical Manual (Eyberg, Chase, Fernandez, & Nelson, 2014) and completing the exercises in the Clinical Workbook (Fernandez, Chase, Ingalls, & Eyberg, 2010) which are available for purchase at www.pcit.org. Researchers should use the DPICS Comprehensive Coding System for Research and Training – 4th Edition (Eyberg, Nelson, Ginn, Bhuiyan, & Boggs, 2013). Primary DPICS codes are described briefly below.

The DPICS "do" and "don't" skills are based on the concept of using play therapy to enhance the relationship between a caregiver and child. Parents are asked to provide a 5-minute, one-on-one, play therapy session with the identified child each day. This daily play session is designed to accomplish many goals, including the following: (1) improving the parent-child relationship, (2) enhancing child self-esteem, (3) giving the caregiver an opportunity to over-practice skills (until they become a habit) that have been shown to be associated with a warm and sensitive parenting style, (4) allowing the caregiver and child to jointly practice emotion regulation skills, (5) encouraging positive communication, (6) learning to redirect disruptive behavior, and (7) teaching prosocial skills to the toddler (e.g., playing appropriately with toys, sharing, being gentle). The overriding principle of this play therapy time is that the child is in the lead of the play. Termed "child-directed interaction" or CDI, the following skills are taught to caregivers to use intensively during a 5-minute daily playtime. In that CDI time, the skills are to be used at a high rate to teach parents to automatically/habitually respond in a sensitive and warm manner to their child's emotional and physical needs. "Do" and "Don't" skills are based on Eyberg and Funderburk (2011).

"Do" Skills

Labeled Praise

A labeled praise is a statement that specifically and positively evaluates an action, quality, or product of the child. While certain descriptive words are considered sufficiently positive to constitute praise (e.g., "good," "great," "wonderful," "like," "proud"), others are not (e.g., "funny," "energetic," "interesting"). Statements such as "Great job drawing your picture," "I love how nicely you are sitting in your chair," and "Thank you for playing gently with the toys" are each considered labeled praise. Praise statements used with toddlers should be kept brief and stated using simple terms. Therapists should encourage parents to repeat the same praise statements (e.g., "Good sitting," "Nice talking," "Thank you for sharing," "I like your gentle hands") on multiple occasions throughout play sessions. Labeled praise has been found to increase the positivity of the parent-child interaction, increase children's self-esteem, and increase the likelihood that the praised action will occur again.

Unlabeled Praise

Conversely, an unlabeled praise statement is a positive, evaluative statement but does not specify the action, quality, or product in reference. For example, unlabeled praise statements may include "good," "thank you," "awesome," or "wow." While unlabeled praises contribute to the positive nature of the interaction, they lead to less behavior change than labeled (specific) praises.

Reflection

A verbal reflection is a statement said in response to a child's initial verbalization that mimics or summarizes the meaning of the child's speech. While many reflections are stated as word-for-word repetitions of a child's speech, a child's noises or sounds can also be reflected. For example:

CHILD: [pointing to a toy car]: "Car!"
PARENT: "You see a car!"

Reflection statements are especially important during interactions with toddlers as such statements reinforce children's speech and help to build a child's vocabulary. The therapist should emphasize to caregivers the importance of reflecting any vocalization including sounds and noises.

Behavior Description

A behavior description is a statement commenting on a child's immediate action. Only positive, appropriate behavior should be described. Behavior descriptions help to expand a child's vocabulary in addition to helping him or her focus on a single toy or activity for an extended period of time. Behavior descriptions are a highly valuable resource for parents when interacting with young children, particularly when children are playing quietly. Given toddler's high need for consistency and predictability, therapists should encourage parents to describe a toddler's repetitive actions despite the replicative nature of such descriptions. For example:

CHILD: [putting blocks in a bucket and dumps them out again and again].
PARENT: "You put the blue block in the bucket, now the red block, now the yellow block. You dumped them out. You put the blue block in the bucket, now another blue block, now a green block. You dumped them out."

Emotion Labeling

While emotion labeling is not a mastery criteria category, it is an important skill for parents to identify and label children's emotions and states of being ("You seem happy", "You look sad", "You're concentrating"). It is also important for a parent to label their own emotions and states of being ("I'm excited to play with you", "I am so tired", "Mommy is getting hungry"). It is helpful for toddlers to be exposed to feeling words so that they can learn to recognize emotions and associate behaviors with corresponding emotional states. Therefore, parental statements regarding the child's emotion or their own emotion are coded in this category. Additionally, use of this skill is intended to increase children's emotional vocabulary, an important step in communication and emotion regulation.

Neutral Talk

Neutral talk includes statements made by the parent that give a sense of flow and connection to the interaction. These are statements that do not describe the behaviors, actions, or feelings of the toddler. Neutral talk is derived from the parent's commentary to the child and include teaching statements made by a parent ("This is a blue car"), sentences that describe what the parent is doing ("My truck is driving up the ramp"), as well as brief words of acknowledgment ("Yes," "Ok," "Sure," etc.).

Other Positive Skills

Although categories such as imitation (physically mimicking a child's action), enjoyment, physical affection, mutual eye contact, use of under-reaction and redirection, animated tone of voice, animated facial expression, and developmentally appropriate play are not quantitatively coded, the therapist should carefully monitor such verbalizations and behaviors to determine if the parent meets the "satisfactory" or "needs practice" criteria at the conclusion of the session or coded sequence.

"Don't" Skills

Questions

A question is an inquisitive statement that requires a verbal response from the child. Questions may be descriptive or informative in nature or may require the child to repeat or further elaborate on previous verbalizations. Descriptive questions may include words such as who, what, where, how, and when. Alternatively, many questions may occur in response to a child's statement whereby the statement is reiterated in the form of a question and thereby prompts a response. Questions tend to lead conversations and can direct a child's actions. Allowing toddlers to lead the play is especially important not only to minimize the chance of disruptive behavior but to reinforce a toddler's curiosity and need for independence and autonomy. For example:

CHILD: "Dat lello."
PARENT: "That's yellow?"

Commands

A command is a statement that requires the child to perform an action. While some commands may be stated indirectly ("Can you get your shoes?"), others may be stated directly ("Please hand me the blocks."). Alternatively, commands may imply that the parent and child will be performing the action together ("Let's put these dolls away."). As with questions, commands also tend to lead an interaction, making the play less reinforcing. Commands also decrease a child's natural self-direction and increase the chance of disruptive behaviors. Commands are also the one category where the toddler's response to the command is examined and assessed into the following three outcome categories:

Comply (CO): the toddler performs the task as stated in the command within 5 seconds.

Noncomply (NC): the toddler does not perform or make any attempt to perform the task as stated in the command within 5 seconds.

No opportunity to comply (NOC): A command is given such a format that the child is unable to comply or attempt to comply within 5 seconds, such as commands that are stated in rapid succession or repeated multiple times before the child can attempt to complete the task, commands that are to be performed in the future, commands given in list format therefore unclear if the child can recall all steps, and commands that cannot be measured through reliable observation such as "Listen," "Wait a second," "Be careful," or calling out the child's name for attention with no further detail.

Critical (Negative) Talk

A critical statement often includes words such as "no," "don't," "stop," "quit," or "not" and thereby indicates disapproval of a child's actions, products, or ideas. Critical talk has been found to decrease a child's self-esteem and provide attention toward negative behaviors, thereby increasing the chance that such behaviors are repeated. Finally, critical talk serves to decrease the rewarding nature of a parent-child interaction and impair a parent-child relationship. Examples of critical talk include "Don't do that," "That's not nice," and "Stop running around."

Mastery Criteria

In order to reach child-directed interaction mastery, a parent must use ten labeled praise statements, ten reflections, and ten behavior descriptions in a 5-minute coded sequence (Eyberg & Funderburk, 2011). An exception occurs if the child is nonverbal or makes fewer than ten verbalizations during the 5-minute coded sequence. In this case, the parent must reflect at least 75% of vocalizations within the time period. Additionally, caregivers must use three or fewer questions, commands, and critical talk statements during the 5-minute sequence. Once the caregiver successfully meets such requirements and it is determined that he or she has satisfactorily implemented the use of imitation, enjoyment, physical affection, redirection, animated tone of voice, animated facial expression, and developmentally appropriate play, the dyad may advance to the parent-directed interaction portion of the treatment (Table 6.1).

Following the coding sequence, the therapist should also determine the caregiver's use of the positive skills (i.e., imitation, enjoyment, physical affection, mutual eye contact, under-reaction and redirection, animated tone of voice/facial expression, developmentally appropriate play style, emotion labeling) in addition to

Table 6.1 Mastery criteria for child-directed interaction-toddler phase related to DPICS Coding in PCIT-T

Category	Mastery criteria
Labeled praise	10
Behavior description	10
Reflection	10* or 75% of child verbalization if child has limited verbal skills/opportunity for reflection
Questions / Commands / Critical (Negative) Talk	Combined ≤3

the caregiver's use of the CARES steps (discussed in detail in Chap. 6) in response to the child's emotion dysregulation. Such coding should inform the therapist of the caregiver's relative strengths and weaknesses in relation to the CDI-T skills and positive categories. Therapists should provide feedback to the caregiver regarding the strengths of the interaction as well as areas for improvement. Such feedback should be provided in the form of a "feedback sandwich" such that an area of strength is presented first, followed by an area of improvement (stated positively), and ending with another positive observation about the caregiver's skills or caregiver-child interaction. An example of a feedback sandwich is as follows: "You did a great job mastering both reflections, 14 total, and behavioral descriptions – I heard 12 of them. The one skill that can still use some attention is Labeled Praise. During coaching, we will focus on noticing everything that your daughter is doing well and praising these behaviors. Overall, your skills look fantastic. You followed her lead beautifully with great imitation and animation in your voice." The coding and subsequent feedback sandwich should be informative, helping therapists focus on one or two areas of improvement during coaching.

Discontinuing the Behavioral Assessment

It is important to note that if during the 5-minute coded interaction, the child becomes emotionally dysregulated and the caregiver appears overwhelmed or incorrectly performs the appropriate emotion regulation procedure, the therapist should stop coding and begin to coach. The coding is suspended in favor of coaching when a struggling parent seems to need considerable support to respond constructively to a challenging situation. For the most part, coding in PCIT-T is provided without interruption. The coding is only suspended in unusual situations in which the caregiver seems confused or hesitant about quickly assisting the child in managing a big emotion.

Developmental Milestones

PCIT-T requires the clinician to have a keen sense of the developmental issues for children in the 12 to 24 months age range. Therapists need to understand the expressive and receptive language capabilities of toddlers, as well as their physical/motor capacities. To coach effectively, the therapist should know the types of activities that are engaging for children of this age, as well as common safety concerns. In PCIT-T, sensitivity to the cognitive, emotional, physical, and behavioral issues of toddlers is key to improving the overall effectiveness of caregivers, including their awareness of their child's strengths, limitations, and developmental level, as well as their skills in responding empathically to their child's needs. Because of the importance of developmental expertise in this model, information about child development is interspersed throughout this book.

A child's cognitive, physical, social, and emotional growth between birth and 12 months of age is rapid and arguably astonishing to all who are witness to such change. By 1 year, many toddlers are beginning to walk, speak in single words, and apply simple cognitive concepts (e.g., cause and effect) to their physical world. However, careful consideration of the wide spectrum of development at this early stage must occur. A child who was born prematurely may fall behind the developmental level of a full-term infant. A child who suffered frequent ear infections during his first year may only use babble in unintelligible sounds rather than clear single words. Emotionally, some toddlers may point to desired objects while others may simply cry. Finally, a toddler's skill level in each developmental area may depend on his or her mood. Variables related to hunger, thirst, sleep, stimulation, and toileting may dramatically impact a toddler's behavior. For example, a typically patient child may become easily frustrated with a complex toy when he is hungry or nap time is nearing. Similarly, a child's culture and environment as either enriched or deprived of resources also powerfully impacts his or her developmental progression. As toddlers move through their second year of life, such advancement continues, and varying levels of progression may become clearer. Likewise, early intervention services (e.g., speech, physical therapy) can powerfully affect children suffering from developmental delay. Therefore, it is critical for clinicians working with this young population to understand typical developmental expectations to not only recognize a child's current abilities but frame treatment goals and scaffold intervention around such an informed framework. The reader is referred to Figs. 6.1, 6.2, 6.3, 6.4, and 6.5 for developmental checklists that provide a more thorough understanding of developmental expectations for toddlers at each stage of development throughout the third year of life. The authors acknowledge the generous contribution of the Centers for Disease Control and Prevention's "Learn the Signs. Act Early" Program who provided permission for these handouts to be used in this book and shared with parents receiving PCIT-T (Centers for Disease Control and Prevention, 2018).

Your Baby at 9 Months

Child's Name   Child's Age   Today's Date

How your child plays, learns, speaks, and acts offers important clues about your child's development. Developmental milestones are things most children can do by a certain age.

Check the milestones your child has reached by the end of 9 months. Take this with you and talk with your child's doctor at every visit about the milestones your child has reached and what to expect next.

What Most Babies Do at this Age:

Social/Emotional

❑ May be afraid of strangers
❑ May be clingy with familiar adults
❑ Has favorite toys

Language/Communication

❑ Understands "no"
❑ Makes a lot of different sounds like "mamamama" and "babababababa"
❑ Copies sounds and gestures of others
❑ Uses fingers to point at things

Cognitive (learning, thinking, problem-solving)

❑ Watches the path of something as it falls
❑ Looks for things he sees you hide
❑ Plays peek-a-boo
❑ Puts things in her mouth
❑ Moves things smoothly from one hand to the other
❑ Picks up things like cereal o's between thumb and index finger

Movement/Physical Development

❑ Stands, holding on
❑ Can get into sitting position
❑ Sits without support
❑ Pulls to stand
❑ Crawls

Act Early by Talking to Your Child's Doctor if Your Child:

❑ Doesn't bear weight on legs with support
❑ Doesn't sit with help
❑ Doesn't babble ("mama", "baba", "dada")
❑ Doesn't play any games involving back-and-forth play
❑ Doesn't respond to own name
❑ Doesn't seem to recognize familiar people
❑ Doesn't look where you point
❑ Doesn't transfer toys from one hand to the other

Tell your child's doctor or nurse if you notice any of these signs of possible developmental delay for this age, and talk with someone in your community who is familiar with services for young children in your area, such as your state's public early intervention program. For more information, go to www.cdc.gov/concerned or call 1-800-CDC-INFO.

The American Academy of Pediatrics recommends that children be screened for general development at the 9-month visit. Ask your child's doctor about your child's developmental screening.

Adapted from CARING FOR YOUR BABY AND YOUNG CHILD: BIRTH TO AGE 5, Fifth Edition, edited by Steven Shelov and Tanya Remer Altmann © 1991, 1993, 1998, 2004, 2009 by the American Academy of Pediatrics and BRIGHT FUTURES: GUIDELINES FOR HEALTH SUPERVISION OF INFANTS, CHILDREN, AND ADOLESCENTS, Third Edition, edited by Joseph Hagan, Jr., Judith S. Shaw, and Paula M. Duncan, 2008, Elk Grove Village, IL: American Academy of Pediatrics. This milestone checklist is not a substitute for a standardized, validated developmental screening tool.

www.cdc.gov/actearly | 1-800-CDC-INFO

Learn the Signs. Act Early.

Fig. 6.1 Developmental checklist: 9 months

Your Child at 1 Year

Child's Name   Child's Age   Today's Date

How your child plays, learns, speaks, and acts offers important clues about your child's development. Developmental milestones are things most children can do by a certain age.

Check the milestones your child has reached by his or her 1st birthday. Take this with you and talk with your child's doctor at every visit about the milestones your child has reached and what to expect next.

What Most Children Do at this Age:

Social/Emotional

❏ Is shy or nervous with strangers
❏ Cries when mom or dad leaves
❏ Has favorite things and people
❏ Shows fear in some situations
❏ Hands you a book when he wants to hear a story
❏ Repeats sounds or actions to get attention
❏ Puts out arm or leg to help with dressing
❏ Plays games such as "peek-a-boo" and "pat-a-cake"

Language/Communication

❏ Responds to simple spoken requests
❏ Uses simple gestures, like shaking head "no" or waving "bye-bye"
❏ Makes sounds with changes in tone (sounds more like speech)
❏ Says "mama" and "dada" and exclamations like "uh-oh!"
❏ Tries to say words you say

Cognitive (learning, thinking, problem-solving)

❏ Explores things in different ways, like shaking, banging, throwing
❏ Finds hidden things easily
❏ Looks at the right picture or thing when it's named
❏ Copies gestures
❏ Starts to use things correctly; for example, drinks from a cup, brushes hair
❏ Bangs two things together
❏ Puts things in a container, takes things out of a container
❏ Lets things go without help
❏ Pokes with index (pointer) finger
❏ Follows simple directions like "pick up the toy"

Movement/Physical Development

❏ Gets to a sitting position without help
❏ Pulls up to stand, walks holding on to furniture ("cruising")
❏ May take a few steps without holding on
❏ May stand alone

Act Early by Talking to Your Child's Doctor if Your Child:

❏ Doesn't crawl
❏ Can't stand when supported
❏ Doesn't search for things that she sees you hide.
❏ Doesn't say single words like "mama" or "dada"
❏ Doesn't learn gestures like waving or shaking head
❏ Doesn't point to things
❏ Loses skills he once had

Tell your child's doctor or nurse if you notice any of these signs of possible developmental delay for this age, and talk with someone in your community who is familiar with services for young children in your area, such as your state's public early intervention program. For more information, go to **www.cdc.gov/concerned** or call **1-800-CDC-INFO**.

Adapted from CARING FOR YOUR BABY AND YOUNG CHILD: BIRTH TO AGE 5, Fifth Edition, edited by Steven Shelov and Tanya Remer Altmann © 1991, 1993, 1998, 2004, 2009 by the American Academy of Pediatrics and BRIGHT FUTURES: GUIDELINES FOR HEALTH SUPERVISION OF INFANTS, CHILDREN, AND ADOLESCENTS, Third Edition, edited by Joseph Hagan, Jr., Judith S. Shaw, and Paula M. Duncan, 2008, Elk Grove Village, IL: American Academy of Pediatrics. This milestone checklist is not a substitute for a standardized, validated developmental screening tool.

www.cdc.gov/actearly   1-800-CDC-INFO

Learn the Signs. Act Early.

Fig. 6.2 Developmental checklist: 12 months (1 year)

Your Child at 18 Months (1½ Yrs)

Child's Name   Child's Age   Today's Date

How your child plays, learns, speaks, and acts offers important clues about your child's development. Developmental milestones are things most children can do by a certain age.

Check the milestones your child has reached by the end of 18 months. Take this with you and talk with your child's doctor at every visit about the milestones your child has reached and what to expect next.

What Most Children Do at this Age:

Social/Emotional

❏ Likes to hand things to others as play
❏ May have temper tantrums
❏ May be afraid of strangers
❏ Shows affection to familiar people
❏ Plays simple pretend, such as feeding a doll
❏ May cling to caregivers in new situations
❏ Points to show others something interesting
❏ Explores alone but with parent close by

Language/Communication

❏ Says several single words
❏ Says and shakes head "no"
❏ Points to show someone what he wants

Cognitive (learning, thinking, problem-solving)

❏ Knows what ordinary things are for; for example, telephone, brush, spoon
❏ Points to get the attention of others
❏ Shows interest in a doll or stuffed animal by pretending to feed
❏ Points to one body part
❏ Scribbles on his own
❏ Can follow 1-step verbal commands without any gestures; for example, sits when you say "sit down"

Movement/Physical Development

❏ Walks alone
❏ May walk up steps and run
❏ Pulls toys while walking
❏ Can help undress herself
❏ Drinks from a cup
❏ Eats with a spoon

Act Early by Talking to Your Child's Doctor if Your Child:

❏ Doesn't point to show things to others
❏ Can't walk
❏ Doesn't know what familiar things are for
❏ Doesn't copy others
❏ Doesn't gain new words
❏ Doesn't have at least 6 words
❏ Doesn't notice or mind when a caregiver leaves or returns
❏ Loses skills he once had

Tell your child's doctor or nurse if you notice any of these signs of possible developmental delay for this age, and talk with someone in your community who is familiar with services for young children in your area, such as your state's public early intervention program. For more information, go to **www.cdc.gov/concerned** or call **1-800-CDC-INFO**.

The American Academy of Pediatrics recommends that children be screened for general development and autism at the 18-month visit. Ask your child's doctor about your child's developmental screening.

Adapted from CARING FOR YOUR BABY AND YOUNG CHILD: BIRTH TO AGE 5, Fifth Edition, edited by Steven Shelov and Tanya Remer Altmann © 1991, 1993, 1998, 2004, 2009 by the American Academy of Pediatrics and BRIGHT FUTURES: GUIDELINES FOR HEALTH SUPERVISION OF INFANTS, CHILDREN, AND ADOLESCENTS, Third Edition, edited by Joseph Hagan, Jr., Judith S. Shaw, and Paula M. Duncan, 2008, Elk Grove Village, IL: American Academy of Pediatrics. This milestone checklist is not a substitute for a standardized, validated developmental screening tool.

www.cdc.gov/actearly   1-800-CDC-INFO

Learn the Signs. Act Early.

Fig. 6.3 Developmental checklist: 18 months

Your Child at 2 Years

Child's Name   Child's Age   Today's Date

How your child plays, learns, speaks, and acts offers important clues about your child's development. Developmental milestones are things most children can do by a certain age.

Check the milestones your child has reached by his or her 2nd birthday. Take this with you and talk with your child's doctor at every visit about the milestones your child has reached and what to expect next.

What Most Children Do at this Age:

Social/Emotional

❑ Copies others, especially adults and older children
❑ Gets excited when with other children
❑ Shows more and more independence
❑ Shows defiant behavior
  (doing what he has been told not to)
❑ Plays mainly beside other children, but is beginning
  to include other children, such as in chase games

Language/Communication

❑ Points to things or pictures when they are named
❑ Knows names of familiar people and body parts
❑ Says sentences with 2 to 4 words
❑ Follows simple instructions
❑ Repeats words overheard in conversation
❑ Points to things in a book

Cognitive (learning, thinking, problem-solving)

❑ Finds things even when hidden under two or three covers
❑ Begins to sort shapes and colors
❑ Completes sentences and rhymes in familiar books
❑ Plays simple make-believe games
❑ Builds towers of 4 or more blocks
❑ Might use one hand more than the other
❑ Follows two-step instructions such as "Pick up your shoes
  and put them in the closet."
❑ Names items in a picture book such as a cat, bird, or dog

Movement/Physical Development

❑ Stands on tiptoe
❑ Kicks a ball
❑ Begins to run

❑ Climbs onto and down from furniture without help
❑ Walks up and down stairs holding on
❑ Throws ball overhand
❑ Makes or copies straight lines and circles

Act Early by Talking to Your Child's Doctor if Your Child:

❑ Doesn't use 2-word phrases (for example, "drink milk")
❑ Doesn't know what to do with common things, like a brush,
  phone, fork, spoon
❑ Doesn't copy actions and words
❑ Doesn't follow simple instructions
❑ Doesn't walk steadily
❑ Loses skills she once had

Tell your child's doctor or nurse if you notice any of these signs of possible developmental delay for this age, and talk with someone in your community who is familiar with services for young children in your area, such as your state's public early intervention program. For more information, go to **www.cdc.gov/concerned** or call **1-800-CDC-INFO.**

The American Academy of Pediatrics recommends that children be screened for general development and autism at the 24-month visit. Ask your child's doctor about your child's developmental screening.

Adapted from CARING FOR YOUR BABY AND YOUNG CHILD: BIRTH TO AGE 5, Fifth Edition, edited by Steven Shelov and Tanya Remer Altmann © 1991, 1993, 1998, 2004, 2009 by the American Academy of Pediatrics and BRIGHT FUTURES: GUIDELINES FOR HEALTH SUPERVISION OF INFANTS, CHILDREN, AND ADOLESCENTS, Third Edition, edited by Joseph Hagan, Jr., Judith S. Shaw, and Paula M. Duncan, 2008, Elk Grove Village, IL: American Academy of Pediatrics. This milestone checklist is not a substitute for a standardized, validated developmental screening tool.

www.cdc.gov/actearly | 1-800-CDC-INFO

Learn the Signs. Act Early.

Fig. 6.4 Developmental checklist: 24 months (2 years)

Your Child at 3 Years

Child's Name   Child's Age   Today's Date

How your child plays, learns, speaks, and acts offers important clues about your child's development. Developmental milestones are things most children can do by a certain age.

Check the milestones your child has reached by his or her 3rd birthday. Take this with you and talk with your child's doctor at every visit about the milestones your child has reached and what to expect next.

What Most Children Do at this Age:

Social/Emotional

- ❑ Copies adults and friends
- ❑ Shows affection for friends without prompting
- ❑ Takes turns in games
- ❑ Shows concern for a crying friend
- ❑ Understands the idea of "mine" and "his" or "hers"
- ❑ Shows a wide range of emotions
- ❑ Separates easily from mom and dad
- ❑ May get upset with major changes in routine
- ❑ Dresses and undresses self

Language/Communication

- ❑ Follows instructions with 2 or 3 steps
- ❑ Can name most familiar things
- ❑ Understands words like "in," "on," and "under"
- ❑ Says first name, age, and sex
- ❑ Names a friend
- ❑ Says words like "I," "me," "we," and "you" and some plurals (cars, dogs, cats)
- ❑ Talks well enough for strangers to understand most of the time
- ❑ Carries on a conversation using 2 to 3 sentences

Cognitive (learning. thinking. problem-solving)

- ❑ Can work toys with buttons, levers, and moving parts
- ❑ Plays make-believe with dolls, animals, and people
- ❑ Does puzzles with 3 or 4 pieces
- ❑ Understands what "two" means
- ❑ Copies a circle with pencil or crayon
- ❑ Turns book pages one at a time
- ❑ Builds towers of more than 6 blocks
- ❑ Screws and unscrews jar lids or turns door handle

Movement/Physical Development

- ❑ Climbs well
- ❑ Runs easily
- ❑ Pedals a tricycle (3-wheel bike)
- ❑ Walks up and down stairs, one foot on each step

Act Early by Talking to Your Child's Doctor if Your Child:

- ❑ Falls down a lot or has trouble with stairs
- ❑ Drools or has very unclear speech
- ❑ Can't work simple toys (such as peg boards, simple puzzles, turning handle)
- ❑ Doesn't speak in sentences
- ❑ Doesn't understand simple instructions
- ❑ Doesn't play pretend or make-believe
- ❑ Doesn't want to play with other children or with toys
- ❑ Doesn't make eye contact
- ❑ Loses skills he once had

Tell your child's doctor or nurse if you notice any of these signs of possible developmental delay for this age, and talk with someone in your community who is familiar with services for young children in your area, such as your local public school. For more information, go to **www.cdc.gov/concerned** or call **1-800-CDC-INFO.**

Adapted from CARING FOR YOUR BABY AND YOUNG CHILD: BIRTH TO AGE 5, Fifth Edition, edited by Steven Shelov and Tanya Remer Altmann © 1991, 1993, 1998, 2004, 2009 by the American Academy of Pediatrics and BRIGHT FUTURES: GUIDELINES FOR HEALTH SUPERVISION OF INFANTS, CHILDREN, AND ADOLESCENTS, Third Edition, edited by Joseph Hagan, Jr., Judith S. Shaw, and Paula M. Duncan, 2008, Elk Grove Village, IL: American Academy of Pediatrics. This milestone checklist is not a substitute for a standardized, validated developmental screening tool.

www.cdc.gov/actearly | 1-800-CDC-INFO

Learn the Signs. Act Early.

Fig. 6.5 Developmental checklist: 36 months (3 years)

References

Abidin, R. R. (1995). *Parenting stress index: Professional manual* (3rd ed.). Lutz, FL: Psychological Assessment Resources, Inc.

Achenbach, T. M., & Rescorla, L. A. (2000). *Manual for the ASEBA preschool forms and profiles*. Burlington, V.T: University of Vermont, Research Center for Children, Youth & Families.

Briggs-Gowan, M. J., Carter, A. S., Bosson-Heenan, J., Guyer, A. E., & Horwitz, S. M. (2006). Are infant-toddler social-emotional and behavioral problems transient? *Journal of the American Academy of Child and Adolescent Psychiatry, 45*, 849–858.

Carter, A. S. (2013). Infant-toddler social and emotional assessment (ITSEA). In F. R. Volkmar (Ed.), *Encyclopedia of autism spectrum disorders* (pp. 1601–1606). New York, NY: Springer.

Carter, A. S., Briggs-Gowan, M. J., Jones, S. M., & Little, T. D. (2003). The infant–toddler social and emotional assessment (ITSEA): Factor structure, reliability, and validity. *Journal of Abnormal Child Psychology, 31*(5), 498–514.

Centers for Disease Control and Prevention. (2018). Learn the Signs. Act Early. Retrieved from https://www.cdc.gov/ncbddd/actearly/index.html

Cox, J. L., Holden, J. M., & Sagovsky, R. (1987). Detection of postnatal depression: Development of the 10-item Edinburgh postnatal depression scale. *British Journal of Psychiatry, 150*, 782–786.

Eyberg, S., Chase, R., Fernandez, M., & Nelson, M. (2014). *Dyadic parent-child interaction coding system (DPICS) clinical manual* (4th ed.). Gainesville, FL: PCIT International.

Eyberg, S., & Funderburk, B. W. (2011). *Parent-child interaction therapy protocol*. Gainesville, FL: PCIT International.

Eyberg, S., Nelson, M., Ginn, N., Bhuiyan, N., & Boggs, S. (2013). *Dyadic parent-child interaction coding system: Comprehensive manual for research and training* (4th ed.). PCIT International.

Eyberg, S., Nelson, M. M., Duke, M., & Boggs, S. R. (2010). Manual for the Dyadic Parent-Child Interaction Coding System. Retrieved from http://www.pcit.org

Eyberg, S., & Pincus, D. (1999). *Eyberg child behavior inventory and Sutter-Eyberg student behavior inventory*. Lutz, FL: Psychological Assessment Resources.

Fernandez, M. A., Chase, R. M., Ingalls, C. A., & Eyberg, S. M. (2010). *The abridged workbook: Coder training manual for the Dyadic Parent-Child Interaction Coding System* Retrieved from Retrieved from http://pcit.phhp.ufl.edu/measures/abridged workbook feb 10.pdf:

LeBuffe, P. A., & Naglieri, J. A. (2003). *The Devereux early childhood assessment clinical form (DECA-C): A measure of behaviors related to risk and resilience in preschool children*. Lewisville, NC: Kaplan Press.

LeBuffe, P. A., & Naglieri, J. A. (2009). The Devereux early childhood assessment (DECA): A measure of within-child protective factors in preschool children. *NHSA Dialog, 3*(1), 75–80.

Mackrain, M., LeBuffe, P., & Powell, G. (2007). *Devereux early childhood assessment infants and toddlers*. Lewisville, NC: Kaplan Early Learning Company.

Robins, D. L., Casagrande, K., Barton, M., Chen, C. A., Dumont-Mathieu, T., & Fein, D. (2014). Validation of the modified checklist for autism in toddlers, revised with follow-up (M-CHAT-R/F). *Pediatrics, 133*(1), 37–45.

Robins, D. L., Fein, D., & Barton, M. (2009). *Modified Checklist for Autism in Toddlers, Revised, with Follow-Up (M-CHAT-R/F)*.

Squires, J., & Bricker, D. (2009). *Ages & stages questionnaires, third edition (ASQ-3)*. Baltimore, MD: Brookes Publishing.

The Devereux Center for Resilient Families. Retrieved from https://www.centerforresilientchildren.org/infants/assessments-resources/devereux-early-childhood-assessment-deca-infant-and-toddler-program/

Chapter 7
Room Setup, Toy Selection, and Special Considerations

Room Setup

Given the developmental stage of the toddler population, the selection of toys and setup of the therapy room are critically important to the success of treatment sessions. In contrast to PCIT, in which caregiver-child interactions often occur at a table, it is recommended that PCIT-T sessions occur while the dyad is seated on the floor. Ideally, the space should be free of tables and chairs or contain only small toddler-size table and chairs for imaginative play to occur. Such procedures increase the child's safety by minimizing the possibility of furniture-related hazards. All outlets should be covered. Any breakable items or items that may be a choking hazard must be removed from the room or placed far out of the child's reach. After a therapist has determined that a child is capable of remaining safe with the inclusion of such items, they may be included for clinical utility. Therapists are strongly urged to place protective caps on the corners of tables to increase safety. Ideally, the floor space may be covered with a colorful rug to increase its welcoming feel. Floor space must be cleaned frequently given the likelihood that young children may place nonfood items in their mouth.

Therapists should refer to the toy selection handout included in this book for specific toy suggestions found at the end of this chapter and reprinted in the CDI-T teaching session-by-session guide. Only a few toys should be placed in the room at the start of session. Toys may be rotated during the course of the session. Toys should be easily manipulated and should not include any small pieces. Therapists may consider items such as sorting toys, a play kitchen, as well as toys with light and sound, particularly to be used to redirect the child. Such cause-and-effect toys assist children with learning skills such as planning and organization, vocabulary development, and fine motor skills. Balls and other items that may inspire throwing behavior should be avoided. Regardless, it is likely that this age group will continue to throw available toys. A box should be provided in which toys may be appropriately placed. Given the likelihood that toddlers will frequently place toys in their

© Springer Nature Switzerland AG 2018
E. I. Girard et al., *Parent-Child Interaction Therapy with Toddlers*,
https://doi.org/10.1007/978-3-319-93251-4_7

mouth, it remains critically important that toys be cleaned and disinfected after each session, with particular detail during cold and flu season.

Toy Selections for Toddler-Aged Clients

Pretend Play Toys

Many toddlers in this stage are experiencing a growing vocabulary and demonstrate an increasing ability to use toys that encourage active pretend play. Toys such as farm sets, baby dolls, little people play sets, kitchen and house items present a wealth of opportunity for caregivers to use animated facial expressions, animated verbal expressions, as well as positive physical touch during play with their toddler. Using pretend play toys can also increase a toddler's exposure to hearing a variety of new vocabulary words and sounds such as caregivers "mooing" for the cow, naming the duck that says, "quack-quack", or describing the bright green peas placed into a pretend pot of soup. Through parent-child engagement in pretend play, a world of make-believe can be role modeled while simultaneously providing fun and learning to a toddler.

Stacking, Drop, and Dump Toys

Most toddlers love to watch items fall to the ground (much to the frustration of caregivers at mealtimes!). This newly developing skill of learning cause and effect is encouraged in play through the use of sorting toys where a piece fits into a certain shape or slot and then falls into a larger container, often with an accompanying sound. Toys that can be stacked and knocked over such as nesting bowls, large soft blocks, and stacking rings may also be used. Some toddlers end to have a repetitive play style (e.g., stack and dump, stack and dump, over and over again). Here, the caregiver has the opportunity to role model surprise and laughter at loud sounds of items falling, to label the colors of the blocks being stacked, to clap and cheer as the toddler looks for the correct sorting toys, and to encourage language by repetition of words such as, "Uh-oh the blocks fell down. Fell down."

Motor Movement Play

Toddlers are full of energy and very active. Play that includes motor movement helps to meet their developmental needs. Toys to assist in motor movement include: learning tables, walkers, push-and-pull toys, crawl tunnels, and ride-on scooters (avoid electronic). Toys to assist with fine motor movement include items that have dials, knobs, and switches that require manual manipulation. Moving parts are often paired with sounds/music and pop-up characters and include cause-and-effect response to buttons pushed, knobs turned, or switches flipped. During motor movement play, caregivers have the opportunity to model and express facial expressions of surprise to pop-up toys, clap and encourage child attempts to push buttons and flip switches, teaching the skill of perseverance. The toddler can gain exposure to a wider vocabulary during motor movement play when the caregiver names the colors of buttons pushed and describes the physical play of a toddler's movement such as moving, up and down, crawling, scooting, pushing, and pulling.

Creative Play

Curiosity and exploration are also milestones of play during the toddler years. Items such as jumbo crayons or "palm crayons" and large sheets of paper allow for body tracing, scribbles, and beautiful works of toddler art. Large empty boxes are a fantastic way to develop imagination and exploration with toddlers as they can be used for games of crawling/walking inside and outside the box, playing hide-and-seek, and opening and closing flaps. Creative play also includes use of music and songs to dance and move during the session and may include simple, sturdy musical play instruments such as xylophones, drums, maracas, and guitars to create their own music. The opportunity for caregivers to continue modeling facial expressions and animated vocal expression, cheering, clapping, and encouraging their toddler's music-making skills, imagination, and exploration are all present with the use of creative play.

Relaxing Play

During periods that require more quiet and relaxation, play items such as board books, bead mazes, peg boards, and wooden peg puzzles are great options to continue the fun of interacting together while engaging in more subdued activities. Board books provide a wonderful opportunity to read aloud to toddlers, name animals, generate animal sounds, point to pictures, and cuddle in close by having the toddler sit on the lap of or very near their caregiver. Bead mazes, peg boards, and wooden puzzles allow for focused sitting play which are helpful activities particularly when a toddler and caregiver are spending time in a waiting room or have limited space for movement. Teaching opportunities continue in relaxing play with labeling colors on the maze bead, describing what the toddler is doing with their hands, and assisting the toddler with turning peg puzzle shapes to fit into the peg board. The running theme for parent enthusiasm continues in this style of play with clapping and cheering when the toddler places puzzle pieces into the correct spot, or when the toddler reaches the end of the maze line with a particular bead, or when the toddler turns the pages of a board book.

Toy Selection

The number of ways to engage in play with a toddler is infinate as noted with the variety of choices previously described. The biggest limitation may be the adult's lost skill to play, be silly, and act young, especially in front of a clinician. Therefore, clinicians need to bring to session a sense of fun, playfulness, and an animated style of engagement to role model these skills for caregivers and to set the precedent regarding expectations for behavior. Additionally, clinicians need to be thoughtful regarding the number of toys selected for play as to not overstimulate the toddler. The clinician must also be aware and provide toys that are a developmental match to the toddler's play level as offering toys beyond the toddler's developmental level may lead to frustration and big emotions. During the initial assessment session, the clinician should seek feedback and guidance from the caregiver regarding the types of toys that hold the toddler's interest in the home environment. Clinicians should also have additional toys to swap in and out of session based on how the toddler responds during play. Table 7.1 provides recommended toys for use in PCIT-T.

Special Considerations for the Toddler Age Group

Scheduling Appointment Times: Naps, Hunger, and Diaper Changing

Scheduling therapeutic appointment times for the toddler age range can be tricky given the ideal time for learning occurs after nap time, once a child is fully awake and after all their basic needs have been met, such as hunger and diaper changing. Caregivers often have busy lives and so it can be a challenge to find times when their schedules overlap with the clinician's appointment openings. Avoid forcing an appointment times during the toddler's typical nap time, as this will only create frustration on the part of the caregiver when the toddler falls asleep in the car on the way to the appointment or struggles to wake from napping once arrived at the office setting. For some families with a less structured daily routine, it may be more challenging to predict when a toddler will require a nap, and clinicians must keep in mind that if the toddler appears cranky and tired at every session, an alternative appointment time may be required.

This same principle holds true for meal times. Toddlers eat multiple small portion sizes throughout the day, and learning during PCIT-T will occur best when hunger has been satisfied before the session begins. Encouraging a parent to meet their

Table 7.1 Recommended toy list for PCIT-Toddlers

Recommended Toy List for PCIT-Toddlers

Pretend Play

Puppets

Farm sets

Chunky train sets

Little People play sets

Kitchen / House sets

Baby dolls & items (doll bed, clothes, stroller)

Large wood / plastic toy vehicles with wheels

Stacking, Drop & Dump Play

Plastic bowls

Nesting toys / stacking rings

Large beads (non-choking hazard)

Soft blocks & cubes

Large Duplo blocks

Shape sorters

Relaxing Play

Board books

Bead Maze

Peg boards

Wooden peg puzzles

Motor Movement Play

Learning tables

Learning walkers

Push & pull toys

Crawl tunnels

Ride on / scoot vehicles

Toys with cause and effect/pop-up

(turn dials, switches, knobs, lids)

Creative Play

Jumbo/Palm crayons & large paper

Large empty cardboard boxes

Music / songs to dance

Simple sturdy musical instruments

child's basic needs is a fundamental component to PCIT-T and so the clinician may choose to encourage the caregiver to pack a small healthy snack every session, to be eaten when needed.

After consuming a meal or snack before arrival or during the PCIT-T session, the natural process of digestion leads to the next item of caregiver preparation, having diaper-changing supplies available. An agency offering PCIT-T should also consider having a diaper-changing station available in their restrooms, as well as a diaper pail for disposal of dirty diapers. Another recommendation for PCIT-T sites is to stock a small emergency supply of various size of diapers for caregivers caught off guard to a toddler's diaper-changing needs, including wipes and diaper cream. This models for caregivers how to be prepared for "diaper blowouts" and may serve as a teaching opportunity for caregivers that might not be aware of how frequently a diaper should be changed or how to identify the early signs of a diaper rash which may explain the fussy mood and irritability of a toddler.

Coaching During Transitions Between Caregivers

Transition periods for toddlers are a common time for them to experience a big emotion. This is often seen during PCIT-T when coaching two caregivers in the same session and may start as early as shifting from the waiting room into the treatment room. During coaching the transition period happens again when switching between the first caregiver and the second caregiver and having the toddler change focus on who is now participating in session with them. The recommendation to ease the transition period is to coach the caregivers implementing the following steps:

1. Have the currently coached parent come in close to the toddler, within touching distance and perhaps rubbing their back while stating, "Now [Daddy] is coming to play with you."
2. The "new" parent enters the room bringing with them upon entry a different toy to serve as a technique to decrease separation problems by using the toy as a distraction.
3. The "new" parent then gives a transitional statement, "[Daddy] is here to play with you," while showing the new toy as a distraction.
4. Both the "new" parent and "old" parent remain in close proximity with a gentle hand placed on the toddler, and then fade the "old" parent out of the room, while the "new" parent begins to play with the toddler.

Teething, Illness, and Growth Spurts

The importance of regularly attended sessions is a key factor to success in treatment as experiential learning and in vivo coaching are guiding principles to create change. The recommendation is to hold PCIT-T sessions twice a week if possible. When children in treatment become ill, have slight fevers due to teething, in general have a case of being "off" due to possible growth spurts, or a poor night sleep, it is imperative to reschedule the PCIT-T appointment as soon as possible. Postponed sessions and gaps in providing live in vivo coaching may contribute to delayed parent skill acquisition and slow momentum of caregiver and toddler learning, prolong the length of treatment, and can create a sense of doubt in the caregiver regarding treatment effectiveness. Therefore, every effort must be made by clinicians to provide consistent and regular treatment. This includes maintaining a flexible schedule to meet the quickly evolving needs of toddlers and their parents.

Referrals to Other Providers

The toddler years are complex, and referrals commonly involve other providers. Typical referrals may include pediatricians, audiologists, ophthalmologists, speech and language pathologists, and regional centers to name a few. Clinicians must be aware of their scope of practice and function within appropriate limits.

Chapter 8
Child-Directed Interaction-Toddler

The basic premise of PCIT-T is centered upon building a strong, positive relationship between a parent and toddler that, in turn, is used to teach young children a variety of emotion regulation, language, and social skills. Similar to standard PCIT, such skills remain the focus of the child-directed interaction portion of the program. Parents learn to use the power of their positive attention to manage and shape young children's behaviors. Such positive attention skills are built in the context of play-based parent-child interactions where parents learn to tune into, predict, and respond to young children's needs and natural cues, thereby preventing difficult behavior. While many of the CDI skills remain consistent between the standard PCIT model and the current adaptation, some are particularly emphasized, given the developmental needs of the population. New skills have also been added, in an effort to enhance the rewarding value of the parent-child interaction and provide a framework for enhancing emotion regulation in both the caregiver and child. Parents practice these skills in a daily, 5-minute play therapy session with the child which is referred to as "special time" (Eyberg & Funderburk, 2011).

© Springer Nature Switzerland AG 2018
E. I. Girard et al., *Parent-Child Interaction Therapy with Toddlers*,
https://doi.org/10.1007/978-3-319-93251-4_8

"Do" Skills

Labeled Praise

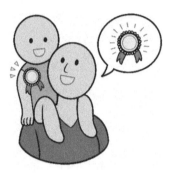

Specific, labeled praise ("Great job playing gently with the toys on the floor," "I love the way that you are keeping your hands to yourself") remains central to the dyad's positive interaction while increasing the likelihood that toddlers will continue to display such behaviors (Eyberg & Funderburk, 2011). In addition to providing toddlers with high-quality language, labeled praise is also used to build children's self-confidence and self-esteem. Positive attention is integral to the warm and nurturing parent-child relationship that serves as a foundation for promoting adaptive behavior in the child. It is likely and expected that certain labeled praise statements, targeting particular behaviors of interest, will be repeated on many occasions throughout a given session and in the course of special play time. Therapists may therefore consider discussing the specific behaviors and accompanying praise statements of particular focus for a given parent-child dyad. It is also expected that praise statements remain short and use language that is developmentally appropriate to the toddler population. Therefore, such praise statements may consist of fewer words and use less complex language as compared to that used with preschool-aged children. While non-specific praise statements are coded, emphasis should be placed on changing such unlabeled praise (e.g., "good job," "thank you") into labeled praise statements. Although such language is expressed as a positive evaluation of a child, little to no behavior change is likely due to the non-specific nature of such statements. For toddlers, labeled praise is made even more effective when given in an animated tone of voice and paired with physical displays, such as back rubs, tickles, high fives, claps, and hugs.

Behavior Description

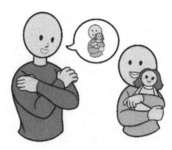

Behavior descriptions (Eyberg & Funderburk, 2011) are an especially useful verbal tool that provides regular, meaningful language to describe the toddler's actions. While some toddlers may be highly verbal in their use of words and sounds, others may remain relatively quiet during play, thereby allowing generous space for the use of descriptive statements. Such statements have been shown to improve children's ability to sustain attention as well as provide high-quality attention for appropriate behaviors (Tempel, Wagner, & McNeil, 2013). Enthusiasm in the context of descriptive statements remains critical both for enhancement and warmth of the interaction as well as the rewarding value of such positive attention. Additionally, behavior descriptions help parents remain focused on their child's play, allowing the dyad to engage in joint attention. Therapists should emphasize the importance of describing children's actions ("You put the man in the box") versus the actions of the toy ("The man went in the box"), as the toy description does not emphasize the child's behavior. Parents are likely to play at the child's developmental level and follow the child's lead when using behavior descriptions as the specific attention is directed to the child's ongoing, second-by-second actions. Similar to many other skills, therapists should remain especially mindful of the complexity of language being used to describe toddler's play. Scaffolding, or the concept of challenging individuals just beyond, without exceeding, their developmental potential, should be used when determining the context of language, relative to the individual toddler's expected level.

Reflection

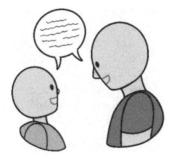

The use of verbal reflection is of critical importance during dyadic interactions between parents and their toddler-aged children. The skill provides reinforcement of verbalizations including words, sounds, and noises (Eyberg & Funderburk, 2011). Toddlers are likely to engage in sensible as well as non-sensible speech. All sounds, especially those of toddlers who are generally quieter by nature, should be reflected. Although verbal reflection may occur by summarizing the meaning of the child's speech, it is developmentally expected and appropriate for parents to repeat toddler's words and noises verbatim. Reflection allows parents to subtly correct a child's grammar and pronunciation by modeling correct speech, without criticism of the child's verbal efforts. Developmental concepts such as egocentrism, or the concept that young children view themselves, and their behaviors, wants, and needs, at the center of their understanding of the world, play a role in the extremely rewarding nature of verbal reflection for toddlers. Similar to praise and behavior description, the enthusiastic quality of such reflection is a critical aspect of the rewarding value of the social interaction.

Emotion Labeling and Emotion Coaching

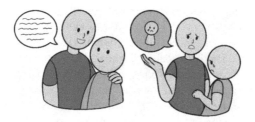

Emotion labeling and emotion coaching represent a novel, yet critical component of CDI-T skills. Improving young children's emotion regulation capacity remains integral to PCIT-T. Within this larger goal lies a smaller goal of increasing children's emotional vocabulary, identification, and understanding. Exposure to a wide variety of emotion labels, beyond basic emotions, is of key importance to increasing such skills in young children, thereby assisting children in the ability to recognize and feel validated for their feelings. Such labeling is to be implemented when it is perceived that children are experiencing a given emotion in the context of play. By labeling children's feelings in the moment that the feeling is experienced, it is expected that children will learn to connect such emotions to the provided vocabulary word, thereby allowing them to identify and appropriately express their emotions in the future. Additionally, parents are encouraged to label their own emotions and states of being while interacting with their child to role model emotional expression and vocabulary. Use of feeling words by parents is likely to increase parents' recognition of their child's emotional states, positively impact their understanding of their emotions on their child and help increase parents' responsivity to their child's emotional and behavioral needs.

There are six primary features of emotion coaching with examples provided in Table 8.1:

1. To describe to the parent the behaviors that you recognize to be associated with an emotion. This assists with a parent tuning into their toddler's cues and increasing the toddler's emotional vocabulary. It allows the parent to be present with their child's emotion without discounting how their toddler feels.
2. To encourage the parent to label the feeling the child is expressing. This also increases the emotional vocabulary of the toddler and assists in the parent tuning into the child's cues. It informs the child that the parent is present and aware of their emotional state.
3. To encourage the parent to show support and interest through CARES. The CARES model is discussed in detail later in this chapter.
4. To reflect and praise if the child uses any emotion labels. As the toddler begins to use emotional vocabulary, the caregiver is to reinforce this positive step through the use of reflection and praise. Use of the reflection skill provides a message to the toddler that they are being listened to and that their words are meaningful to the parent. The process of adding praise to the child after the reflection is to reinforce the use of emotional vocabulary and to build the self-esteem of the toddler. Praise, as discussed earlier, adds warmth to the relationship of the parent and toddler dyad.
5. To have the parent model, the use of feeling words, by expressing their own feelings. This provides observational learning for the toddler and helps the toddler understand how to react to emotions based on the parent response.
6. To praise the parent when they use feeling words and vocabulary. Through the use of praise to the parent, the coach is reinforcing the targeted skill of emotion labeling. The more parents are praised for a particular skill, the more likely they are to incorporate that skill outside therapeutic sessions.

Table 8.1 Six features of emotion coaching utilized in PCIT-T and example emotion coaching statements

Emotion coaching feature	Examples of emotion coaching statements
Describe to parent the behaviors that you recognize to be associated with an emotion	"Do you see how he is tensing up his muscles? Looks like he is getting frustrated and angry"
	"She has a big smile on her face. I think she might be feeling proud"
	"He jumped away from the toy. Looks like he felt surprised by that noise"
	"She is shaking a little and moving in for comfort. She looks a little fearful"
Encourage parent to label the feeling	"Can you label the emotion for her?"
	"Say, you seem a little sad about the puppy"
	"What do you think she is feeling right now? Can you label it for her?"
	"Let her know that she looks happy about completing that tower"

(continued)

Table 8.1 (continued)

Emotion coaching feature	Examples of emotion coaching statements
Encourage parent to show support and interest through CARES	Parent actions include:
	Physically moving in closer to the child
	Providing positive, gentle touch to the child
	Gaining mutual eye contact with the child
	Reassuring the child that the parent is there
	Parent offers to assist and help as needed versus taking over and doing for the child, thus taking time to problem-solve and teach
Reflect and praise if child uses any emotion labels	Child: "I'm mad at you mommy." Coach: "Say, good job using your feeling words. You are mad at mommy right now. I'm here. I am happy to help"
	Child: "I scared." Coach: "You're scared. That happened with the big sound. Nice job telling daddy your feelings. I'm here. We're both ok."
Parent models the use of feeling words, by expressing their own feelings	"This toy is hard to fix. I am feeling frustrated"
	"I am feeling proud that we cleaned up all the toys"
	"I am worried that you might fall off that chair"
	"I feel happy today because we get to play together"
Praise parent when they use feeling words	"Great job talking about feelings"
	"I like how you showed your child how to talk about anger"
	"Nice job labeling his emotion there"
	"You're setting a great example for how to handle emotions"
	"Good job for helping him understand the relationship between his feelings and his behaviors"

"Don't" Skills

Questions

Given the rule of allowing children to lead the play during the child-direction interaction portion of PCIT-T, skills that detract from the child's natural agency over play should be avoided. Specifically, the use of questions, commands, and critical statements should be kept to a minimum. Questions may begin with words such as "who," "what," "where," "why," and "how," or conversely, attempted reflections or behavior descriptions may turn into questions when the parent's voice inflects upward at the end of the phrase (e.g., "You are helping the kitty?"). Both types of questions should be avoided as they, often unintentionally, place demands on children with the expectation of a verbal answer (Eyberg & Funderburk, 2011).

Commands

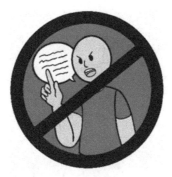

Commands may occur in the form of direct (e.g., "Please hand me the block.") or indirect (e.g., "Can you hand me the block?") demands in which a subsequent behavior is expected. Like questions, command statements may decrease the positivity of an interaction and direct the child's play, thereby increasing the chance that difficult behaviors may occur. Subsequently, if a child does not respond to a given demand, a negative interaction between the parent and child may ensue (Eyberg & Funderburk, 2011).

Negative Talk/Critical Statements

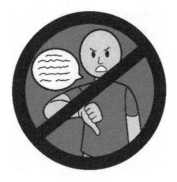

Finally, negative or critical speech may decrease children's self-esteem and sense of agency over the environment in which they naturally desire independence. Words indicative of critical speech include "no," "don't," "stop," "not," and "quit." In addition to providing attention for undesirable behaviors, the overuse of such phrases may decrease their potency when children are engaging in unsafe or dangerous behaviors. Taken together, the "don't" skills should be kept to minimal levels during in-session and Home Therapy Practice times in an effort to increase the parent's awareness of such statements and thereby increase the warmth and positivity of the parent-child relationship (Eyberg & Funderburk, 2011).

Other Positive Skills

Enjoyment, Animation, and Enthusiasm

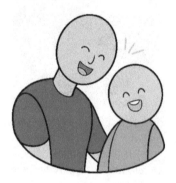

Although the importance of displaying enjoyment and enthusiasm should arguably be emphasized during play with children of all ages, it remains especially critical during play with toddlers. Signs of enjoyment, including an enthusiastic, animated tone, animated facial expressions, variability in the parent's voice, use of sounds (e.g., animal noises, nonsensical sounds), clapping, and smiling, elevate the reinforcing power of the PRIDE skills. Such sounds are especially important with the toddler population given the variability in receptive language abilities. Therefore, such enjoyment naturally increases the rewarding value of spoken language regardless of the child's cognitive comprehension. Additionally, explicit enjoyment and enthusiasm also increases the positive, engaging quality of the interaction, thereby increasing the warmth of the relationship. Toddlers are more likely to remain engaged in an interaction that is perceived as fun and, therefore, sustain attention on the given task (Eyberg & Funderburk, 2011).

Physical Affection

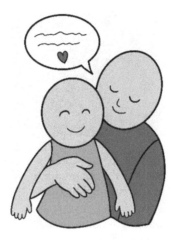

Similar to the importance of enjoyment, animation, and enthusiasm, physical affection is a critical aspect of warm relationships. Affection creates connection between people and serves as a natural bonding agent. Affection and physical touch increases the reinforcing value of praise and can help orient a child's attention toward or away from a given task. Touch can also serve as a physiological calming agent, particularly during times of distress. It may come in the form of rubbing a child's back, giving a "high five," hugging, holding, rocking, or cuddling. As it is important for touch to occur in a way that feels natural to a particular parent, therapists should consider speaking to caregivers about their preferred methods for using touch to show physical affection. Naturally less affectionate parents may need more directed coaching on how and when to express physical touch, while overly affectionate parents may benefit from guidance regarding giving their toddler developmentally appropriate levels of independence. Therapists may then explicitly point out the impact of such touch on children during live coaching, thereby reinforcing its value to the parent and the dyadic relationship. For example, a coach may point out to the parent that a particular touch encouraged the child to sit on the parent's lap or that a well-timed hug helped the child to soothe quickly when frustrated. Such observations should be noted to parents to reinforce their appropriate use of the skill.

Mutual Eye Contact

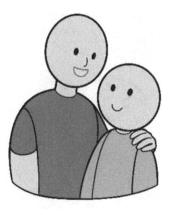

Mutual eye contact between a parent and child is a sign of connection and joint attention between two people. Joint attention assists a child in orienting toward a given stimulus and contributes to engagement integral to the implementation of the child-directed interaction skills. Mutual eye contact and joint attention play an integral role in helping to form the positive parent-child bond built in the child-directed interaction phase of the intervention. Parents can be coached to look directly into their child's eyes when speaking and to use smiles and exaggerated facial expressions while sustaining eye contact. Games like "peek-a-boo" can encourage parents to use eye contact in an animated fashion to bond with their children.

Play at Child's Developmental Level

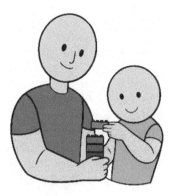

While use of behavioral descriptions and imitation assist parents in playing at a child's developmental level, the concept should be emphasized throughout PCIT-T. Playing at a child's developmental level supports the foundational concept of following the child's lead during the child-directed interaction portion of PCIT-T.

The use of scaffolding, or challenging children in play just beyond the area in which they are comfortable, should be a constant theme of parent's play and therapist's coaching. Such developmental considerations are likely to vary considerably among children depending upon their chronological age, emotional, physical, social, and language development. Such skills are also likely to change throughout the course of PCIT-T, so constant anecdotal assessment of the child's developmental abilities should be conducted during observation and coaching. By scaffolding play, children learn skills and abilities just beyond those at their current developmental level. However, playing at a toddler's developmental level may feel repetitive and under-stimulating for some parents, particularly those who do not feel naturally connected to their child. Therapists must remain especially mindful of the types of toys provided in the environment from which the child and parent's play originates. If provided toys are developmentally advanced or inspire play over and above the child's level, reconsideration should occur. Additionally, if parents or children become bored by the use of the same toys, dyads may have difficulty engaging in developmentally appropriate play. Coaches should be especially mindful of instances in which the parent intentionally or unintentionally may begin to play at a level far above that of the toddler-aged child. Such instances are likely to cause children to decrease their natural initiation. Additionally, some may cease playing all together which, in turn, may lead to the experience of big, negative emotions.

Imitation

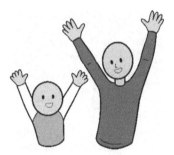

Finally, the critical importance of imitation should be emphasized as a primary area of intervention throughout PCIT-T. Young children, in particular, learn fundamental concepts such as cause and effect as well as basic play and social skills via the imitation of others. Imitation allows parents to remain focused on play at the toddler's developmental level by following the toddler's lead. Finally, imitation provides natural reinforcement for and approval of toddlers' appropriate behavior, thereby increasing the likelihood of such behaviors in the future (Eyberg & Funderburk, 2011).

CARES Skills

Similar to the PRIDE skills, the CARES model is an acronym to symbolize the use of five critical skills to be implemented by parents when their toddler-aged children experience big, difficult-to-manage emotions. CARES skills provide a clear guide to recognize and respond to children's cues of emotional distress. Therefore, such skills assist parents and therapists to model and teach emotion regulation skills while also teaching children appropriate coping skills to manage such emotions. Although instances in which all skills are used may occur, there are times in which only some skills may be applicable. The CARES steps may be used in any order as appropriate to the situation and are often implemented simultaneously. Table 8.2 provides the caregiver handout that explains the CARES Emotion Regulation Skills for Toddlers.

Come In

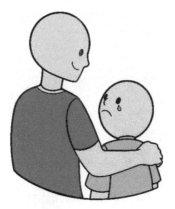

The "C" stands for the concept of coming in close to the child. During this step, therapists should coach parents to physically move into close proximity to the child, a necessary step of the implementation of subsequent CARES skills. Such physical movement communicates messages of warmth and responsivity, as well as physical and emotional availability. A calm demeanor during implementation of this step is critical so as to avoid emotional escalation on the part of the child or parent. A calm presence also models effective emotion regulation skills.

Table 8.2 CARES emotion regulation skills for toddlers

PCIT-T: Emotion Regulation for Toddlers

CARES

Steps Provided in Any Order & Often Simultaneously

Picture Icon		Skill	How & Why Use This Skill?
	C	**Come In**	• Move your body physically close to child • Make movements calm and slow • By moving closer child sees you are present and available to them • Increases child sense of reliability with the caregiver
	A	**Assist Child**	• Help child problem solve current issue • Establishes early teaching experiences • Perform with child versus doing for child Example: (child) starts to fuss when unable to sort toy (parent) slowly turns toy while child remains holding toy to show placement in toy sort
	R	**Reassure Child**	• Creates opportunity for increased trust • Verbal statement child will be taken care of by caregiver Example: (parent) "It's ok, Mommy/Daddy is here." (parent) "I've got you, you're alright."
	E	**Emotional Validation**	• Label child's feeling being expressed • Creates sense of understanding & support • Helps to build emotional vocabulary Example (parent) "I know it's sad/frustrating when…" (parent) "You're proud/happy because…"
	S	**Soothe (voice/touch)**	• Provides sense of safety & security • Gives physical cues everything is ok • Model for child relaxed & calm demeanor Example (parent) Give cuddle to child or soft caress (parent) Use quiet, lulling tone of voice

Provide **REDIRECTION** after CARES

Use toys with sounds for distraction
Note if child tired, hungry, wet and address

Move to different area/location
Increase facial and verbal animation

Assist

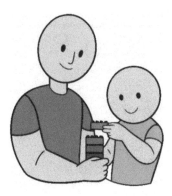

The "A" stands for assist, in which parents should physically assist the child with his or her difficulty at hand. Preferably, therapists may assist parents in scaffolding the desired task and thereby enable the child to solve the difficulty on his or her own. Child-directed interaction skills should continue to be used during this time to encourage the child and continue to orient his or her attention toward the task. Upon successful completion, high levels of specific, enthusiastic praise should be provided. However, if scaffolding does not quickly result in the child's independent task completion, the parent should complete the task for the child. Should the parent consistently need to complete such tasks, consideration regarding the developmental level of the provided toys should occur. This "assist" step helps to alleviate children's frustration by reducing the difficulty of tasks or solving such problems altogether. Subsequently, such parental responsivity helps to improve the parent-child bond by increasing feelings of trust and warmth in the parent-child relationship.

Reassure Child

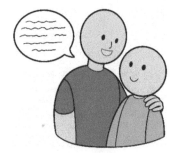

The "R" stands for Reassure Child, in which the parent should verbally state the concept that they are physically present, and their needs will be met (e.g., "Mommy is here to help."). It is critical that such Reassure Child is done in a calm and soothing tone of voice, thereby allowing toddlers with limited receptive language skills to also feel comforted by these words. Such verbal expression communicates feelings of care and acknowledgment of the child's feelings. Additionally, these words naturally convey hope for resolution of the dilemma through the parent's nurturing actions.

Emotional Validation

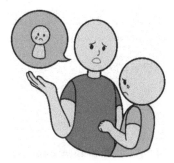

Next, the "E" stands for emotional validation, as the parent labels the emotion being experienced by the child. Active labeling of feelings models complex emotional vocabulary, a critical step within the broader context of emotion regulation. By labeling the child's emotion, parents communicate their validation of the child's emotional state. In turn, such emotional recognition increases the chances that upon gaining the appropriate expressive language skills, children will be more likely to identify, describe, and understand their own emotional state and those of others in the future. Although it is likely that core emotional descriptions such as happy, sad, scared, and angry will be offered, more complex states such as disappointment, surprise, frustration, boredom, and excitement should also be incorporated into such descriptions, as appropriate to promote expansion of emotional vocabulary for both the parent and child.

Soothe

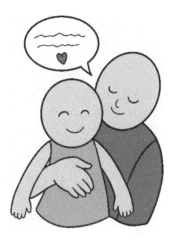

Finally, the "S" stands for soothe the child with voice and touch. While the concept of positive touch is emphasized throughout the current intervention, it remains critical within the CARES model. Physical touch assists children in physiological relaxation while also promoting feelings of closeness and responsivity between parents and their children. While touch may occur in the form of rubbing or patting the child's back, stroking his or her head, or picking up the child and rocking him or her, such positive touch naturally communicates messages of care, comfort, and connection between a parent and child. Therapists should discuss forms of touch that feel natural to the parent and child and incorporate coaching surrounding such touch into session. Additionally, therapists should point out the effect of touch upon the parent-child relationship as well as the child's ability to regulate his or her emotions.

Redirection After CARES

Immediately after implementing CARES, the caregiver is instructed to enthusiastically describe a toy or fun play activity in order to redirect the child toward a type of play that will further encourage emotion regulation. To summarize, the steps of handling a big emotion involve coming in closely and calmly, assisting the child, reassuring the child that the parent is there to help, validating the child's emotional experience, soothing the child with words and touch, and finally engaging the child in a fun activity through enthusiastic distraction and redirection procedures.

Parallel Process of CARES

In PCIT-T, the CARES steps are primarily discussed with regard to parents' implementation of the model for their children; however, emphasis is also placed upon the parallel process that naturally occurs as the therapist models and assists parents in implementing the steps for themselves, particularly during the presence of their own big emotions. In an effort to increase the parents' awareness of their emotions and their effect upon the toddler-aged child, it is recommended that parents practice diaphragmatic breathing exercises prior to engaging in play. The CARES steps for adults are as follows: "C" = Check Cognitions, Clue into Yourself, "A" = Assist Self with Relaxation, "R" = Reassure Self with Positive Self-talk, "E" = Emotional Awareness and Acceptance, and "S" = Sensitive and Soothing Thoughts and Behaviors.

Should strong parental emotions arise, particularly during moments of child distress, the therapist should remind parents to be kind to themselves, reflect upon feelings, and continue to develop awareness of their cognitions (the "C" step). Next, parents should assist themselves in managing their feelings by using relaxation steps such as deep breathing and cognitive distraction (the "A" step). Therapists should also reassure parents that they have the skills and knowledge to manage their emotions and the situation at hand. Positive self-talk may be used to decrease maladaptive thoughts (the "R" step). Next, parents should recognize and validate their own feelings. Techniques such as mindfulness may be useful in identifying and accepting, rather than judging their emotions (the "E" step). Finally, therapists may help parents soothe themselves by prompting them to speak to themselves in a calm voice and use relaxation strategies (the "S" step).

Outside the therapy session, it should be noted that it is not possible or expected that parents will utilize the CARES steps in response to every instance of the toddler's emotion dysregulation throughout the day. Instead, emphasis should be placed on the implementation of such skills during the five-minute play practice at home, with the expectation that regular practice will make these skills more automatic (habitual). Therapists should provide empathy regarding the fact that despite learning such valuable skills, consistent implementation of the skills is exhausting and may detract from the toddler's ability to learn self-regulation, frustration tolerance, and self-control skills, also imperative to successful emotion regulation. The expression of such empathy may help decrease feelings of guilt when the parent is unable to implement CARES skills every time a child is distressed throughout the day and night. Finally, instances may arise in which the child clearly desires space away from the parent. Careful thought should be put toward recognizing and complying with the child's request for distance/autonomy and whether to use the full CARES model within this context. Many times, recognition and compliance with requests for autonomy demonstrate attentive understanding toward a child's feelings. However, at other times, a parent and therapist may identify a child's need for assistance with emotion regulation despite the child's cues indicative of a desire to distance from the parent (e.g., pushing a parent away). Toddlers can have ambivalent or contradictory needs for both closeness and distance at the same time. The therapist should assist parents in reading and interpreting complex emotions and behaviors in the toddler. During sessions, the therapist can use "trial and error" coaching to determine the timing of when to have the parent come in closer with CARES and when to give the child some space before implementing the standard CARES approach. Table 8.3 provides the caregiver handout that explains the CARES Emotion Regulation Skills for Adults.

Behavior Management Skills

Skills of Under-Reaction and Redirection

In contrast to the CARES steps, instances may arise in which a child is *not* experiencing a big emotion but engages in minor misbehaviors while remaining calm seen during interactions of cause and effect (e.g., tossing the cup off the table and then looking at the parent or turning a light switch off and on while looking at the parent). Although it is emphasized in the current model that a toddler's experience of difficult behaviors and emotions is not typically indicative of negative

Table 8.3 CARES emotion regulation skills for adults

PCIT-T: Emotion Regulation for Adults

CARES

Picture Icon		Skill	How & Why Use This Skill?

	C	**Check Cognitions, Clue into Yourself**	• Before beginning special time with your toddler recognize:
			  o your thoughts/reason why you are spending time together
			  o the feelings you bring into play
			  o how your body language demonstrates your current style of engagement

	A	**Assist Self**	• If not emotionally ready for play implement relaxation techniques to help refocus energy:
			  o deep breathing
			  o quick shower
			  o progressive muscle relaxation
			  o call to supportive system

	R	**Reassure Self**	• Parenting presents challenges and no one technique works for all children therefore use:
			  o positive self-talk
			  o remind yourself of tender moments
			  o foresee future events that will take place with your child bringing joy

	E	**Emotional Awareness**	• Toddlers and babies are remarkably good at sensing emotions. They seem to track and respond to stress. • Special time allows for fun and connection to be experienced when we engage in play with positive thoughts and emotions.
	S	**Sensitive & Soothing**	• Similar to using a soothing voice with your toddler, be kind and sensitive to yourself in how you reassure yourself and the tone of your own self-talk. Remind yourself learning is a process of trial and error, plotting and adjusting courses as you go.

Steps Provided in Any Order & Often Simultaneously

> The more **EMOTIONAL REGULATION** we can create in ourselves the greater the benefit to our children.

attention-seeking but rather difficulty with emotion regulation. There are specific instances in which attention-seeking plays a role in the behavior. In those instances when a toddler is engaging in a maladaptive behavior to provoke a reaction from the caregiver, the use of under-reaction and redirection is warranted in an effort to decrease the chance of their reoccurrence. Such under-reaction may involve a minor pulling away of attention by the parent in which the parent breaks eye contact and simply looks away from the child's behavior for a few seconds. A more overt form of under-reaction may occur by turning the parent's body away from the child.

The ability to initiate provocative, attention-seeking actions that would warrant the use of under-reaction is likely to increase as the toddler ages. During under-reaction, the parent may intentionally look away from the child and refrain from speaking about the behavior. The parent may also choose to remove the object in use and quickly replace it with a toy that by nature inspires more appropriate play. The parent should refrain from speaking about the undesirable behavior. Then, the parent may implement the skill of redirection by enthusiastically playing with and describing a toy. Toys with lights, sounds, and moving parts may be especially useful during redirection. It is likely that by this point, the child's attention will have been redirected elsewhere, and the parent may be able to quickly return to the use of PRIDE skills. Given that CARES is the preferred response in the presence of the child's big emotions, under-reaction and redirection are most commonly used when the child's emotions are regulated, and they are calmly testing the parent's likelihood of reacting to a given behavior. In other words, big emotions are not typically occurring during the under-react and redirect process. However, should such big emotions occur when coaching the parent to under-react and redirect, the therapist should switch to coaching the parent in the CARES skills. In addition to the use of redirection following the implementation of under-reaction, redirection should also be implemented if it appears that a child is becoming bored or is no longer interested in a given activity (e.g., by walking away from the parent). Upon reinitiation of play, the PRIDE skills should be used to reinforce the child's return to the play.

Dangerous and Destructive Behaviors

Although the majority of young children's negative behaviors involve instances of emotion dysregulation without dangerous and destructive behaviors, such concepts may co-occur. Given safety concerns and possible perpetuation of dangerous and destructive behaviors, additional attention toward these behaviors is warranted, despite the presence of emotion dysregulation. First and foremost, prevention of such behaviors remains critical. Therefore, careful consideration should be given to designing the environment to minimize such behaviors. PCIT-T's approach to dangerous and destructive behaviors is consistent with the child attachment litera-ture's conceptualization that the parent is the "bigger, stronger, wiser and kind one" (Powell, Cooper, Hoffman, & Marvin, 2014), which teaches children to access parents as a source of comfort and safety.

Aggression and self-injurious behaviors represent two common dangerous behaviors in toddler-aged children. Following such behavior in PCIT-T, a brief, yet assertive, limit-setting procedure is implemented (i.e., holding the child's hands

Table 8.4 PCIT-T Aggression and self-injury limit-setting technique

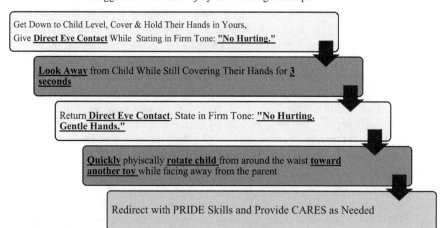

and positioning the child away from the parent), whereby the child is quickly prevented from engaging in the behavior. After a few seconds of limit setting, it is critical that the caregiver then provides enthusiastic redirection to reorient the child's attention and engages him or her in appropriate play. Such firm attention remains in direct contrast to the presence of enthusiastic, high-quality attention provided during the absence of such behavior, sending a message to the child that the behavior is unacceptable. If, after the procedure, there is a reoccurrence of aggression or self-injury, the procedure should be repeated. Table 8.4 outlines the steps to coach a parent through aggressive or dangerous behaviors.

An exception for the aggression procedure is when the child escalates to extreme levels of emotional and behavioral dysregulation (e.g., thrashing, kicking or head banging) that preclude the parent from simply holding the toddler's hands. In these cases of extreme emotion dysregulation, the parent should be instructed to pick up, rock, and soothe the child, while the parent is either standing or sitting on the ground. In such cases, it is likely that implementation of a minor hand-holding procedure is likely to perpetuate, rather than diminish, the presence of the aggressive behavior, as intended. Therefore, emphasis is placed on the child's clear inability to regulate his or her emotions, and physical assistance is warranted. In cases in which the child and parent both demonstrate mutual difficulty regulating their emotion, the therapist may consider entering the room to support and coach the parent in the physical presence of the parent and child.

Crucial to coaching is teaching a parent how to implement preventative measures prior to a toddler's emotional dysregulation. A preventative approach includes looking for early cues to interrupt dangerous or destructive behaviors before they begin. Early toddler cues are noted by increased tension in muscle tone, facial grimaces, toddlers vocalized frustration, and physically swatting away toys and objects. Theses cues are often present prior to head banging or hitting. These concerns highlight the need for assessing early child cues in all areas by both the clinician and parent. Through coaching one goal is to have the parent begin to see the buildup of cues. Clinical success is noted that once a parent begins to use new language and states, "he needs my help", mentioning the child's emotion by use of emotion labeling prior to being coached. More information regarding emotion coaching is provided in CDI-T Chap. 8.

In addition to physical aggression, toddlers commonly engage in toy throwing. While the use of under-reaction and redirection procedures is likely to resolve instances in which such behavior is low in intensity, not accompanied by a big emotion, and primarily based in a cause-and-effect-like game, a big emotion may accompany other instances. When a big emotion does accompany such behavior, parent responsivity is critical to assisting the child in regulating his or her emotions. In such cases, the child should be physically moved away from the thrown toy, thereby naturally redirecting the child to a new, immediate environment. If the toy must be taken away from the child, a new, safe toy should be given to the child, while enthusiastic redirection occurs. Finally, if emotional escalation continues to occur, the therapist may coach the parent to physically remove toys from the play area and place such toys out of the child's sight while simultaneously implementing the CARES model.

In addition to physical aggression, property destruction, and toy throwing, other behaviors that require parental guidance are also likely to occur. For example, toddlers may climb on furniture, should such items be present. When possible, furniture should be taken out of the room or the parent may strategically place his or her body in front of the furniture to minimize the likelihood of climbing. It should be expected that toddlers will place toys in their mouth. In addition to regular toy cleaning, any small toys that are mouthed should be removed, and redirection should quickly occur. In such cases, a replacement toy may be provided. If toddlers attempt to touch off-limit items (e.g., electrical outlets, parent's purse), parents should physically move the child away from the item, and redirection should occur. Similarly, if a child becomes frustrated by a toy that is over his or her developmental level, the item may be removed, and the child redirected. Finally, if a child becomes bored by a given set of toys, the therapist may consider entering the room with new toys, or the parent may redirect the child by demonstrating a novel use of a toy already present in the space.

Coaching Considerations During CDI-Toddlers

Readers should reference coaching considerations previously discussed in Chap. 2 ("philosophy of coaching") for a critical, broad-based understanding of coaching philosophy. Similar to the core foundation of the child-directed phase of PCIT and PCIT-T, child-directed interaction coaching is warm, supportive, encouraging, and skill-based. Many of the coaching categories that focus on increasing parents understanding of their toddler's behavior is similar to the concept of "reflective functioning," discussed in attachment literature, which impacts emotion regulation. Parents are learning to divide their attention between listening to and incorporating feedback while playing with and implementing CDI-T skills with their child. Therapeutic rapport is built through CDI-T coaching. Given that parental skill acquisition may occur at varying speeds, it is critical that parents in CDI-T feel supported and understood throughout the process. Relationship building takes time. Beyond the quantitative skills (e.g., praise, reflection, description), positive (qualitative) skill use (e.g., imitation, enjoyment, physical affection, mutual eye contact) remains critically important to successful CDI-T implementation. When interactions are going well, CDI-T coaching should be viewed as a rhythmic exchange between the parent and therapist. Brief, consistent feedback should be provided after each parent verbalization. When the parent accidently uses an avoid skill, the therapist should ignore its use, wait for a positive skill to be used, and praise its use. At times, a gentle correction may be provided without use of the words "no," "don't," "stop," "quit," and "not." Following CDI-T sessions, therapists should provide parents with praise for skill use and its subsequent effect upon the child. Discussion regarding areas of improvement including clarification of skills and goals for the upcoming week of Home Therapy Practice should occur. Depending on children's moods, such discussion may also occur via phone shortly following the session. Additional information and guidance regarding coaching can be found in Appendix A at the conclusion of this book.

In addition to emotion coaching statements seen in Table 8.1 and the various categories of coaching statements presented in Table 8.5, it is often common for a clinician to recognize and coach caregivers who may experience dysfunctional cognitions about themselves, or their child. Given that thoughts, feelings, and behaviors are all intricately connected, it is clinically relevant for a PCIT-T coach to address a parent's maladaptive thoughts. Through live coaching the PCIT-T clinician assists the parent in reframing their dysfunctional cognitions and helps the parent implement the use of positive self-talk with the goal to improve the parent-child relationship. Table 8.6 provides commonly experienced dysfunctional cognitions and sample coaching statements.

Table 8.5 A selection of PCIT-T coaching categories and example coaching statements

Labeled praises	• Good job showing him you understand what he wants
	• I like how you came close to him
	• You are doing a great job of calming him down
	• Nice work being so sensitive to his needs
	• Great work labeling his feelings
	• Good work commenting on his eye contact
	• Good job being available and labeling the emotion
	• Wow, that's great that she is showing you that she needs your help
	• That's a great way to assist her
	• You set a very clear limit, well done
	• I love how you redirected him with a noisy toy
	• Your enthusiastic voice is making it fun for him, well done
	• Your close positioning is perfect for letting her know you're available
	• I am so impressed how quickly you are calming him now congratulations
Directives	• You can acknowledge his feelings
	• He needs you to come in close and help him calm down
	• You need to reassure him
	• I want you to tell him "mummy is here for a cuddle"
	• He needs your help, so move in close
	• Show him you're available for him by some physical contact
	• You can tell her that you like it when he lets you help him
	• You need to set a gentle clear limit
	• I want you to say in a gentle voice, "No hurting"
	• Please distract him with a noisy toy
	• You need to say: We need to use gentle hands
Observations	• It's hard for him when he can't get what he wants
	• Your calm voice and closeness is very reassuring for him
	• I can see he is more settled now and ready for a cuddle
	• He knows you are there to help him as he is more peaceful now
	• That's going to teach her that she can count on you
	• He's not ready yet, please stay close
	• Your close positioning is perfect to help keep him calm
	• It's great to see you come in close to help him with his emotions
	• You have worked so hard to develop your skills and it is really paying off
	• You are using the calming skills so confidently, it is really working
Education	• Nice reflecting, that will help her with her speech
	• Good describing, it helps him focus
	• By being close you're letting him know you are there for him
	• Your modeling gentle play helps him to learn how to be gentle
	• By labeling his feelings and helping him you have avoided a tantrum
	• Being close and those little pats keeps him calm
	• She is talking a lot because of your Behavioral Descriptions
	• Your special time together is making him so happy and content
	• I can see you are enjoying those cuddles and he can too

(continued)

Table 8.5 (continued)

Praise the child category	• She's so clever with those shapes • He is so sweet the way he always gives you the blocks • I can see lots of beautiful smiles today, what a happy boy • Love how he looks into your eyes so lovingly • She is leaning into you and is feeling very safe • What a cutie. She is sharing • She has a great laugh • He is so good at giving cuddles

Selective ignoring of parental mistakes	• Parent Using lots of questions:
	  Coach – Good making that a positive statement
	• Parent unsure what to do:
	  Coach – You can distract him with a noisy toy. Wow you got him playing again
	• Parent not joining in the game:
	  Coach – You can show her how to share by copying what she is doing with the toy. Great job imitating her game
	• Parent taking over the game:
	  Coach – Let her lead. Fantastic job following her lead
	• Parent unsure what to say:
	  Coach – You can tell her what you like that she is doing; follow-up with wonderful label praise
	• Child is fussy:
	  Coach – He needs your help and to be close. Beautiful job calming him down

Table 8.6 Common dysfunctional cognitions and coaching healthy cognitions in PCIT-T

Dysfunctional cognition	Healthy cognition
"I'm a terrible parent"	"My child is displaying some especially challenging behaviors, and I don't know how to manage them quite yet"
"My child hates me"	"My child says and does things that make me sad when he is upset"
"At this rate, she's going to grow up to be a real disappointment to me"	"I'm so glad that we are addressing these behaviors now so that the world will be able to see all of her amazing strengths and not just these difficult behaviors"
"She's doing this on purpose to irritate me"	"She is still learning to express how she is feeling in an appropriate way"
"He was born this way and he'll never change"	"He is strong-willed and that trait will serve him well when he wants to get a good job 1 day!"
"This treatment won't work"	"I've tried therapy before, but this one seems different. I need to give it a chance"
"Nothing calms him down"	"He is very difficult to soothe, but this new approach is designed to help children just like him"
"I'll never be able to get him to sleep"	"He hasn't been sleeping as well as I'd like, but this treatment will help him soothe himself so that I can sleep better too"

(continued)

Table 8.6 (continued)

Dysfunctional cognition	Healthy cognition
"She will never be potty-trained"	"It might take her a little longer to be potty-trained than other kids, but we'll get there"
"When he's like this, nothing works"	"His emotions feel overwhelming for both of us sometimes"
"She loves to get me mad"	"She has a difficult time calming herself down when she is upset. That's why we're getting help."
"I can't do this positive parenting stuff"	"This feels so foreign to me. Maybe it'll feel more natural after some practice"
"She is never good. She misbehaves constantly."	"It feels like she misbehaves all day, but we actually do have some positive moments. Maybe I'm just having a hard time noticing them"
"I tried the special play once, and it didn't work"	"We tried something similar to this once but maybe some of the differences in this new program will be exactly what we need."
"I should be more patient, like all the other parents"	"I've had to manage some difficult behaviors that make it especially hard to be patient."
"I will never be able to master these skills"	"These skills are really challenging. I think I need more practice in order to master them"
"The damage is done. I've already messed her up for life"	"We've had some negative interactions, but she is still young, and we're learning new, healthier ways to get along"
"He's going to grow up to be hateful, just like his father"	"I see some similarities between him and his father, but there are still lots of time to help him learn ways to cope when he's upset"

References

Eyberg, S., & Funderburk, B. W. (2011). Parent-child interaction therapy protocol. Gainesville, FL: PCIT International.

Powell, B., Cooper, G., Hoffman, K., & Marvin, R. (2014). *The circle of security intervention: Enhancing attachment in early parent–child relationships*. New York: Guilford Press.

Tempel, A. B., Wagner, S. M., & McNeil, C. B. (2013). Behavioral parent training skills and child behavior: The utility of behavioral descriptions and reflections. *Child & Family Behavior Therapy, 35*(1), 25–40.

Chapter 9
Parent-Directed Interaction-Toddler

Parent-Directed Interaction-Toddler Overview

It is well known within the child development literature that authoritative parenting, which includes fundamental aspects of warmth and positivity, while clearly enforcing control and discipline, has been found to lead to highly positive outcomes for children (Baumrind, 1978). Therefore, similar to standard PCIT, the parent-directed interaction-toddler (PDI-T) component of the intervention remains integral to teaching children, and their parents, the necessary skills to assist children in learning to listen, regulate their emotions, and in turn, develop self-control. Unlike standard PCIT, however, the nuances of toddlers' emotional, cognitive, physical, and social abilities place them in a markedly different developmental place as compared to preschool-aged children. The current implementation of parent-directed interaction skills, named parent-directed interaction-toddler (PDI-T), is thus conceptualized within the toddler's developmental framework. Additionally, it is recognized that such abilities, even among toddlers of the same chronological age, are likely to vary greatly. Therefore, it is expected that clinical judgment will be carefully exercised during implementation of the PDI-T procedures.

The most fundamental aspect of PDI-T lies in the basic understanding that the procedure is meant to teach listening skills, rather than implement negative consequences for noncompliance. In standard PCIT, it is assumed that the preschool- or school-aged child may intentionally defy authority to delay or escape completion of the undesirable demand. Toddlers, however, remain in the process of learning the necessary abilities to comply with demands, including language comprehension, sustained attention, and social awareness. Therefore, noncompliance in its standard sense is better conceptualized as a lack of applicable listening skills. In turn, such skill deficits lead to the increased provision of appropriate opportunities to learn such skills. In PDI-T, listening skills are taught using a guided compliance procedure, commonly used in applied behavior analysis (ABA), to help children of varying abilities learn to follow instructions. The rules of effective commands remain

© Springer Nature Switzerland AG 2018
E. I. Girard et al., *Parent-Child Interaction Therapy with Toddlers*,
https://doi.org/10.1007/978-3-319-93251-4_9

foundational to the appropriate implementation of the procedure and are therefore taught first. Similar to standard PCIT, commands should be stated directly and in a neutral tone of voice, given one at a time, specific, and provided with explanations only prior to the command or following compliance. Overall, commands should be used only when necessary.

Three additional rules have been and are emphasized within the context of toddler's developmental abilities. First, commands should be limited to only a few simple concepts (e.g., "Please hand me ___." "Please sit down."). Prior to implementation, parents are asked to rank order a short list of developmentally appropriate commands in order from most to least likely to lead to child compliance. Then, commands are taught in the same order to maximize the child's chance of success. Progress through each command only occurs following mastery of the chosen concept. The commands provided encompass an appropriate range of toddler's developmental abilities and are likely to be useful in the daily lives of young children and their parents. Next, a positive, physical touch and clear, physical gestures must be used in conjunction with the provided command. A physical touch (e.g., touching the child's back) is used to assist in gaining the child's attention, while gestures help children orient toward stimuli necessary for completing the desired listening exercise. Finally, the close proximity between the parent and child is emphasized as a critical aspect of teaching listening skills to toddlers. This includes caregivers providing eye contact to the child during the command process while getting down to the child's level. The caregiver does not force the child to engage in eye contact but rather models providing eye contact as part of the process of verbal communication. This critical skill is fundamental to the success of the listening procedure by emphasizing the parent's physical role in teaching listening skills. Listening practice is also limited to when the child is in a good mood. A maximum of three commands per PDI-T coaching session are implemented, if appropriate, and during the PDI-T parent-child home therapy practice the same limitation of three commands total is followed. Emphasis is placed on providing opportunities to teach listening skills versus drilling a toddler with multiple commands, much like older children learning to spell their name small periods of practice are provided and revisited in manageable daily doses.

Guided Compliance Steps

Next, each step of the guided compliance procedure is described: "Tell," "Show," "Try Again," and "Guide." These four steps provide the structure to teach listening skills and allow rehearsal of listening skills to occur for toddlers, keeping in mind a maximum practice of three commands per day with use of the Tell-Show-Try Again-Guide procedure. Additionally, optimal learning conditions are needed prior to the start of the Tell-Show-Try Again-Guide procedure; therefore, should the child be sick, teething, hungry, or have other basic needs at the time of PDI-T coaching listening skills no commands shall be provided and the Tell-Show-Try Again-Guide procedure will not be implemented.

Tell

"Tell," the initial step of the listening procedure, uses a verbal command to communicate the desired action. Using simple language, the behavior is paired with a physical gesture (e.g., pointing repeatedly) to visually orient the child to the action. To enhance the child's comprehension, the gesture should be repeated constantly throughout the five-second window following the initial command. Oftentimes, a distracted or otherwise engaged toddler will naturally orient to the desired action via the gesture during the course of the five-second process. The parent should be silent during this time frame. Additionally, the importance of a full, five-second window following delivery of the command is emphasized. Similar to standard PCIT, young children need quiet time to cognitively process and begin to act upon spoken words. If the child completes the command during the designated five-second window, an enthusiastic labeled praise and warm, positive touch should be provided. The positive touch is particularly emphasized in the current adaptation as such actions serve to enhance the positive value of the praise as well as feelings of warmth within the relationship.

Show

The second step, "show," uses physical modeling to demonstrate the desired action to the child. Within the step, the parent repeats the command along with the words "like this". The parent then physically completes the command prior to placing the object back in its original location. It is then expected that the toddler replicates the parent's modeled actions. A silent, five-second window with repeated gestures orienting the child to the desired behavior is then provided. The procedure is meant to complement toddler's cognitive comprehension of spoken language with a visual display of the intended behavior. Upon compliance, an enthusiastic labeled praise and warm, positive touch should be provided. Should listening not occur, the procedure progresses onto a third step.

Try Again

The "try again" step is a novel adaptation within the current protocol added based on anecdotal accounts of young children appearing confused by the parent's initial completion of the original command in the previous step. Therefore, the step provides parents with an additional opportunity to reiterate the expectation that the child, rather than the parent, should independently complete the desired demand. A verbal prompt of "your turn" is simultaneously provided prior to the reiteration of the original command. Repeated gestures, along with a five-second window of silence, are provided. Upon compliance, an enthusiastic labeled praise and warm, positive touch should be provided. Should listening not occur, the procedure progresses to a fourth, and final, step.

Guide

The final step, labeled "guide," is used to physically assist the child in the completion of the original demand. The words "Daddy (or Mommy, Grandma, etc.) will help you" are provided prior to the reiteration of the original command. The parent then gently guides the child's hand, by placing their hands over the child to guide and complete the original command. The procedure concludes with the words "That's [original command]." It is assumed that the child does not possess the necessary understanding and skills to complete the demand, and thus, the final step is used to teach the child how to complete the demand. A behavior description is provided to clarify and teach the skill of listening. A labeled praise may follow the behavior description. The PRIDE skills are then used to redirect the child back to appropriate child-led play. Should emotion dysregulation occur, the CARES model should be implemented (Table 9.1).

Language Encouragement

A final, novel aspect of the PDI-T procedure includes the use of procedures meant to encourage the use of language. Toddlerhood falls within a critical period in which children's language abilities are in the beginning states of acquisition. Additionally, toddlers with sufficient language use such skills to assist them in appropriately getting their needs met, rather than resorting to procedures indicative of emotion dysregulation. It is emphasized that current language encouragement procedures are never to be used in a punitive or otherwise forced fashion. If a child does not yet possess spoken language, this procedure should not be utilized, and instead, verbal reflection of the toddler's sounds should be a primary focus of treatment. Additionally, the current procedure should only be used when a toddler is calm and reasonably capable of managing his or her emotions during implementation.

The language encouragement procedures of PDI-T are based on studies of language acquisition in applied behavior analysis (Hansen & Shillingsburg, 2016; Kelley, Shillingsburg, Castro, Addison, & LaRue, 2007; Lerman, Parten, Addison,

Table 9.1 PCIT-T teaching listening/compliance skills (PDI-T) Tell-Show-Try Again-Guide flow chart

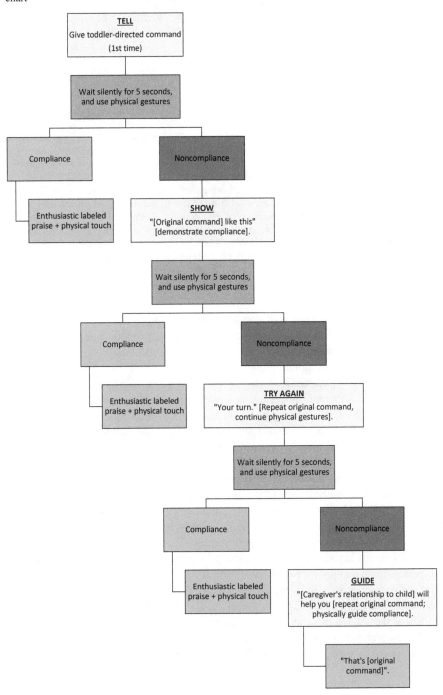

Vorndran, Volkert, & Kodak, 2005). Highly technical language skills from applied behavior analysis have been greatly simplified in PDI-T so that parents can be coached to mastery on one or two basic procedures to encourage language in their toddlers throughout the day. Below is an excerpt from Kelley et al. (2007) based on the work of Lerman et al. (2005) that describes the research base for PDI-T:

> Lerman et al. (2005) suggested four verbal responses or operants described by Skinner that are relevant for early language training: echoics, tacts, mands, and intraverbals. Each of these verbal operants are occasioned and maintained by specific antecedents and consequences. Echoics are occasioned by a verbal stimulus that is similar in form to the response and are maintained by generalized reinforcement. For example, a therapist may say, "say 'truck'"; the child responds, "truck"; and the therapist may deliver praise (e.g., "Good job saying truck!"). Tacts are occasioned by a nonverbal stimulus and are also maintained by generalized reinforcement. For example, a therapist may hold up a picture of a dog; the child responds, "dog"; and the therapist may deliver praise (e.g., "Good job saying dog!"). Mands, on the other hand, are occasioned by a motivating operation (Laraway, Snycerski, Michael, & Poling, 2003), such as deprivation of a preferred stimulus, and are maintained by contingent access to a specific consequence. For example, a child may say "juice" after a period of time of not having juice; contingent on the response "juice," a therapist may provide juice. Finally, intraverbals are occasioned by verbal stimuli that are dissimilar in form to the response and are maintained by generalized reinforcement (like echoics and tacts). For example, a therapist may say, "What's juice for?"; the child may respond, "drinking"; and the therapist may deliver praise (e.g., "Good job answering correctly!"). (Kelley et al., 2007, p.431)

Because we are working with parents who do not have a background in behavioral theory, we have eliminated the technical vocabulary in PDI-T. Yet, the parent is essentially taught simple tacts and mands, along with reflection of sounds/words and praise for speech, to encourage language. The CDI-T phase establishes the foundation for the language acquisition skills, as the daily play therapy sessions increase the reinforcement of parental attention, as well as the reinforcement of toy play, by teaching parents to use stimulating positive attention during play interactions. The tacts and mands can then be used more successfully in the second phase, PDI-T, as the child is motivated to receive parental praise when using words to obtain desired objects.

Language encouragement procedures are to be implemented during the course of play, when the toddler naturally desires an object. At this time, a verbal prompt requesting the object is modeled by the parent (e.g., "Say cup," "Say car please"). Upon an approximation of verbalization, the child is rewarded with an enthusiastic labeled praise and the presence of the object. Similar to listening procedures, a five-second window is provided following the prompt in an effort to allow the child time to comprehend and produce a verbalization. If no verbalization has occurred following the five-second window, the item is provided, and the parent repeats the desired verbalization (e.g., "Cup. This is a cup."). The procedure is meant to foster and enhance the child's natural use of language abilities during natural instances in which an approximation toward language is likely to occur. Language encouragement procedures are reserved for the PDI-T portion of the program due to the likelihood that parents and the therapist are highly aware of the child's emotional and behavioral cues indicative of emotion dysregulation, as no language encouragement procedures are used when a child is dysregulated. Finally, it is also expected that parents have developed the ability to praise effectively and enthusiastically. Such skills following language approximation or production remain integral to the toddler's likelihood of language use.

PDI-T Mastery

Similar to standard PCIT, PDI-T skills are interwoven within a high proportion of CDI-T skills in a standard PDI-T session. Finally, a parent is considered to have mastered PDI-T when he or she is able to demonstrate the use of 75% effective commands and 75% effective follow-through to effective commands during a five-minute coded sequence at the beginning of a PDI-T session. Additionally, parents must also demonstrate satisfactory implementation of language encouragement procedures, as well as the CARES model and the CDI-T procedure for dangerous and destructive behaviors if needed.

Coaching Considerations During PDI-Toddler

Readers should reference coaching considerations previously discussed in Chap. 2 "philosophy of coaching" for a critical, broad-based understanding of coaching philosophy. Although the foundational premise of PDI-T coaching remains highly positive and supportive in nature, PDI-T coaching differs from CDI-T coaching in its direct use of line-fed statements to the parent (e.g., say "Please hand me the block. Now, stay quiet and point to the block."). See Table 9.2 for a PDI-T coaching example of Tell-Show-Try Again-Guide sequence. By this point, it is likely that therapeutic rapport will be well established, and the parent will have mastered child-directed interaction skills, thus allowing increased parental independence during non-listening focused interactions. During listening procedures, therapists and parents should remain attuned to the child's mood and determine the implementation of such tasks accordingly. Variables such as illness, teething, and lack of sleep may dramatically impact a toddler's mood and may cause the treatment team to refrain from the use of listening procedures and solely concentrate on implementation of the CDI-T skills during a PDI-T session. Such flexibility speaks to the broad premise that listening practice should be seen as a fun, learning activity rather than one associated with noncompliance and consequences. Enthusiasm and facial animation

Table 9.2 PDI-T coaching example of Tell-Show-Try Again-Guide sequence

Individual	Coaching/parent statement given
Therapist	"In a minute, we will give him the first command. We will start with our *"Tell"* step. You will say, 'mommy has no toy. Please hand me the car,' as you mentioned earlier that 'hand me' commands are easiest. Go ahead and push the other toys out of the way to prevent distractions. Pull the car close to you. That's it. Now get his attention by touching him on the knee. Good. Look him right in the eyes and say, 'please hand me the car.' Hold your hand out. Point to the car and point to your hand. Stay quiet and keep pointing."
Parent	"Please hand me the car." (parent points to car and points to her hand)
Child	Keeps playing and does not comply
Therapist	"Wait quietly and keep pointing for the 5 s. One, two, three, four, five. Okay, we now will go to the *"Show"* step. Tell him 'please hand me the car like this.' Show him how to put the car in your hand. Now put the car back where it was. Keep pointing to the car and pointing to your hand. Stay quiet and point."
Parent	"Please hand me the car like this." (parent puts the car into her own hand and then sets it back down. She points to the car and points to her hand)
Therapist	"Great job showing him how to do it. Now just continue to point to the car and to your hand. Stay quiet. One, two, three, four, five."
Child	Keeps playing and does not comply.
Therapist	"Okay. We need to move to our *"Try Again"* step. Say, 'your turn. Please hand me the car.' Then stay quiet and point."
Parent	"Your turn. Please hand me the car." (parent points to car and points to her hand)
Child	Walks away. Does not comply with the command
Therapist	"Okay. He did not comply. So, we need to move on to our *"Guide"* step. Bring the car with you and move closer to him. Get down on his level. Stay calm and quiet while you guide him. Say, 'mommy will help you hand me the car.' Then take his hand in yours and pick-up the car together. Gently guide him to put the car in your open hand."
Parent	"Mommy will help you hand me the car." (parent guides the child hand to put the car into her hand)
Child	Cooperates with the physical guidance
Therapist	"Because he needed a guide, we will use a behavior description first. Say, 'you put the car in mommy's hand.' Now you can give a labeled praise, 'good helping Mommy.'"
Parent	"You put the car in mommy's hand, good helping Mommy."
Therapist	"Great job teaching him how to listen. I love how you stayed calm during the guide. Now follow his lead. Use your nice PRIDE skills and let him lead the play."

should be consistently applied throughout PDI-T. Toddlers may smile and laugh during listening practice as a result of its fun, game-like application. In contrast to traditional PDI, PDI-T must be applied from a more flexible perspective. Natural intuition should be used during the five-second wait time in between listening steps. For example, if it is clear that the toddler is processing the initial command or has a history of delayed initiation, additional time should be provided beyond the five-second window to accommodate for his or her individual needs. The use of developmentally appropriate demands is highly important and may vary dramatically among toddlers of similar ages. Overall, coaching in PDI-T may include more directive line feeding, but listening practice must be conducted in a fun, game-like manner when the child demonstrates emotional readiness to learn such new skills and listening practice is limited to three commands per PDI-T coaching session and PDI-T Home Therapy Practice. Additional information and guidance regarding coaching can be found in Appendix A at the conclusion of this book.Throughout PDI-T, the therapist works with caregivers on understanding the developmental need of toddlers to develop independence and sense of control. As such, parents are encouraged to practice listening skills sparingly (during the 5 minute listening practice at a maximum of three attempts and only occasionally during the rest of the day). Whenever possible, caregivers should avoid control battles with toddlers, and opt instead for providing choices, using indirect commands, and providing gentle physical guidance to assist with listening throughout the day. Our goal is to help parents set the toddlers up for success and celebrate their emerging ability to follow directions.

References

Baumrind, D. (1978). Parental disciplinary patterns and social competence in children. *Youth and Society, 9*, 238–276.

Hansen, B., & Shillingsburg, A. M. (2016). Using a modified parent-child interaction therapy to increase vocalizations in children with autism. *Child & Family Behavior Therapy, 38*(4), 318–330.

Kelley, M. E., Shillingsburg, A. M., Castro, J. M., Addison, L. R., & LaRue, R. H. (2007). Further evaluation of emerging speech in children with developmental disabilities: Training verbal behavior. *Journal of Applied Behavior Analysis, 40*(3), 431–445.

Laraway, S., Snycerski, S., Michael, J., & Poling, A. (2003). Motivating operations and terms to describe them: Some further refinements. *Journal of Applied Behavior Analysis, 36*, 407–414.

Lerman, D. C., Parten, M., Addison, L. R., Vorndran, C. M., Volkert, V. M., & Kodak, T. (2005). A methodology for assessing the functions of emerging speech in children with developmental disabilities. *Journal of Applied Behavior Analysis, 38*(3), 303–316.

Chapter 10
Conclusions

In summary, PCIT-T is a promising evidence-based treatment intervention that integrates behavior and attachment theories in order to meet the unique developmental needs of toddlers. PCIT-T emphasizes instruction and coaching of emotion regulation skills with regard to the parent, child, and the dyadic interaction. With the help of a skillful coach, parents learn to recognize and respond to their own emotional reactions, model such reactions for their children, and recognize the impact of their emotions and behavior on their young children's emotions and behavior. As parents feel calmer, they are better able to assist their children in managing their own emotions and accompanying behaviors, skills that will greatly benefit children socially and academically. As treatment progresses, such dyadic interactions and strategic coaching help parents to read children's cues and become more sensitive to their needs, thereby improving the parent-child bond. Following mastery of child-directed and parent-directed interaction toddler skills, select life-enhancement topics are chosen to help parents apply such skills to unique real-life situations (e.g., feeding, diapering, nap time). Given toddlers' rapidly changing development, an intricate awareness of developmental milestones is encouraged throughout treatment.

The Art and Heart of Coaching PCIT-Toddlers

While PCIT-T is a manualized, technique-driven treatment program, the spirit of the intervention should not be forgotten. PCIT-T is, at its core, a strength-based program that aims to improve the attachment relationship between parents and children. The relationship between the coach and parent is also an attachment relationship and as such is a pivotal ingredient in the process of change. The PCIT-T coach must therefore possess not only a high level of technical skill in order to successfully implement the techniques outlined in this book; they must also have an adequate grasp of attachment theory and practice, and they must embody the personal

© Springer Nature Switzerland AG 2018
E. I. Girard et al., *Parent-Child Interaction Therapy with Toddlers*,
https://doi.org/10.1007/978-3-319-93251-4_10

attributes and relationship-based skills that the program seeks to foster in parents. This includes the ability to reflect on and manage difficult emotions, to be calm and empathic in the face of difficult emotions or relationship dynamics, and to respond sensitively to meet the emotional needs of the parent and child. Clinical work of this nature with parents and young children can be complex and challenging, and so it is essential that PCIT-T is delivered within the context of a supportive team environment and that the therapist participates in regular reflective supervision.

Training Requirements for PCIT-Toddlers

As the field of infant mental health continues to grow, the developers of PCIT-T are keenly aware that the training need for clinicians will be varied. Therefore, three different training tracks to develop competency in delivery of PCIT-T are outlined.

1. PCIT standard-trained clinicians (all competencies completed) seeking additional training to implement adaptation of PCIT-Toddlers

    (a) Required 2-day (16 h) training provided by a PCIT-T developer (Girard, Wallace, Kohlhoff, Morgan, & McNeil, 2018) and/or authorized PCIT-T trainer as approved by the PCIT-T developers
    (b) Case consultation with a PCIT-T trainer through delivery of two completed PCIT-T cases including both CDI-T and PDI-T portions of treatment via a live trainer model and/or tele-health and/or telephone contact, dependent on status of PCIT-T trainer, which begins post 2-day training through duration of PCIT-T delivery through graduation of cases

2. Clinicians seeking both PCIT standard training and PCIT-Toddlers training

    (a) Meet all training requirements for certification as a standard PCIT therapist per PCIT International, see PCIT International website for most current guidelines (http://www.pcit.org/therapist-requirements.html) and/or meet all training competencies required by UC Davis PCIT Training Center (Urquiza, Zebell, Timmer, & McGrath, 2015), and see UC Davis website for most current guidelines (https://pcit.ucdavis.edu/wp-content/uploads/2013/01/3_competencieschecklist-v4-numbered-1.pdf)
    (b) Additional, required 2-day (16 h) training provided by a PCIT-T developer (Girard, Wallace, Kohlhoff, Morgan, & McNeil, 2018) and/or authorized PCIT-T trainer as approved by the PCIT-T developers
    (c) Case consultation with a PCIT-T trainer through delivery of two completed PCIT-T cases including both CDI-T and PDI-T portions of treatment via a live trainer model and/or tele-health and/or telephone contact, dependent on status of PCIT-T trainer, which begins post 2-day training through duration of PCIT-T delivery through graduation of cases

3. <u>Clinicians seeking only PCIT-Toddlers training</u>

   (a) Required 5-day (40 h) training provided by a PCIT-I certified trainer (i.e., Master Trainer, Level 2 Trainer or Level 1 Trainer) who is also a PCIT-T developer (Girard, Wallace, Kohlhoff, Morgan, & McNeil, 2018) and/or authorized PCIT-T trainer as approved by the PCIT-T developers

   (b) Case consultation with a PCIT-T trainer through delivery of two completed PCIT-T cases including both CDI-T and PDI-T portions of treatment via a live trainer model and/or tele-health and/or telephone contact, dependent on status of PCIT-T trainer, which begins post 2-day training through duration of PCIT-T delivery through graduation of cases

PCIT-T Website

PCIT-T training requests and additional information regarding PCIT-T training requirements maybe found at http://www.pcit-toddlers.org/. The developers of PCIT-T are in the discussion phase of developing a roster system for clinicians who have gone through training.

The toddler years are an exciting, sensitive period in which lifelong changes can occur, for both parents and their young children. The formation of this book has fueled our existing passion for working with this exciting age group. We hope that you will enjoy this book as much as we have enjoyed its creation.

Section II provides the PCIT-T session-by-session guide for treatment intervention.

References

Girard, E., Wallace, N., Kohlhoff, J., Morgan, S., & McNeil, C. (2018). *Parent-Child Interaction Therapy for Toddlers (PCIT-T)*. Retrieved from PCIT-Toddlers.org.

Parent-Child Interaction Therapy International (2018). Therapists Requirements retrieved from http://www.pcit.org/therapist-requirements.html.

Urquiza, A., Zebell, N., Timmer, S., & McGrath, J. (2015). *PCIT: Sample course of treatment manual for traumatized children*. Unpublished Manuscript.

Part II
Parent-Child Interaction Therapy with Toddlers Clinical Manual: A Session-by-Session Guide

Chapter 11
Treatment Overview and Implementation of the Current Protocol

Parent-Child Interaction Therapy-Toddlers (PCIT-T): Improving Attachment and Emotion Regulation is a novel treatment approach adapted from Parent-Child Interaction Therapy, an evidence-based parent-training treatment for children with behavior problems. The current approach is designed to be used with toddlers between the ages of 12 and 24 months, a stage when problem behaviors often manifest. As previously noted, the approach may be used as a preventative tool designed to improve parenting skills, improve child behavior and emotion regulation abilities, and strengthen the parent-child bond. However, the treatment should not be used with (1) children or parents in the middle of medical procedures that prevent them from consistently utilizing treatment strategies and regularly attending sessions and (2) any caregiver with a sexual perpetrator history, whether a substantiated case or not. Clinical judgment is critical to determining whether a given family is appropriate for PCIT-T based on characteristics of the parent, child, and family situation. The rationale for not providing PCIT-T to any caregiver with a history or alleged history of sexual perpetration is to prevent skills implemented during the course of treatment which improve the relationship between a parent and child to be used as possible grooming techniques that may foster abuse.

The following section of this book aims to provide clinicians with a session-by-session guide to treatment delivery. However, implementation of the model should not occur without its accompanying in-person training; see Chap. 10 under Training Requirements for PCIT-Toddlers. Additionally, some basic knowledge, affinity, and understanding of attachment theory and implementation should be part of the clinician's repertoire.

All treatment guidelines, coding sheets, and paper-based materials are provided and can be photocopied for therapeutic use. Session outlines, examples, and scripts are provided within each session description to enhance clarification of the procedures used and improve treatment integrity. Similar to PCIT, therapeutic discretion should be used prior to therapeutic advancement through treatment sessions. It is expected that PCIT-T clinicians will have a previous theoretical understanding as well as clinically based practice in the delivery of PCIT prior to

© Springer Nature Switzerland AG 2018

E. I. Girard et al., *Parent-Child Interaction Therapy with Toddlers*,
https://doi.org/10.1007/978-3-319-93251-4_11

implementation of PCIT-T. It is expected that PCIT-T clinicians obtain clinical training, case experience, and competency achievement in standard PCIT prior to implementing PCIT-T as outlined in Chap. 10, Section Training Requirements for PCIT-Toddlers. Finally, it is also expected that all procedures recommended in the current treatment will be reviewed and approved by a therapist's respective agency.

Chapter 12
Pretreatment Interview and Assessment Session

The pretreatment interview and assessment session are designed to gain a thorough qualitative and quantitative understanding of a family's presenting concerns, including baseline levels of child behavior problems and developmental abilities, parent skills and emotional concerns, and the quality of the parent-child interaction. Ideally, therapists should problem-solve the best time for a family to attend the session, based on a range of child variables (e.g., nap/feeding time). The therapist may also prompt the parent to bring snacks and familiar objects to help the child remain occupied during the initial interview. To accomplish these goals, clinicians should conduct a thorough clinical interview with the child's caregiver(s) as well as administer a range of standardized assessment measures (outlined below). It is assumed that therapists will follow all initial confidentiality procedures including necessary releases of information, limits to confidentiality, and video/audio recording agreements. Both the parent and child should be present for the initial interview to allow the clinician to conduct standardized and naturalistic behavior observations. In some cases, the assessment may be completed in one session, but in other cases, due to variables such as childcare responsibilities, insurance and agency-based requirements, and family variability in progression through the assessment protocol, it may be necessary to conduct the assessments across the context of two distinct sessions. Given the extended nature of the session, breaks may also be necessary (e.g., to take the child for a walk, feed the child). Upon the conclusion of the assessment, the clinician should have gained enough information to determine the appropriate fit (e.g., the family will be able to commit to consistent, weekly sessions; the ability to complete daily "Home Therapy Practice") between the current treatment plan and the presenting difficulties in the context of the child's developmental abilities. It is important to note that, as described above, room setup is critical to the success of the session and safety of the child.

Developmentally appropriate toys, separate from those to be used for the standardized behavior observation, must be provided, and all potentially dangerous materials (e.g., outlets, cords, small objects) must be safely covered or placed out of the child's

© Springer Nature Switzerland AG 2018   125
E. I. Girard et al., *Parent-Child Interaction Therapy with Toddlers*,
https://doi.org/10.1007/978-3-319-93251-4_12

reach. The therapist and parents may consider joining the child on the floor throughout the course of the interview to easily reach the child and attend to his or her needs. In some cases, clinicians may be able to have the child cared for by an additional family member or member of the clinic staff in an adjoining or nearby space.

Session Preparation Items

1. Intake interview form
2. DPICS-T coding sheet
3. Required assessment measures:

   (a) DECA-I, DECA-T OR BITSEA
   (b) DPICS

4. Optional assessment measures:

   (d) PSI – Short Form
   (e) EPDS
   (f) ASQ
   (g) CBCL
   (h) M-CHAT-R/F

Session Goals

1. Conduct clinical interview.
2. Administer standardized assessment measures.
3. Determine the fit between the family's needs and the current treatment approach.

Note The procedures in the current session may need to be accomplished over the course of two sessions depending on the child's behavior, logistics, and parent's efficiency in completing session tasks.

Session Outline

1. **Bring family into the developmentally prepared space for the child.**
2. **Provide parents with a summary of the intake and initial assessment process.**

   (a) *Sample Script: "During our time today, we will do our best to complete the initial interview, where we will discuss your primary concerns as well as gain a thorough understanding of your child's developmental and medical history. I will also ask you to complete some paper and pencil questionnaires asking about your child's behavior and development. Since every child and family is different, this information will help us to better understand the difficulties your child and family are experiencing in the context of his or her background. It is normal for some parents and caregivers to minimize or downplay their concerns at first - we want you to include as many concerns you've had even if it's been awhile since you've had to deal with it. During an assessment, more information is better than a lack of information. Finally, if time permits, I'd like to do some behavior observations of your child's behavior during a few specific play situations with you. First, I will have you play with your child while following his or her lead and playing along with him or her. Then, I will have you take the lead and try to get [child's name] to play what you want to play. Finally, I'll have you prompt [child's name] to help you clean up the toys. We understand that it may not be possible to complete all of these procedures today and if that is the case, then we will schedule another time for your family to return soon. If you feel that your child needs a break at any time today, to have a snack, get his or her diaper changed, or take a walk, please let us know. We want you and your family to feel as comfortable as possible here today. At the end of the assessment process, I will use all of the information that we have gathered to decide if PCIT-T is the best fit for your family."*

3. **Complete the pretreatment intake interview with parents.**

   (a) If the child is present, ensure that the child is occupied with developmentally appropriate toys, snacks, and activities. In addition to information concerning the child's behavior and reasons why the family is seeking treatment at the present time, it is essential that clinicians gather information related to the child's previous history with early intervention and behavior services, should it exist.

   (b) A conversation related to the parent's philosophies and beliefs about parenting should also occur. Therapists may ask parents about how they were raised as well as effective and ineffective parenting strategies that they observe their friends, neighbors, and peers are using. This conversation should include a discussion of the parent's ability to regulate his or her own emotions during the child's times of emotion dysregulation.

   (c) A conversation related to effective and ineffective methods of discipline used, where they learned these methods, and their thoughts on such methods should also occur. This helps the therapist build rapport and provides the therapist with valuable information related to the appropriate fit between the family and use of the PCIT-T treatment model.

   (d) Following the aforementioned discussion, therapists should gather all additional background information including but not limited to:

      (i) Referral source
      (ii) Family constellation (those living in the home and other significant individuals in the child's life along with their names and ages).

(iii) Birth history (prenatal history/complications present/substances consumed, birth history/complications present, child's birth weight, post-birth hospital experience including length of time in hospital/complications present)

(iv) Medical history (any medical illnesses, injuries, hospitalizations, previous or current medical diagnosis)

(v) Medication history (medications previously and currently consumed, dosage, time/frequency administered, purpose)

(vi) Developmental history/ages in which milestones have been achieved (motor, speech, toileting)

(vii) Sleep routine (sleep schedule, sleep difficulties, typical mood upon waking).

(viii) Feeding routine (feeding schedule, feeding difficulties)

(ix) Educational information (including daycare placement – type of setting, number of children in class, number of teachers, age range of class, any behavioral concerns in the daycare environment).

(x) Childcare information (who babysits or provides care to child if caregivers at work, have a doctor's appointment, or night out/date night)

(xi) Child strengths (personal strengths, areas in which the child excels, activities that he or she enjoys)

(xii) A thorough summary of current behavior concerns and how such concerns have evolved over time (e.g., problem behavior has become more frequent/intense)

(xiii) Any other family stressors/complications/changes that have occurred or are currently occurring that may impact the child's behavior

4. **Initiate three DPICS observations (verbatim instructions are provided below).** Code all verbalizations according to DPICS coding rules. Additionally, determine the parent's skill with regard to positive skills and fulfillment of the CARES model during any moments of child emotion dysregulation.

Important guidelines If two parents or caregivers are present, each should complete his or her own behavior observations. Ideally, each parent should conduct the observations privately, without observation by the other parent. When possible, observations should be conducted on a small rug or blanket on the floor with selected developmentally appropriate toys to increase child safety. Guidelines for each situation may be given over a bug-in-the-ear walkie-talkie device particularly when it is suspected that the therapist's guidance may otherwise affect the child's behavior (e.g., slightly older children). Guidelines may be provided in person for younger toddlers.

(a) **Child-Directed Interaction Script** "In this situation, tell [child's name] that he/she may play with whatever he/she chooses. Let him/her choose any activity he/she wishes. You just follow his/her lead and play along with him/her" (Eyberg & Funderburk, 2011, p.13). Begin to time a 5-minute warm-up period prior to formally using the DPICS to code the 5-minute situation.

(b) **Parent-Directed Interaction Script** "That was fine. Now we'll switch to the second activity (Eyberg & Funderburk, 2011, p.13). Redirect [child's name] to play with a different toy in the room that you have chosen and see if you can get [child's name] to play with you." Begin to time and DPICS code the 5-minute situation.

(c) **Cleanup Script** "That was fine. Now please tell [child's name] that it is time to clean up the toys (Eyberg & Funderburk, 2011, p.13). Help him/her put all the toys in their containers and all the containers in the toy box [or designate location]." Begin to time and DPICS code the 5-minute situation.

5. **Debrief DPICS observation**

Discuss the parent's impression of any similarities and differences between the situations and the child's typical behavior in similar situations.

6. **Ask parent(s) to complete paper and pencil assessment measures.** Such measures may also be sent home with the family and returned at the next session if appropriate. Assessment measures include (also shown in Table 12.1):

(a) The Devereux Early Childhood Assessment (DECA)

   (i) DECA-Infant (ages 12–18 months)
   (ii) DECA-Toddler (ages 18–36 months), OR

(b) The Brief Infant-Toddler Social Emotional Assessment (BITSEA)

Optional Measures: The Ages and Stages Questionnaire (ASQ); the Child Behavior Checklist (CBCL); the Modified Checklist for Autism in Toddlers, Revised, with Follow-Up™ (M-CHAT-R/F); the Parenting Stress Index – Short Form (PSI-SF); and the Edinburgh Postnatal Depression Scale (EPDS).

Table 12.1 List of required and optional measures implemented over the course of treatment in PCIT-T

Required measures	Optional measures
The Devereux Early Childhood Assessment (DECA) • DECA-Infant (ages 12–18 months) • DECA-Toddler (ages 18–36 months)	The Ages and Stages Questionnaire (ASQ)
The Brief Infant-Toddler Social Emotional Assessment (BITSEA)	The Child Behavior Checklist (CBCL)
The Dyadic Parent-Child Interaction Coding System (DPICS)	The Modified Checklist for Autism in Toddlers, Revised, with Follow-Up™ (M-CHAT-R/F)
	The Parenting Stress Index – Short Form (PSI-SF)
	Edinburgh Postnatal Depression Scale (EPDS)

7. **Clinician completes Dyadic Parent-Child Interaction Coding System (DPICS) and records outcomes to corresponding skills tracking graphs.**

   (a) Child-Led Play (CLP) baseline; Relationship Enhancement Tracker for CDI-T skills
   (b) Parent-Led Play (PLP) baseline; Listening/Compliance Tracker for PDI-T skills
   (c) Cleanup (CU) baseline; Listening/Compliance Tracker for PDI-T skills

8. The therapist should provide the family with empathy and support with regard to the presenting concerns, optimistic hope for the impact of treatment on such concerns, and praise for taking the steps to make positive changes in the child's life and the life of their family. Talk to parents about the feedback and didactic focus of the next session in which only adults should attend. Assist the family in problem-solving any barriers to obtaining childcare. In extenuating circumstances, when childcare is unavailable, the family can be allowed to bring the child; however, problem-solving regarding ways to occupy the child (e.g., use of iPad/electronics) should occur. Finally, timing of future sessions in the context of the child's sleep and feeding schedule should also be discussed.

9. **Complete integrity checklist: PCIT-T assessment session.**

Integrity Checklist: PCIT-T Assessment Session

 As you view the session, place a checkmark under the appropriate column, Yes (Y), Not Applicable (NA) or No (N). List these totals in the appropriate blanks below the table. See expanded session outlines for more information on each item. (Integrity checklist and directions are based on Eyberg & Funderburk, 2011).

Integrity Checklist: PCIT-Toddlers Pre-Treatment Assessment Session		
Client & Caregiver:		
Therapist Conducting Session:		
Checklist Completed By:		**Date:**

	ITEMS	Y	NA	N
1	Prepares developmentally appropriate and safe space and model PCIT-T skills while supporting the caregivers to enter the room			
2	Provides caregivers a summary of the intake and initial assessment process			
3	Explains limits of confidentiality and appropriate consents completed			
4	Completes pre-treatment intake interview			
5	Sets room for DPICS observation and attends with each caregiver separately			
6	Gives instructions for Child-Led Play Situation (verbatim)			
7	After warm-up, gives a prompt to continue Child Led Play			
8	Codes CDI for exactly 5 minutes			
9	Gives instructions for Parent Led Play (verbatim)			
10	Codes PDI for exactly 5 minutes			
11	Gives instructions for Clean-up (verbatim)			
12	Codes Clean-up for exactly 5 minutes			
13	Asks caregiver if each situation was typical			
14	Gives brief supportive feedback about observations			
15	Caregiver completes assessment measures			
16	Records outcomes in corresponding skills tracking graphs			
17	Provides empathy, support and optimism to caregivers			
18	Discusses future appointments and goal of that session			
19	Clinician provides label praise to caregiver for their positive parenting skills and child's strengths			
20	Supports dyad as required during to exit of session and models CDI-T skills			
	TOTALS			

Therapist comments about session

_____

_____

_____

Integrity checker comments about sessions:

_____

_____

_____

Integrity = $\dfrac{\text{Yes Total}}{\text{Yes Total} + \text{No Total}}$ = _____ %

Length of session = _____ minutes

Handouts and Forms

PCIT-T Pre/Post DPICS Assessment for Therapist

Child Name/ ID _____ Date:_____

Assessment: □ **PRE**   □ **POST**   Coder:_____

Parent: □ Mother   □ Father   □ Other _____

Situation: □ **Child Lead Play**   □ **Parent Lead Play**   □ **Clean Up**

Start Time:_____   End Time:_____

Do Skills		Tally Count	TOTAL
Neutral Talk			
Emotion Labeling			
Behavioral Description			
Reflection			
Labeled Praise			
Unlabeled Praise			
Don't Skills		Tally Count	TOTAL
Question			
Direct	Comply (CO) Tell-Show-Try Again		
Command	Non-Comply (NC) Guide		
(DC)	No Opportunity (NOC)		
Indirect	Comply (CO) Tell-Show-Try Again		
Command	Non-Comply (NC) Guide		
(IC)	No Opportunity (NOC)		
Negative Talk			

Big Emotion Present?	YES	NO	# Tally	

CARES Skills Used	CIRCLE ONE			NOTES
Come In	Satisfactory	Needs Practice	N/A	
Assist Child	Satisfactory	Needs Practice	N/A	
Reassure Child	Satisfactory	Needs Practice	N/A	
Emotional Validation	Satisfactory	Needs Practice	N/A	
Soothe	Satisfactory	Needs Practice	N/A	

Coach caregiver through any missed step (if needed) in the moment, **INCLUDING** getting on the microphone during the 5 minutes of DPCIS Coding.

Positive Skills	Circle One		NOTES
Imitate	Satisfactory	Needs Practice	
Show Enjoyment	Satisfactory	Needs Practice	
Physical Affection	Satisfactory	Needs Practice	
Mutual Eye Contact	Satisfactory	Needs Practice	
Animated Tone of Voice	Satisfactory	Needs Practice	
Animated Facial Expressions	Satisfactory	Needs Practice	
Play Style at Developmental Level	Satisfactory	Needs Practice	

Bx Management Skills	Circle One			NOTES
Skill of Redirection	Satisfactory	Needs Practice	N/A	
Skill of Under Reaction	Satisfactory	Needs Practice	N/A	
Limit Setting - 'No Hurting'	Satisfactory	Needs Practice	N/A	

Relationship Enhancement Tracker of
CDI-Toddlers Skills

Session #	Baseline CLP								
Date									
Home Therapy Practice									
7	X								
6	X								
5	X								
4	X								
3	X								
2	X								
1	X								
0	X								
Labeled Praise									
10+									
9									
8									
7									
6									
5									
4									
3									
2									
1									
0									
Reflection									
10+									
9									
8									
7									
6									
5									
4									
3									
2									
1									
0									
Behavior Description									
10+									
9									
8									
7									
6									
5									
4									
3									
2									
1									
0									

Relationship Enhancement Tracker of CDI-Toddlers Skills

Session #	Baseline CLP								
Date									

Emotion Labeling

10+									
9									
8									
7									
6									
5									
4									
3									
2									
1									
0									

Question/Command/Critical Statement

10+									
9									
8									
7									
6									
5									
4									
3									
2									
1									
0									

CARES

Satis-factory									
N/A									
Needs Improv.									

Other Positive Skills
(Imitate, Enjoy, Affection, Eye Contact, Animation, etc.)

Satis-factory									
N/A									
Needs Improv.									

Redirection and Under-Reaction

Satis-factory									
N/A									
Needs Improv.									

Limit-Setting "No Hurting"

Satis-factory									
N/A									
Needs Improv.									

Listening/ Compliance Tracker of
PDI-Toddlers Skills

Session #	Baseline PLP	Baseline CU							
Date									
PDI-T Home Therapy Listening Practice									
7	X	X							
6	X	X							
5	X	X							
4	X	X							
3	X	X							
2	X	X							
1	X	X							
0	X	X							
Effective Direct Commands									
100%									
90%									
80%									
70%									
75%									
60%									
50%									
40%									
30%									
20%									
10%									
0%									
Consistent Follow Through									
100%									
90%									
80%									
75%									
70%									
60%									
50%									
40%									
30%									
20%									
10%									
0%									
Child Compliance Behavior*									
100%									
90%									
80%									
75%									
70%									
60%									
50%									
40%									
30%									
20%									
10%									
0%									

*Compliance Behavior is calculated by task completion during the
PDI-T sequence of "Tell", "Show" or "Try Again."

Reference

Eyberg, S., & Funderburk, B. W. (2011). Parent-child interaction therapy protocol. Gainesville, FL: PCIT International.

Chapter 13
Child-Directed Interaction-Toddler Teach Session

Decades of research on the child-directed interaction portion of PCIT has shown an increase in the positivity of parent speech and the frequency and quality of child speech, as well as a decrease in child behavior problems and parent stress levels (Eisenstadt, Eyberg, McNeil, Newcomb, & Funderburk, 1993; Lieneman, Brabson, Highlander, Wallace, & McNeil, 2017). The primary goal of the child-directed interaction-toddler teach session is to teach parents the specific skills used in the child-directed phase of PCIT-T. Unlike standard PCIT, the child-directed interaction portion of PCIT-T encompasses the majority of the treatment approach. Behavior management skills used in the current phase have been uniquely tailored to match toddlers' developmental level and emotion regulation needs and fulfill the primary aims of the current treatment.

Given the volume of material covered in this session, it is strongly advised that the parent attend this session without the child (or bring another caregiver to assist with the child during the didactics). Although only a single session is dedicated to teaching caregivers the CDI-T skills, ongoing practice and discussion of such skills are provided throughout subsequent coaching sessions. The CDI-T teach session is estimated to take between 60 and 90 minutes. It is recommended that the teach didactic be held in one session to avoid delay of treatment delivery with the parent and toddler, and parents will learn as they go, via live in vivo coaching. Accompanying handouts for the current session are included. The basis for much of the material in chap. 13 is related to the CDI Teach Session of Eyberg and Funderburk (2011).

Note Developmental tip of the day cards are provided in Appendix H at the conclusion of this manual. Clinicians have the option of using these cards at the end of each session to assist parents to develop a better understanding of the special developmental needs of toddlers. As the cards are optional, therapists may use their clinical judgment to determine if a particular parent is likely to benefit from this type of instructional material. Additionally, clinicians should only use the cards when the family has the time and resources to engage in a discussion at the end of the session. If the child is bored or fussy, or the parent or therapist is in a hurry, or there are too many other issues to discuss at the end of the session, the clinician should save that tip of the day discussion for another session.

Session Preparation Items

1. Visual transition aide card
2. Necessary handouts and coding sheets

   (a) "Do" skills (PRIDE)
   (b) "Don't" skills
   (c) CARES for toddler and CARES for adult
   (d) Teaching your child about feelings from birth to age 2
   (e) Recommended toy list
   (f) Response to aggression
   (g) Home Therapy Practice sheet
   (h) DPICS-T Coding sheets
   (i) Relationship Enhancement Tracker of CDI-Toddlers Skills

3. Selected toys

Session Goals

1. Provide the parent(s) with feedback regarding the results of the clinical outcome measures administered in the previous session.
2. Provide the parent(s) with a brief understanding of PCIT-T. Include the expected setup of treatment sessions.
3. Inform parents of the goals of the child-directed interaction skills as well as the rationale behind teaching such skills prior to the implementation of compliance skills.
4. Teach parents about the parallel process between the therapist, parent, and child as well as the impact of such process on treatment.
5. Discuss the importance of the parent-focused self-care model and its role in treatment success.
6. Teach parents the "don't" skills along with the rationale for the use of each.
7. Teach parents the "do" skills along with the rationale for the use of each.
8. Teach parents what a "big emotion" is for a toddler and how to manage "big emotions" with the skills of CARES, redirection, and under-reaction and the rationale behind the use of such techniques for the toddler age group.
9. Discuss the importance of regular attendance and Home Therapy Practice to the success of the intervention.
10. Conclude with an opportunity for the parents to reflect upon the potential impact of such skills upon their child and family and ask questions.

Session Outline

1. **Provide parents with a brief summary of PCIT-T.**

   Sample Script: "Parent-Child Interaction Therapy-Toddlers is a treatment adapted from Parent-Child Interaction Therapy, an evidence-based treatment for children with disruptive behavior difficulties. PCIT-T uses similar principles to PCIT but is uniquely adapted to the developmental needs of toddlers. PCIT-T is concentrated on accomplishing three primary goals throughout the course of treatment: improving caregiver skills, improving child behavior, and improving the quality of the caregiver-child relationship. Furthermore, a primary focus of the treatment lies in improving toddlers' ability to regulate their emotions while decreasing parents stress levels and improving parents' developmental under-standing of their child and his or her behavior.

   The treatment is divided into two primary phases, child-directed interaction-toddler (CDI-T) and parent-directed interaction-toddler (PDI-T). The first phase, CDI-T, is primarily focused on using a set of skills designed to increase the positivity and warmth of caregiver-child interactions and how to respond to your child should he or she become emotionally dysregulated. The second phase, PDI-T, is primarily focused on teaching listening skills designed to increase your child's compliance to your directions, as well as helping your child to use his or her words (instead of disruptive behavior) to express feelings and needs.

   Since we know that children learn best through play, the entire intervention will take place in the context of play-based interactions between you and your child. In an effort to increase the natural feeling of the interaction, you and your child will be alone in the therapy room. I will be sitting in an adjoining room and speaking to you through a bug-in-the-ear device. The reason for coaching out of room is to allow you as the parent to be the primary source of comfort to your child, for your child to clearly hear your voice, and to limit any distraction or unnatural interactions from occurring should I be in the room with you."

2. **Describe the nature of the current session and the expected course of future sessions.**

   Sample Script: "Today, we will begin by checking in on any changes or major events that came up during the past week, reviewing the results of the assess-ment measures and behavior observations that you completed during the last session. Then, I will teach you the specific skills that will be the focus of the CDI-T/Relationship Enhancement phase of treatment. Sessions are designed to teach you to use play therapy, emotion regulation, and behavior analysis skills when you give the therapy to your child at home. The 'Home Therapy Practice' therapy sessions are short, just 5 minutes per day, but the success of this program is entirely dependent on your ability to consistently give your child the treatment sessions at home. Future sessions will be completely dedicated to practicing these skills with your child while I coach you as you play with him or her.

After each session, I'll assign some Home Therapy Practice, as mentioned earlier, so that the skills can feel even more natural to use with your child in your everyday lives. Each time you and your child come in, I will watch you and your child play while I sit quietly to see how you are progressing to meeting what we call mastery levels of the skills. By mastering the skills, we mean that you essentially will have many of the skills that therapists use when they work with toddlers. You will become an expert at meeting the many needs of children in the toddler age range. After you've reached this mastery level, we will have another session like this where I will teach you the skills used in the compliance and language training stage of this treatment."

3. **Check in on any major changes that may have occurred since the previous session. Ask the parent to think of an example of one time during the previous week where he/she felt connected to his/her child or noticed a strength in his/her child.**

    (a) If the parent exhibits difficulty finding a time when he/she felt connected to his/her child, ask the parent to think of a moment when he/she noticed a strength of the child (e.g., physically strong, smart, funny, compassionate).

    "Tell me about a time that you really enjoyed your child, felt connected to your child, when you and your child were "in sync," when you laughed, or experienced a special bonding time where you felt like you "clicked.[1]"

4. **Review the results of the previously completed standardized assessment measures and behavior observations.**

    (a) Begin the feedback discussion by pointing out the child's strengths observed during the observation.
    (b) Discuss areas of foreseeable growth/improvement.
    (c) Conclude by reiterating areas of strength and the fit between the current model and the difficulties being experienced by the parent and child.

5. **Describe the rationale behind teaching CDI-T before PDI-T.**
    Sample Script: "CDI-T is primarily taught before PDI-T because the CDI-T skills will improve your child's emotion regulation abilities and increase the likelihood that your child will naturally comply with your requests. You will be able to better understand and manage many of your child's behaviors with the foundational skills that you will learn and practice in CDI-T before the compliance phase of the treatment. Much of this is done by improving the already positive relationship that you have built with your child by way of focusing on you following his or her lead during play and shaping his or her behavior by increasing the positivity of your attention. The skills of CDI-T are based on what we know about the power of play therapy. You will be asked to use these new skills in a 5-minute play therapy session each day at home."

---

[1]This question was informed by Parent Development Interview (PDI; Slade, 2005).

6. **Discuss the unique benefits and challenges associated with behavioral treatment with toddlers.**

   Benefits:

   (a) Very young children are still in the process of learning how to play, behave, and manage their emotions.

   (b) Toddlers are changing very quickly. Clear differences in their developmental abilities can be seen on a week-to-week basis, and therefore, the impact of intensive, early treatment can have a profound positive effect upon their emotional, social, intellectual, and behavioral abilities for years to come.

   (c) Early intervention programs similar to this one have been shown to enhance and stimulate processes such as language development.

   (d) Given the unique nature of the current treatment, it is likely that parents will retain their use of skills as the child continues to grow.

   Challenges:

   (a) Young children often experience emotions in intense ways. Such big emotions may be expressed as difficult behaviors.

   (b) Young children often have not yet developed the cognitive and language abilities necessary to appropriately manage and control such emotions in ways that older children and adults might.

   (c) Therefore, attempting to verbally reason with and cognitively understand the reasons why young children tend to become very upset can be especially difficult.

   (d) The combination of young children's developing language and emotional abilities as well as the intensity of such emotional expressions can be stressful for parents and caregivers to manage.

   (e) Such stressful, intense situations may negatively affect parents' emotion regulation abilities, making it more difficult to meet the needs of their young children.

7. **Discuss the concept of the parallel process between the coach, parent, and child with regard to emotion regulation.**

   (a) Children learn how to regulate their emotions/feelings, in part, by watching the ways that the adults in their environment regulate their own emotions.

   (b) As [child's name]'s [relationship of the caregiver to the child], your emotions and behavior have a big impact on how [child's name] feels and behaves.

   (c) So, throughout the therapy process, I'll be modeling good emotion regulation techniques for you as I coach you through some of the difficult emotional situations, so that you can be modeling these techniques with [child's name]. This is called the parallel process. We'll all work as a therapy team to help [child's name] learn to manage his/her emotions.

   (d) When difficult situations arise, I'll coach you through using some relaxation techniques that will likely be really helpful in decreasing your stress level and in turn, these techniques will benefit both you and your child.

8. **Explain and practice the diaphragmatic breathing relaxation technique.**

(a) One of these techniques is called diaphragmatic or deep breathing. Deep breathing may sound simple, but when you are stressed, it's a great way to help your body physically relax so that your mind can relax too.

(b) Let's practice this technique now so that you'll understand what I mean. These steps will be the exact same steps that we follow when you are in session with [child's name].

> **Step One:** Move to a comfortable position, either seated in a chair or on the floor.
> **Step Two:** Place one hand on your stomach. Take a slow, deep breath in.
> **Step Three:** Exhale slowly while pushing your stomach outward.
> **Step Four:** Repeat the process two to three times.

9. **Explain the use of cognitive strategies during coaching to help the parent better manage his or her emotions.**

(a) We know that thoughts, feelings, and behaviors are all intricately connected.

(b) By changing thoughts, we can in turn affect your feelings and behaviors, particularly during stressful moments when you are helping [child's name] to better manage his/her emotions.

(c) We'll also use cognitive/thinking strategies to help you catch and change any maladaptive thoughts that you may be experiencing. I'll help you challenge those cognitions during coaching using techniques such as positive self-talk. Positive self-talk will help you reframe thoughts that you may be having so that you too can better manage your emotions.

(d) For example, if [child's name] is having a tantrum, a parent may think, "This is overwhelming. I don't know what to do and it feels like this will never end." We may reframe the thought as, "This feels overwhelming now but my coach is here to help me through it. I'm helping [child's name] learn to cope with his/her emotions. It will be over soon."

10. **Explain the "don't" skills along with the rationale for each (Eyberg & Funderburk, 2011).**
Sample Script: "Now we are going to discuss some of the 'don't' or 'avoid' skills. These are skills that we are going to try to minimize during interactions with your child as they have been found to increase the negativity of interactions and may lead to negative behavior."

(a) **Commands**

(i) When we use an indirect command we are asking a child to do something, which is often understood as being given a choice (e.g., "Can you put your shoes on?").

(ii) When we use a direct commands we are telling a child to do something (e.g., "Please hand me the cup").

(iii) Commands increase the potential of negative interactions should noncompliance occur.

(iv) Commands lead the play.

(b) **Questions**

(i) Place demands on children by requesting an answer, which in turn could lead to negative behavior.

(ii) Detract from the positivity of an interaction by leading the conversation and guiding the play.

(c) **Negative/Critical Speech**

(i) May lead to increases in negative behavior by providing attention to inappropriate behavior.

(ii) May negatively impact a child's self-esteem

(iii) Can damage an interaction by decreasing warmth and positivity

11. **Ask the parent to recall all "don't" skills. Clarify any remaining questions.**

12. **Explain the "do" skills along with the rationale for each (Eyberg & Funderburk, 2011).**
Sample Script: "Now we are going to discuss some of the 'do' skills, or skills that we want to emphasize during interactions with your child as they have been found to increase the positivity of interactions and can help improve children's behavior. Conveniently, the first letter of each skill contributes to the word 'PRIDE' and thus, the skills are often collectively described as the PRIDE skills."

(a) **[Labeled] Praise**

(i) A specific, positive, evaluative statement commenting on an attribute or product of the child

- Labeled praise: "Thank you for playing so nicely with the toys"
- Unlabeled praise: "Good job!" "Awesome!" "Super!"

(ii) Increases the positivity of the interaction

(iii) Reinforces positive behavior thereby increasing the possibility that such behavior continues

(iv) Can help increase a child's self-esteem

(b) **Reflection**

(i) An immediate, verbal reiteration of a child's speech. Such speech may include sounds, words, or phrases and may be repeated verbatim or paraphrased while preserving the meaning of such speech.

- Child: "Big truck!"
- Parent: "You have a big, blue truck!"
- Child: [playing with a train set]: "Choo, Choo"!
- Parent: "Choo, Choo"

      (ii) Increases the quality and frequency of the child's speech.

     (iii) Demonstrates approval and validation of appropriate verbalizations.

     (iv) Enables the child to lead verbal communication.

(c) Imitation

      (i) Imitation includes mimicking or copying a child's immediate, appropriate behavior.

- Examples: The child is playing with the trains, and the parent plays with the trains as well. The child begins to clap his hands. The parent imitates such behavior by clapping her hands.

     (ii) Allows children to lead the play by mimicking appropriate behaviors

     (iii) Expresses approval of chosen activities.

     (iv) Teaches appropriate play skills.

      (v) Encourages developmentally appropriate interactions.

(d) Description

      (i) Behavior descriptions are a specific explanation of a child's immediately completed action. In contrast to a labeled praise, behavior descriptions do not include a positive, evaluative word.

     (ii) Behavior descriptions serve as a running commentary on a child's immediate actions.

- Behavior description: "You are running the train on the track." "You picked up two blocks." "You put the man on the castle."

     (iii) Helps maintain a child's attention on a task.

     (iv) Exposes a child to meaningful vocabulary.

      (v) Provides attention to appropriate behaviors thereby indicating approval.

     (vi) Allows the child to lead the play.

(e) Enjoyment

      (i) Enjoyment indicates a mutually rewarding experience between the parent and child.

     (ii) Indications of enjoyment may include smiling; clapping; laughing; use of an upbeat, enthusiastic voice; and eye contact.

     (iii) Increases the rewarding value of the play, particularly important for the toddler age group.

     (iv) Keeps children interested in play.

      (v) Helps to create a warm, happy connection between parents and children.

     (vi) Enhances the reinforcing value of any praise, reflective, or descriptive statement.

(f) Emotion Labeling

      (i) Verbal description and labeling of the child's observed emotion, as well as the parent's labeling of their own emotion

(ii) Increases emotional vocabulary of child and caregiver

(iii) Demonstrates the caregivers awareness of child's emotional presentation and their own presentation

(iv) Helps prepare caregiver for use of CARES if signs of emotional dysregulation present

- **Step One: Provide an introductory phrase.**
  - "You seem..."
  - "You look..."
  - "Your face looks..."
  - "Your body looks..."
  - "You are..."

- **Step Two: Insert the corresponding emotion label.**
- Emotion Glossary:
  - Upset
  - Frustrated
  - Confused
  - Cross
  - Worried
  - Mad
  - Sad
  - Happy
  - Scared
  - Excited
  - Tired
  - Hungry

Examples:

Child: (smiling and clapping after placing toy into sorter)
Parent: "You look proud of yourself."

Child: (child looks afraid, runs to parent, and gives parent a hug)
Parent: "You had a fright."

Child: (yawning and rubbing their eyes)
Parent: "You seem tired and ready for a nap."

Child: (slapping the floor with toy when they cannot open it)
Parent: "You're frustrated" + provide CARES.

(g) **Other Positive Skills:** Due to the developmental need of toddlers in addition to the PRIDE skills, other physical behaviors need to be demonstrated by the caregiver to improve their child's learning and understanding of social interactions.

NOTE: Therapists should model each of the following positive skills, provide examples, and have the parent give examples and practice each one.

These include:

(a) **Physical Affection**

  (i) Positive touch (e.g., hugs, rubbing a child's back, clapping for a job well done) adds warmth to the relationship.
  (ii) Develop a sense of trust and caretaking within the dyad.
  (iii) Demonstrates to child how to engage physically with others.

(b) **Skill of Redirection**

  (i) De-escalates the possibility of a child's misbehavior by providing a distraction or new focal point of interest
  (ii) Requires finely honed observation of child's behavior to interrupt a possibly negative interaction
  (iii) **Example:**

  Child: Begins to loudly bang two pots together.
  Parent: Looks away, pushes buttons on the toy police car, and begins to drive it around the room, while saying, "Here comes the police car. I'm going to drive really fast!"

  Child: [comes to join the parent].
  Parent says: "Thanks for coming to play! It's your turn with the car now."

(c) **Animated Tone of Voice**

  (i) Vocal dexterity catches a toddlers' attention and holds their interest longer than monotone speech patterns.
  (ii) Enthusiastic tones make play sound fun and more exciting.

(d) **Animated Facial Expressions**

  (i) Facial dexterity catches toddlers' attention and holds their interest longer than an expressionless face.
  (ii) Improves eye contact and adds visual interest for child to look at caregiver.

(e) **Play Style at Developmental Level**

  (i) Though rolling a ball on the ground may not be exciting for an adult, for a toddler, it's a new world of exploration.
  (ii) Repeating play themes and repeating words provide multiple opportunities for a toddler to hear how things are described and increases their understanding of the world around them.

(f) **Mutual Eye Contact**

  (i) Occurs when the parent's and toddler's eyes meet, creating a moment of connection and nonverbal communication of being together.
  (ii) The moment signifies an emotional connection between the parent and child, foundational to the development of social communication.

    (g) **Under-reaction**

        (i) An active parenting strategy to minimize reinforcement of a particular behavior by looking away from the toddler and keeping a neutral facial expression when a toddler is attempting to entice engagement from adults (e.g., dropping food off a high chair and looking at the parent with an engaging grin).

       (ii) Used in the absence of a "big emotion".

      (iii) Often combined with enthusiastic redirection.

      (iv) Can be followed by a labeled praise for the positive opposite behavior.

13. **Ask the parent to recall all "do" skills. Clarify any remaining questions.**

14. **The therapist should model all "do" skills while allowing the parent to play the role of the child. Switch roles. Only provide the parent with positive feedback regarding the use of any PRIDE skills used during the role-play.**

15. **Ask the parent how he or she believes his or her child will behave during interactions in which these skills are used. Provide the parent with the "do" and "don't" skills handout.**

16. **Discuss how children typically react to CDI-T, and introduce the parent to the specialized behavior management strategies that will be used. The following is a sample script and should not be read verbatim to the parent.** *Sample Script: "The type of attention that children receive during CDI-T is highly rewarding. Very few demands are placed on them and appropriate behavior is highly reinforced with enthusiastic social attention. Therefore, children typically behave very well in CDI-T. However, it is possible that difficult behaviors and upsetting emotions may arise. A big emotion is a change in the child's behavior, and it often includes crying, whining, or yelling, that appears to indicate an overwhelming emotional reaction that is difficult to control. The big emotion often includes anger and frustration. It grows in intensity and might include a demand for immediate parent access or a strong rejection of the parent (e.g., pushing away the parent). Big emotions involve a change of facial expression and vocalizations beyond simple crying, whining, or yelling and may include physical aggression, destruction of property, flailing, arching the back, falling to the floor, and even unusual behaviors such as turning to the corner, freezing, withdrawing, or self-injury. If and when such emotions occur for your child, we will respond to them in very specific ways. The goal of these unique strategies is to help children develop the necessary emotion regulation skills that will help them to be successful and learn the skills that they can use to help themselves. The techniques to improve emotion regulation skills can be recalled through the use of an acronym that spells the word "CARES."*

It is important to note that the steps of CARES occur in response to the presence of upsetting emotions and may be provided in any order. At times, only a subset of the CARES steps may be needed for a particular big emotion (e.g., "assist" may not be necessary if the child is not working on a task). It is likely that children may need assistance in regulating both positive and negative emotions. Particularly when parents are first learning to conduct the CARES steps, it is possible that the therapist may need to enter the room to support the parent in managing his or her own emotion regulation during CARES implementation. It is critical that therapists also help parents observe children's cues and intervene using the CARES model in assisting children of this age quickly before the child's emotions and behavior feel out of control. Although there seems to be a lot of steps, each step is done quickly, and often, simultaneously. The words used are clear and simple in an effort to help the child feel supported and quickly recover from the upsetting situation. Finally, the CARES model is only implemented in response to behaviors that are NOT dangerous or destructive (e.g., physical aggression, self-injurious behaviors). We will talk shortly about how we will respond to behaviors that fall into this dangerous category."

17. **Explain and discuss each component of the CARES model.**

   (a) **Come in (calmly and close)**

      (i) The parent should physically move to be in close proximity to the child.

      (ii) Demonstrates parental warmth, responsiveness, and availability.

   (b) **Assist**

      (i) The parent should physically assist the child with the particular problem/issue occurring, ideally by scaffolding the situation to allow the child to independently complete the desired task.

      (ii) If such assistance does not quickly result in success and emotional relief, the parent may complete the task for the child being mindful the parent does not consistently take over by assisting when not warranted.

      (iii) Helps to reduce the child's negative emotions by taking away/solving the problem/issue.

   (c) **Reassure**

      (i) Parent should make a verbal statement to the child that they will be taken care of.

      (ii) Such verbalizations should be done in a calming, warm, and comforting tone.

      (iii) Communicates to the child that the parent is there to support and nurture them.

   (d) **Emotional validation**

      (i) Parent labels the emotion being experienced by the child.

      (ii) Teaches emotional vocabulary and range of emotions beyond happy, sad, and mad.

      (iii) Communicates to the child that their feelings are valid and noticed.

      (iv) Helps the child to understand their inner experiences/make sense of their emotions.

(e) **Soothe (the child with voice and touch)**
  (i) Parent provides soft, gentle touch and words to child.
  (ii) This is a form of scaffolding offering physical and emotional comfort and support.

Examples and Applications of the Model:

CARES Vignettes: Early Stages of CDI-T
The following vignettes provide examples of directive, clear coaching to allow scaffolding with the caregiver as they learn the CARES model. This coaching technique is often implemented in the early stages of CDI-T coaching. Over the course of PCIT-T less directive coaching and more prompting of CARES skills should take place as the caregiver increases their knowledge base and confidence in the use of the CARES model throughout the full course of treatment.

George
An 18-month-old George is enjoying special time with his mother in CDI 1 and suddenly decides that he wants to leave the room. He tugs at the door and starts to cry.

The coach says, "He wants to leave the room. You can acknowledge his feelings."

His mother says, "I know you want to go, but we are still having special play" [EMOTIONAL VALIDATION], to which the coach says "Good job showing him that you understand what he wants."

George then falls to the ground and thrashes around, screaming loudly. The coach observes, "It's hard for him when he can't get what he wants. He needs you to come in and help him to calm down." George's mother positions herself next to George on the floor [COME IN] and says gently, "I know you want to go but we haven't finished playing" [EMOTIONAL VALIDATION].

The coach says "I like how you came to his side calmly and close. This is very calming for him. He needs you now to reassure him." The mother says, "It's okay, mommy's here when you want a cuddle" [REASSURE].

The intensity of George's emotion peaks and then starts to subside, evident by a reduction in his crying and thrashing. The coach observes, "He's starting to calm down now. He needs you to soothe him with physical contact." She reaches out to George and rubs his back, repeating, "I am here if you want a cuddle" [REASSURE; SOOTHE]. The coach says, "Wow, you are doing such a great job calming him down. He's becoming more settled. He's ready for a cuddle now."

George starts to take some big slow breaths and sobs slowly. She picks him up calmly and cradles him in her arms [COME IN]. The coach says, "I really like how you are being so sensitive to his needs."

While she is cuddling George, she rocks from side to side and says in a soft, calm voice, "Mommy is here" (REASSURE; SOOTHE]. George initially resists the embrace at which point she continues to rock him calmly. The coach says "I like your calm voice and cuddle – that is really helping to calm him down. He knows that you are there to help him." George soon relaxes and becomes calm.

The coach says "I love how you are able to calm him down with your soothing voice and touch. Now it's time to distract him with a toy and return to special play." The mother picks up a noisy train and starts to play with it. George soon joins in [RETURN TO SPECIAL PLAY].

Sarah

A 20-month-old Sarah has been engaged with her father for 15 minutes in special play when she starts to get restless while attempting to put a large saucepan in a small toy oven. Sarah starts to growl, whine, and become rough with the saucepan.

The coach says, "Sarah's getting frustrated because she can't get the saucepan in the oven. Let her know that you know how she's feeling." The father says, "I know it's frustrating, darling" [EMOTIONAL VALIDATION]. The coach says "Great work labeling her emotion. Now it's time to move in closer to her." The father kneels next to Sarah and gently puts his hand on her back [COME IN; SOOTHE]. The coach says "Good coming in close. That physical touch is helping her to calm down. Now you can assist her with the saucepan." The father says to Sarah in a soft voice "You're trying to put the saucepan in the oven but it's too big. Daddy's here to help" [SOOTHE; ASSIST; REASSURE]. The coach says "Great job being available for Sarah. That's going to teach her that she can count on you."

Sarah looks to her father and holds the saucepan up to him, indicating that she wants help. Coach comments, "Wow, that's great that she's showing you that she needs help. You can tell her that you like that." The father says, "Thank you for asking Daddy for help." The coach says "Nice labeled praise."

The father then offers Sarah a smaller saucepan [ASSIST]. The coach says, "That's a great way to assist Sarah. That's going to help her with her problem-solving skills." Together, they resume special play [RETURN TO SPECIAL PLAY].

18. **Discuss the application of the CARES model to the parent as a technique to help *the parent better regulate his or her emotions while working with the child.***

    Sample Script: "Given that managing the big emotions of young children can be a particularly difficult and, at times, frustrating task, it will also be important for us to have a common language to check in on and discuss your emotions. I'll be using the same model for myself. That way, we can all be sure that we are setting [child's name] up for success when teaching him/her how to manage his/her emotions in the best way we know how. Let's talk about how we will apply the CARES model to us as adults."

    (a) **C: Check cognitions, clue into yourself** – before beginning special time with your toddler, recognize:

        (i) Your thoughts/reason why you are spending time together.
        (ii) The feelings you bring into play.
        (iii) How your body language demonstrates your current style of engagement.

(b) **A: Assist self** – if not emotionally ready for play, implement relaxation techniques to help refocus energy:

  (i) Deep breathing.
  (ii) Quick shower.
  (iii) Progressive muscle relaxation.
  (iv) Call to supportive system.

(c) **R: Reassure self** – parenting presents challenges, and no one technique works all the time for all children all of the time; therefore:

  (i) Use positive self-talk.
  (ii) Remind yourself of tender moments experienced.
  (iii) Foresee future events that will take place with your child bringing joy.

(d) **E: Emotional awareness**

  (i) Toddlers and babies are remarkably good at sensing emotions. They seem to track and respond to stress.
  (ii) Special time allows for fun and connection to be experienced when we engage in play with positive thoughts and emotions.

(e) **S: Sensitive and soothing**

  (i) Similar to using a soothing voice with your toddler, be kind and sensitive to yourself in how you reassure yourself and the tone of your own self-talk. Remind yourself learning is a process of trial and error, plotting and adjusting courses as you go.

19. **Note that it is expected that the parent will be unable to implement the CARES model in response to every instance of a toddler's emotion dysregulation throughout each day.**

(a) Express empathy regarding the fact that being overly attentive to every little sign of distress could be exhausting for the parent.
(b) Note a parallel goal of teaching children to self-soothe, develop frustration tolerance, and self-control abilities.
(c) Simultaneously, there may be times in which the child verbally or physically indicates that he or she desires space away from the parent during moments of emotion dysregulation. Parents can gauge the balance between allowing the child space (particularly if it was requested) and full or partial implementation of the CARES model.
(d) Emphasize the primary focus of implementation of the CARES model during the 5 minutes of at-home therapy practice.

20. **Have the parent play the child. Tell the parent to become upset with a given toy. Demonstrate use of the CARES model with the parent. Switch roles.**

21. **Explain the additional use of under-reaction and redirection (See Table 13.1 for further details about when to use the CARES model versus under-reaction and redirection).**

Sample Script: "In addition to the CARES model, the use of redirection is an integral aspect of behavior management as it teaches critical emotion regulation skills to toddlers. Redirection uses enthusiastic verbalizations or toys to distract the child from an activity or a dysregulated state to engage in an appropriate behavior. Like the CARES model, it is critical that parents recognize and quickly respond to children's signs of distress, particularly when the situation is not easily remedied by the parent (e.g., by helping to fix the toy causing frustration)."

Step 1: Parent notices child's emotional and behavioral distress quickly and determines one of the following: (a) the situation cannot be remedied quickly or at all or (b) the caregiver has previously attempted to remedy the situation and the child's distress continues. Additionally, the parent should under-react to any non-dangerous, negative behaviors that arise (e.g., child is yelling, stomping, flailing arms) by slightly turning his or her head or body away from the behavior in order to avoid looking or speaking to the child.

Step 2: The parent begins to enthusiastically describe his or her own play, particularly with toys that include lights and sounds. Toys with sound effects may also be used in the place of or in addition to verbal description of play.

Step 3: When the child begins to play with the new item or joins the parent in appropriate play, the parent may implement CARES, if necessary, or begin using the PRIDE skills.

Situational Example: After playing with provided toys for approximately 15 minutes, child tosses the toy that he had been playing with, walks around the room, and cries.

The parent determines that the child might be bored with the toy that he was playing with. The parent then pushes buttons on a different toy that spins around, lights up, and plays music. The parent says, "Wee! Wow, I see the lights and the cars spinning around and around! This is fun!" The child, now calm, gets up, joins the parent, and pushes the same buttons on the toy. The parent (resuming the PRIDE skills), rubs the child's back and says, "Good job pushing the button!"

Table 13.1 Distinguishing between the use of the CARES model versus under-reaction and redirection

CARES Model *Only*	Under-React and Redirection *Only*
• An emotion is being experienced (e.g., frustration, anger, sadness, excitement, happiness, pride) and needs to be labeled in order to teach or soothe child • Such big emotions may be accompanied by difficult behaviors	• A big emotion is not being experienced, and therefore, CARES steps are not necessary • Redirection is used to divert the child's attention and prevent emotions from escalating • Parent should under-react to behavior Example: Child begins to play with outlet covers; parent pushes buttons on toy with sound effect to redirect and distract child from previous activity

22. **Have the parent play the child. Tell the parent to become bored while playing with a specific toy. Model the use of redirection for the parent. Ensure that all three steps are included. Switch roles.**

23. **Explain the steps for responding to dangerous and destructive behaviors in this phase of the intervention.**

Sample Script: "In CDI-T, we try to minimize the chance that dangerous or destructive behavior arises by allowing the child to direct the play and providing the child with high quality attention for appropriate behavior. We also attempt to recognize and help these young children remedy instances of emotion dysregulation early in an effort to prevent higher level negative behaviors. We also set up the therapy room in a developmentally appropriate way, minimizing the chances that children will engage in dangerous behaviors (e.g., climbing on tables). However, should dangerous or destructive behaviors arise, we have a specific way in which we would like you to manage such behaviors."

(a) **Discuss procedures in response to physical aggression. Explain to the parent the child-development-based rationale for why the specific procedure and wording were chosen.**

    (i) Physical aggression in very young children is not uncommon.

    (ii) Such aggression may occur toward another and even toward oneself (e.g., head banging, face slapping, arm/hand biting; refer back to Chapter 8 under section "Behavior Management Skills").

    (iii) The child attachment literature says that the parent is the "bigger, stronger, wiser one" (Cooper, Hoffman, Marvin, & Powell, 1998), which teaches children to access parents as a source of comfort and support.

    (iv) Physical aggression is seen as a signal that the child's needs are not being met and the child has not learned appropriate ways to express such emotions.

    (v) It is important to teach young children, early on, appropriate coping skills to manage their big emotions while simultaneously shaping such negative behaviors toward behaviors that will be acceptable in the preschool or daycare setting.

    (vi) We must remain calm but serious when responding to such behaviors.

    (vii) The specific wording used in this procedure was selected for its simplicity and overlap with what [child's name] will likely hear in other settings, like daycare or school. These words will be used to teach [child's name] clear limits and only used in the context of this procedure in order to make them stand out and unique to these high-level, dangerous situations.

    (viii) Allows consistent wording when child is hurting a person versus toys, and enables a blanket rule for life – no hurting anyone or anything.

    (ix) Engage the parent in a discussion about any physically aggressive behaviors that [child's name] displays.

Sample Script: "Some level of physical aggression in children [child's name]'s age is developmentally typical and sometimes occurs when children of this age are experiencing a difficult emotion. This physical aggression may occur towards another person or towards the self. The child attachment literature says that the parent is the "bigger, stronger, wiser one", which teaches children to access parents as a source of comfort and support. Physical aggression is seen as a signal that the child's needs are not being met and the child has not learned appropriate ways to express such emotions. Even though some aggression is typical in children this age, this is a critical time to shape such behaviors and help them learn more appropriate ways to communicate and cope with these feelings so that they can be successful in daycare or pre-school.

It is important that we remain calm, but serious, when managing these behaviors so as not to accidently reinforce their occurrence. Your ability to under-react to [child's name]'s aggression and redirect his/her attention is the foundation of these steps but now, we will expand on these skills even further. The specific wording used in this procedure was selected for its simplicity and overlap with what [child's name] will likely hear in other settings, like daycare or school. These words will be used to teach [child's name] clear limits and only used in the context of this procedure in order to make them stand out and unique to these high-level, dangerous situations. This procedure allows consistent wording when the child is hurting a person versus toys, enables a blanket rule for life - no hurting anyone or anything. Have you seen [child's name] exhibit aggression? When does such aggression that occur? How have you typically managed such aggression in the past? Now, I'll teach you a series of clearly defined steps in order to manage these types of behaviors.

Response to Aggression (Toward Another or Oneself) Steps

STEP 1 [child hits parent]: Parent should get down to child level, cover and hold their hands in yours, and give *direct eye contact* while stating in firm tone: *"no hurting."*

STEP 2: *Look away* from child while still covering their hands for *3 seconds*.

STEP 3: Return *direct eye contact,* and state in firm tone: *"No hurting. Gentle hands."*

STEP 4: Let the child's hands go.

STEP 5: *Quickly physically rotate the child* from around the waist toward another toy and facing away from the parent.

STEP 6: Redirect with PRIDE skills and provide CARES as needed.

STEP 7: Praise the child for rejoining the parent.

**Therapists should demonstrate this procedure with the parent (perhaps using a large stuffed animal or doll) to ensure understanding and answer any questions prior to continuing on with the session. Emphases are given to the parent to look for behavioral cues related to child frustration and therefore attempt to prevent aggression before it escalates out of growing frustration. When aggression does occur, consistency in the parental response is key.

*If **repeated aggression** occurs and if higher-level emotion (e.g., screaming) **is not present**, repeat this model two or three times.

Exception:

(a) If repeated aggression occurs and a higher level of emotion and behavioral dysregulation such as thrashing/attacking parent/self-injurious (e.g., head banging, arm/hand biting) behavior is present, the child may need to be picked up and soothed in a rocking motion.

(b) For safety reasons, if the child is highly dysregulated, this may need to be done, while the parent is sitting with the child on the ground. If the child is safe to be carried or moved, the parent could consider taking the child to a new environment (e.g., a walk down the hall). The therapist may consider entering the room to support the parent.

Jordan

A 22-month-old Jordan comes into the session cranky and crying. While the coach is talking to the mother at the start of the session, Jordan lashes out at his mother, hitting and kicking her in the shins. Jordan's mother appears unsure about what to do. She turns to the coach and says, "this behavior has been happening all morning."

The coach says, "It's not okay for Jordan to hurt mommy. You need to set a gentle limit. Take his hands in yours and say in a firm but gentle voice 'No hurting'." The mother does this, and the coach says, "Great job setting that limit. Now look away for three seconds and then make direct eye contact and again state in a firm voice, 'No hurting'." Finally, now say, "Gentle hands." The mother does this to which the coach responds, "Well done for saying that in such a calm voice. Now quickly rotate Jordan around the waist towards another toy, making him face away from you." Jordan's mother does this and attempts to distract him with a noisy toy, but Jordan falls to the ground, screaming and thrashing. The coach says "I love the way you tried to redirect him into play. He's just not ready yet. Let him know that you are there for a cuddle when he is ready." The mother says, "I am here when you want a cuddle" [REASSURE]. The coach says, "Well done for letting him know that you are there for him. That is going to help him calm down. Now position yourself next to him but in a place where you can't get hurt." The mother sits on the floor next to Jordan [COME IN], but he violently pushes her away. The coach says, "It was great to see you coming in close to Jordan, he's still feeling angry. You can validate that emotion for him." The mother says "It's okay that you're still angry. I am here when you are ready." [EMOTIONAL VALIDATION; REASSURE]. The coach says "Great job letting him know that you understand his feelings and that you are there for him. Now it's time for you to calm yourself down with some deep breaths." The mother uses deep breathing to calm herself down and then in a calm, soft voice says, "I am here when you are ready" [SOOTHE]. The coach says, "Good work being there for him and using your adult CARES skills to remain calm." Jordan's emotions soon begin to de-escalate. The coach comments "He's becoming calmer because you have assisted him to regulate his emotions."

The mother smiles and positions herself closer to Jordan and again says, "I'm here when you're ready for a cuddle" [COME IN; REASSURE]. The coach says, "It's lovely to see you coming in close and giving him reassurance." This time Jordan doesn't push her away, and she scoops him up in her arms and cradles him [COME IN; SOOTHE]. The coach observes, "Wow, he's really feeling safe in your arms."

She holds him close to her body and continues to rock from side to side. Jordan starts to whimper and the intensity of his emotion reduces. They soon resume play again, with Jordan sitting on his mother's lap [RETURN TO SPECIAL PLAY].

Throwing Toys It is critical that therapists coach parents to intervene early based on a predetermined motivational purpose of the toy-throwing behavior. Toy throwing might occur for a variety of reasons including boredom, lack of constructive play skills, attention-seeking, stimulation-seeking, fatigue, and venting of frustration/anger. When toy-throwing behavior occurs, we attempt to prevent or minimize behavioral escalation, primarily through enthusiastic redirection. Given that toy throwing is not conceptualized as aggression to self or attempt to purposefully harm others, the steps for handling toy throwing are as follows:

STEP 1: Under-react to toy-throwing behavior as any attention or reaction may result in a cause-and-effect-like game.

STEP 2: Implement CARES model. Redirection should be quickly implemented. Therapist should state: "He needs your help."

STEP 3: When possible, take child away from the thrown toys rather than taking the toy away from him/her.

STEP 4: If a toy must be removed from a child's hands, the caregiver should immediately distract the child by replacing the toy with a novel toy while enthusiastically describing the item or demonstrating its function.

STEP 5: If none of the previously noted steps are effective and toy throwing persists or becomes dangerous, toys may be removed from the play area or placed out of reach and out of sight. Following toy removal, the parent should continue to use redirection. The therapist may consider entering the room to provide a replacement toy and to aid the parent in redirection, if necessary.

24. **Engage the parent in discussion of any dangerous or destructive behaviors that they may expect from their child in this phase of treatment.**

    (a) Problem-solve ways in which to prevent such behaviors (e.g., choosing specific toys that the child enjoys, choosing an appointment time that does not interfere with nap/meal time).

25. **Explain the concept of active, Home Therapy Practice of the skills for 5 minutes each day.**
    Sample Script: "One importance piece of this intervention is practice of the skills that we discussed must occur in the home as a form of play therapy each day, regardless of the child's behavior that day. This practice should only occur for approximately five minutes in which time you are focused on using all of the skills that we discussed today. This practice will help improve your child's behavior in the home setting, improve your use of the skills, and help your relationship with your child to grow even stronger. At the end of Home Therapy Practice sessions, in this phase of the treatment, I don't want you to clean up the toys or tell your child to clean up the toys as this can lead to negative behavior. Instead, I want you to use your redirection skills to help your child to move on to

a different activity away from the toys. During our second phase of treatment we will focus on listening skills to help with clean up. Each week, I will give you a sheet where I want you to check off that you completed Home Therapy Practice and note any difficulties that arose so that we can talk about them in session."

26. **Discuss and problem-solve any barriers that might interfere with the parent's ability to complete Home Therapy Practice sessions with his or her child. If it is clear that the family is unable or unwilling to complete Home Therapy Practice, therapists should consider the use of another intervention method with the family.**

27. **Review key points for Home Therapy Practice:**
    (a) Location in the home where the practice will be completed.
    (b) Parent's response to dangerous/destructive behavior during Home Therapy Practice (i.e., response to aggression procedures discussed previously).
    (c) Home Therapy Practice should be strictly limited to a 5-minute time period.
    (d) No clean up should be expected following at-home therapy practice sessions. Instead, upon the conclusion of the practice, the parent should distract the child with a new activity (e.g., swinging in their swing, bouncing in the bouncer).
    (e) Appropriate toys available for practice.

28. **Discuss the types of toys to be used during CDI-T Home Therapy Practice:**
    (a) Minimal, carefully selected toys should be used.
    (b) It is integral that such toys are safe and developmentally appropriate to be used with the child (e.g., no small pieces, complex aspects).
    (c) Toys should be clean and easily disinfected as mouthing toys is common.
    (d) Toys that include lights, sounds, and aspects that inspire cause-and-effect-based learning are encouraged.
    (e) Balls and other items that may lead to throwing, destructive, or highly active behavior should be avoided.
    (f) Potentially messy items such as playdoh, paints, and markers given the time-limited 5 minutes of practice should also be avoided.

29. **Provide parents with the following handouts:**
    (a) "Do" and "don't" skills (PRIDE)
    (b) CARES for child and adult
    (c) Handout from CSEFEL: Teaching Your Child About Feelings (Vanderbilt University Center on the Social and Emotional Foundations for Early Learning, 1999)
    (d) Recommended PCIT-T toy list
    (e) Responding to dangerous and destructive behaviors
    (f) Home Therapy Practice sheet

30. **Complete Integrity Checklist: CDI-Toddler Teach Session**

Integrity Checklist: CDI-Toddlers Teach Session

 As you view the session, place a checkmark under the appropriate column, Yes (Y), Not Applicable (NA) or No (N). List these totals in the appropriate blanks below the table. See expanded session outlines for more information on each item. (Integrity checklist and directions are based on Eyberg & Funderburk, 2011).

Integrity Checklist: PCIT-Toddlers CDI Teach Session			
Client & Caregiver:			
Therapist Conducting Session:			
Checklist Completed By:	Date:		

	ITEM	✓	NA	X
1	Spends a few minutes checking in on any changes or major events			
2	Discusses feedback from assessment, confirm that PCIT-T is appropriate and identify caregiver's expectation and clarify any incorrect expectations			
3	Gives overview of PCIT-T			
4	Explains the structure of therapy sessions			
5	Explores if there has been a time in the past week when they felt connected or noticed a strength in their child			
6	Reviews standardized assessment measures and behavior observations			
7	Explains why CDI phase is taught first			
8	Discusses unique benefits and challenges associated with behavioral treatments with toddlers			
9	Discusses concept of the parallel process between coach, parent, and child in regard to emotional regulation			
10	Explains and practices the diaphragmatic breathing technique			
11	Explains the use of cognitive strategies during coaching to help the parent manage their emotions			
12	Explains the "Don't skills": Avoid commands, Avoid questions, Avoid Criticism using rationale and examples			
13	Engages caregivers in recalling the "Don't skills"			
14	Explains the "Do" skills along with the rationale and examples for each			
15	P stands for praise: Give your child labeled praises for positive behavior			
16	R stands for reflect: Reflect your child's appropriate talk			
17	I stands for imitate: Imitate your child's appropriate play			
18	D stands for describe: Describe the positive things your child is doing			
19	E stands for enjoy: Enjoy special time with your child			
20	Introduces Emotional Labeling: giving examples			
21	Discusses other Positive Skills: Physical Affection, Skill of redirection, Animation of voice, Animation of facial expressions, Mutual Eye contact			
22	Explains and practice Under Reaction			

23	Engages caregivers in recalling the PRIDE skills			
24	Asks the caregiver how they believe their child will respond and introduce to the caregiver the specialized behavior management strategies (CARES)			
25	Explains each component of the CARES model: Come In (calmly and close), Assist, Reassure, Emotional Validation, Soothe			
26	Discusses the application of the CARES model			
27	Discusses the fact that the CARES model does not need to be implemented in response to every instance of child dysregulation throughout the day			
28	Role-plays CDI-T with each caregiver the CARES model, Under-React and Combination of both			
29	Explains the use of redirection			
30	Explains the procedure for physical aggression			
31	Discusses with the caregiver what behaviors they may expect from their child			
32	Explains how to set up and end the CDI-T home therapy practice (no clean-up in this phase)			
33	Discusses barriers, regular, consistent treatment attendance and problem solve as required			
34	Asks caregivers specifically what toys they will use			
35	Emphasizes the importance of practicing CDI-T for 5 minutes everyday			
36	Asks caregivers to decide what time of day, and what room in their house, they will use for their daily practice			
37	Provides CDI-T handouts, Do/Don't Skills, CARES, Teaching Feelings, Dangerous/Destructive Behavior, Home Therapy Practice and Suggested Toy List			
	TOTALS			

Therapist comments about session

_____

_____

_____

Integrity checker comments about session

_____

_____

_____

Integrity =   <u>Yes Total</u>   = _____ %
            Yes Total + No Total

Length of session: _____minutes

Handouts and forms

PCIT–T Do Skills: Relationship Enhancement

P.R.I.D.E.

Picture Icon		Do Skill	Why Use This Skill?
	P ●	**Praise** Behavior	• Increases behavior you like • Brings connection to relationship • Models positive social skills • Increases self-esteem Examples: While clapping hands say: 　　"Great sharing!" "Beautiful music!" 　　"Awesome talking!"
	R ●	**Reflect** Speech	• Shows child you're paying attention • Allows for word pronunciation • Increases chance for child to add more Examples: (child) "ba ba" (parent) "ba, ba, ball" (child) "lello one." (parent) "Yellow block."
	I ●	**Imitate** Play	• Gives your approval of child's play • Child starts to model your behavior • Teaches child how to interact • Helps child feel important Examples: (Copy their physical movements) (child) puts arms up (parent) puts arms up (child) scoots on floor (parent) scoots on floor
	D ●	**Describe** Behavior	• Describes child's body in action • Teaches organization & ideas • Increases child's focus on task • Slows down an active child Examples: "You're making music." 　　"You're softly petting the dog." 　　"You're hugging the baby doll."
	E ●	**Enjoy** Time Together	• Providing physical affection adds warmth in the relationship • Using animated facial expressions & animated tone of voice keeps play fun • Models positive emotions Examples: Smiling & laughing together. 　　Making eye contact & clapping. 　　Giving a pat on the back or a hug.

PCIT–T Don't Skills: Relationship Enhancement

Picture Icon	Don't Skill	Why Avoid This Skill?
	Q • Questions	• Interrupts the play • Takes over the activity • Often irritating for child • Answer maybe unknown Examples: "What color is this?" "What are you making now?" "Do you want me to help you?"
	C • Commands	• Playing is a time child can lead • Commands place parent in charge • Minimize negative interaction Examples: "Look what Mom has." "Try using this block." "Let's play with this toy."
	C • Criticizing	• Can impact child's self-esteem • Creates an unpleasant interaction • Doesn't work to stop bad behaviors • Often increases criticized behavior Examples: "You're being naughty." "I don't like it when you scream." "Sugar pie, no, it doesn't go there."

AVOID: NO - DON'T - STOP - QUIT - NOT
unless a DANGEROUS or DESTRUCTIVE behavior is occurring

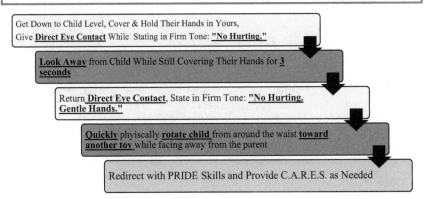

Get Down to Child Level, Cover & Hold Their Hands in Yours,
Give **Direct Eye Contact** While Stating in Firm Tone: **"No Hurting."**

Look Away from Child While Still Covering Their Hands for **3 seconds**

Return **Direct Eye Contact**, State in Firm Tone: **"No Hurting. Gentle Hands."**

Quickly phyisically **rotate child** from around the waist **toward another toy** while facing away from the parent

Redirect with PRIDE Skills and Provide C.A.R.E.S. as Needed

PCIT-T: Emotion Regulation for Toddlers

C.A.R.E.S.

Steps Provided in Any Order & Often Simultaneously

Picture Icon		Skill	How & Why Use This Skill?
	C	**Come In**	• Move your body physically close to child • Make movements calm and slow • By moving closer child sees you are present and available to them • Increases child sense of reliability with the caregiver
	A	**Assist Child**	• Help child problem solve current issue • Establishes early teaching experiences • Perform with child versus doing for child Example: (child) starts to fuss when unable to sort toy (parent) slowly turns toy while child remains holding toy to show placement in toy sort
	R	**Reassure Child**	• Creates opportunity for increased trust • Verbal statement child will be taken care of by caregiver Example: (parent) "It's ok, Mommy/Daddy is here." (parent) "I've got you, you're alright."
	E	**Emotional Validation**	• Label child's feeling being expressed • Creates sense of understanding & support • Helps to build emotional vocabulary Example (parent) "I know it's sad/frustrating when…" (parent) "You're proud/happy because…"
	S	**Soothe (voice/touch)**	• Provides sense of safety & security • Gives physical cues everything is ok • Model for child relaxed & calm demeanor Example (parent) Give cuddle to child or soft caress (parent) Use quiet, lulling tone of voice

Provide REDIRECTION after C.A.R.E.S.

Use toys with sounds for distraction
Note if child tired, hungry, wet and address

Move to different area/location
Increase facial and verbal animation

PCIT-T: Emotion Regulation for Adults

C.A.R.E.S.

Picture Icon		Skill	How & Why Use This Skill?

	C	**Check Cognitions, Clue into Yourself**	• Before beginning special time with your toddler recognize:
			   o your thoughts/reason why you are spending time together
			   o the feelings you bring into play
			   o how your body language demonstrates your current style of engagement

	A	**Assist Self**	• If not emotionally ready for play implement relaxation techniques to help refocus energy:
			   o deep breathing
			   o quick shower
			   o progressive muscle relaxation
			   o call to supportive system

	R	**Reassure Self**	• Parenting presents challenges and no one technique works for all children therefore use:
			   o positive self-talk
			   o remind yourself of tender moments
			   o foresee future events that will take place with your child bringing joy

	E	**Emotional Awareness**	• Toddlers and babies are remarkably good at sensing emotions. They seem to track and respond to stress. • Special time allows for fun and connection to be experienced when we engage in play with positive thoughts and emotions.
	S	**Sensitive & Soothing**	• Similar to using a soothing voice with your toddler, be kind and sensitive to yourself in how you reassure yourself and the tone of your own self-talk. Remind yourself learning is a process of trial and error, plotting and adjusting courses as you go.

Steps Provided in Any Order & Often Simultaneously

> The more **EMOTIONAL REGULATION** we can create in ourselves the greater the benefit to our children.

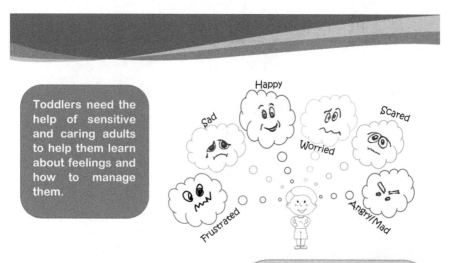

Toddlers need the help of sensitive and caring adults to help them learn about feelings and how to manage them.

Toddlers are wonderfully curious and enthusiastic about learning how to master new skills. Often with great determination they will try to dress or feed themselves, stack blocks, climb onto a chair without help, use a remote control. They love to explore and discover how things work. They have a natural desire to want to have some control over their world.

As your toddler is experimenting with the word 'No' or how to gain new skills, they are learning how to manage their emotions. They learn to do this through their experiences with sensitive and caring adults.

Helping your toddler recognise and manage their emotions is important as it will help your toddler with making friends, schooling and developing of a positive self-esteem.

CARES

C Come in calmly and get close to your child.

A Assist your child when they have a problem.

R Reassure using statements that let your toddler know that you are there for them.

E Emotional validation to support your toddler by stating what emotion your toddler is experiencing.

S Soothe with your voice and touch.

As a parent you may, at times, feel unsure about how best to help your toddler with their emotions. CARES is a simple set of tips which have been found to be very useful in helping young children develop self-regulation. Young children learn the quickest and the strongest from the examples they are shown by the people that care for them. When strong emotions are on display, by your toddler, it may feel really hard to do any of the tips. However, the more you are aware of your own feelings and stop and manage your own strong feelings the better you become at putting the tips into action. The more you try the different tips with your toddler, the more confident you will become in recognising the best approach for all the different emotions your toddler is experiencing. For example; your toddler might be trying to put on a sock and they are getting frustrated. You might move in closer and say "it can be frustrating putting on socks". Stay close and give them some space to keep trying. Notice if they might need some extra help, say "mummy can help if you like".

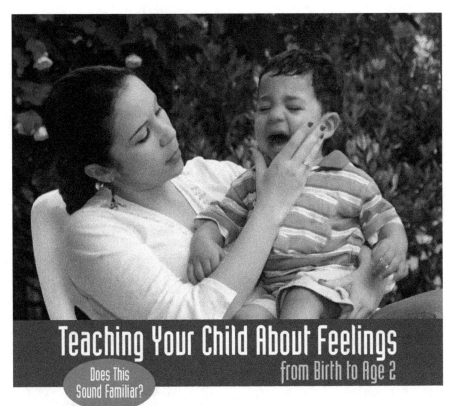

Teaching Your Child About Feelings
from Birth to Age 2

Does This Sound Familiar?

Damon (6 months) and his sister Karenna (20 months) have arrived at their grandmother's house for the day. Even though this has been the morning routine for a few months now, Damon cries and cries when his mother leaves. He is almost inconsolable, and it takes a great amount of time and comforting for him to calm down. Meanwhile, Karenna is pulling on her Granny's arm. She wants to play with her doll stroller but it is in the closet and she can't turn the knob. She is not happy about waiting for her grandmother's attention. Karenna swats her little brother, stamps her feet, and pulls on the doorknob with all her might.

What would you do if this happened in your home? Would you be feeling a little frustrated with one or maybe even *both* children? Or would you be able to hang on to that little piece of calm inside yourself and find the strength to soothe both your little ones?

The Focus

Young children experience many of the same emotions adults do. Children can feel angry, jealous, excited, sad, silly, frustrated, happy, and worried. The difference is that very young children—ages birth to 3—often lack the self-control and language skills to express their strong feelings in ways that adults find acceptable. Instead, babies and toddlers communicate strong emotions through their sounds and actions. For example, Damon cried to show how difficult it was saying good-bye to his mother. Big sister Karenna used her body—swatting, stamping, and yanking—to show her frustration with waiting and her desire for the doll stroller.

The Center on the Social and Emotional Foundations for Early Learning   Vanderbilt University   vanderbilt.edu/csefel

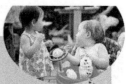

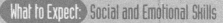

What to Expect: Social and Emotional Skills

Sometimes it is hard to imagine that very young babies are actively learning all the time, especially when they seem to spend most of their time sleeping, spitting up, or dropping strained carrots off the side of the high chair. However, these early years are a critical time of learning for babies and toddlers. They are developing a foundation of social-emotional skills that they will build on for the rest of their lives. Here is a table that highlights the social-emotional skills your child is learning and practicing at different ages. You can use this information to track how your child is growing and changing from birth to age 3.

GREENSPAN'S ESSENTIAL DEVELOPMENTAL STAGES		
Developmental Goal	Age Range	What's Happening?
1 *Stage One:* Being Calm and Interested in All the Sensations of the World	Approximately birth to 3 months	Your baby is: • learning how to be calm, how to accept soothing and comfort from a loved caregiver. • learning to feel secure and interested in the world around him. • trying to organize the information he is receiving from his senses.
2 *Stage Two:* Falling in Love	Approximately 2 to 10 months	Your baby is: • becoming more focused on parents and other persons and things outside herself. • expressing emotional reactions of her own (e.g., smiles and frowns). • expressing pleasure in others' company.
3 *Stage Three:* Becoming a Two-Way Communicator	Approximately 3 to 10 months	Your baby is: • purposefully using gestures (facial expressions, actions, and sounds) to communicate. • responding to others' gestures with gestures of his own. • realizing that he can use sounds and gestures to get his needs met by loved caregivers.
4 *Stage Four:* Learning to Solve Problems and Discovering a Sense of Self	Approximately 9 to 18 months	Your baby is: • learning to solve problems, like how to stack blocks in a tower. • communicating in increasingly complex ways, using language, expressions, and gestures. • learning what to expect from others, based on interactions and experiences with parents and caregivers. • developing a sense of self.
5 *Stage Five:* Creating Ideas	Approximately 16 to 36 months	Your toddler is: • becoming skilled in symbolic thought (e.g., labeling images with words: "Cookie!"). • using verbal means to communicate needs and desires. • engaging in pretend play. • learning to recognize and communicate her feelings. • learning to understand others' feelings.

(Greenspan 1999)

Good Habits to Get Into

From birth to age 2, parents and caregivers have a big part to play in helping children learn about feelings. The most important thing they can do is meet their babies' needs, love and nurture them, and comfort them when they are upset. This type of responsive care helps very young children build a strong, loving relationship with the adults who care for them. Feeling safe and secure, loved and nurtured, is the biggest and most important ingredient for a child's healthy social-emotional development.

There are other things that you can do to help your baby or young toddler begin to learn about feelings and how to express them. These are all good habits to develop while your child is young so that they become part of your everyday interactions and routines.

- **Think about your child's temperament,** or the way in which she approaches and reacts to the world. Temperament influences how intensely your child experiences feelings (like frustration or anger) and how easily she can calm down. A child who has strong feelings and reactions might have a harder time learning to control her emotions. Strong feelings probably feel even bigger and more overwhelming to her. On the other hand, a child who is easy going and allows changes or disruptions to "roll off her back" will probably have an easier time. Think about your own temperament. There is no "right" or "wrong" way to be. But paying attention to your own and your child's temperament gives you important information about each of your preferences. You can learn how to adjust or match your caregiving to meet your child's needs and help her grow and learn.

- **Talk about feelings.** At first, babies and young toddlers will probably not understand when you say, "I can see you are angry because Jessie knocked your blocks over" or "You are so sad that your balloon flew away." It might even feel a little silly to talk to a tiny baby about his feelings. But this is an important part of helping your child learn to identify and describe his emotions. When you use feeling words over and over as your child grows, he will eventually come to understand what you mean. As your child's language skills develop, he will start to use these words on his own.

- **Be a role model for expressing strong feelings in healthy ways:** "I just spilled your cup of juice all over the floor! I am feeling really frustrated. I think I am just going to close my eyes and count to five before I clean up." Through your words and actions, you can show your child how to manage strong feelings and recover. And when you are having a hard time, it's okay to make sure your children are in a safe place and give yourself a couple of minutes to calm down. You are modeling self-control and showing that sometimes you need a break, too.

Practice Makes Perfect

Children from birth to age 2 are learning a lot about relationships, feelings, soothing, and self-control. Here are some activities and strategies you can use with your child to help him or her begin to understand these big ideas:

From Birth to 18 Months

- **Keep your baby close.** Put on some of your favorite music, pick up your baby, and gently sway to the beat. Gaze into your baby's eyes, smile at her, and hold her next to your body. Leave the infant carrier in the car sometimes and hold your baby instead as you walk through the mall or visit a friend. Cuddle and nuzzle your baby during some one-on-one time before bed. Shared moments like these help build a strong bond between the two of you.

- **Read or tell stories about feelings.** Choose books with brightly colored illustrations or pictures and not too much text. Stories help your baby begin to understand emotions like frustration, anger, pride, and joy. As you read, point to the faces in the book and say, "She looks excited. He looks surprised." As your child grows, you can ask: "Who is sad on this page?" When he is able to talk, you can ask, "How is that baby feeling?"

- **Make baby-safe puppets.** Cut some pictures of babies and adults from magazines or catalogs. Choose pictures that show a range of emotions. You can also use family photos. Glue these to sturdy cardboard. If you'd like, you can cover them in clear contact paper so your baby can drool on them! Let your baby choose a face to look at. Let her look at the picture for as long as she'd like. Talk about the picture as your baby gazes at it: "That baby is crying. He is sad." Or, "That baby is laughing. He is happy to play with his puppy."

- **Play peek-a-boo.** Beginning at about 6 to 9 months, babies really enjoy peek-a-boo. Label your baby's feelings as you play: "Uh oh, where's Mommy? Here I am—Peek-a-boo! Are you surprised? Are you happy to find Mommy?" Games like peek-a-boo are also ways you can practice separations, reassuring your child that "I might go away, but I come back."

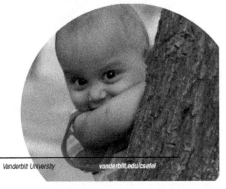

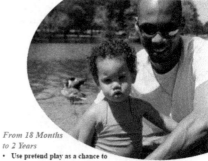

- **Look in the mirror.** Babies don't really know it's them in the mirror until they are about 2 years old. But you can help them become familiar with their own faces by making baby-safe mirrors part of your play. As the two of you look at your reflections, point to your smile and say, "I am so happy. I am happy because I love being here with you!"
- **Watch to see how your child responds to sounds and textures.** Use different sounds (rattles, toy pianos, shakers) and textures (towel, blanket, a square of lace, a piece of sandpaper, etc.) during playtime with your baby. Watch how your child responds. What does he like? Dislike? How much stimulation is too much for him? How do you know when your baby has had enough playtime (does he cry, look away, fall asleep, etc.)? Information like this helps you understand his needs and make him feel safe and comfortable.
- **Help your child recover when feelings get overwhelming.** How does your child like to be soothed? You can try swaddling, or snugly wrapping your baby in a blanket. Giving your baby a pacifier to suck, rocking, and singing can also help soothe little ones. For children over age 1, a cuddly stuffed animal or special blanket can comfort and calm them. Does your toddler need time alone to calm down? A firm hug or cuddle time, a change of scenery, a chance to jump up and down, or some physical play can also help toddlers recover. When you help soothe your young child, you are not "spoiling." Instead, you are teaching your child that she can depend on you. Children are also learning what to do to make themselves feel better when they get overwhelmed—a lifelong skill.
- **Know that your baby senses how you are feeling.** Research has shown that babies watch their loved ones very closely and respond to the feelings of the people around them. They know when you are upset, angry, stressed, or worried, even when you are trying very hard to hide it. They can feel your arms holding them differently when you are stressed and they are able to recognize that although you are smiling, your eyes are sad. So it's very important to take care of yourself so that you can take good care of your baby and help him feel safe, secure, and loved.

Taking Care of Yourself

We all feel stressed and overwhelmed at times. Thinking about what makes you feel calmer and more relaxed gives you an idea of what you can do when the going gets rough. You might try asking a trusted adult to watch your child for a little while so you have some time to yourself; exercising; writing in a journal; talking to a friend, counselor, or home visitor; or connecting with other parents. When you are a parent, it can be easy to forget that you need to be nurtured, too. But you do! Parenting can be hard work at times and all parents need and deserve support.

From 18 Months to 2 Years

- **Use pretend play as a chance to talk about feelings.** Your young toddler is just beginning to play pretend. You can help her develop this important skill by using a doll or stuffed animal in your play. Ask your child, "Doggie is sad because he fell down and got a bump. What can we do to make Doggie feel better?" This helps your child think about others' feelings, a quality called "empathy."
- **Make a homemade book about feelings.** Toddlers love looking at photos of you, themselves, and their friends. Snap some photos of your child when he is happy, silly, tired, excited, etc. Glue each photo to a piece of sturdy paper or cardboard. Write a feeling word under the photo, punch holes in the pages, and tie together with yarn. Let your child "read" the book to you and tell you how he is feeling in each photo.
- **Use songs to practice feeling words.** Your child's language is just beginning to take off, so give her a fun way to practice by changing the words to songs like "When You're Happy and You Know It." Try adding new verses like, "When you're angry and you know it, stomp your feet," "When you're sad and you know it, get a hug," "When you're cranky and you know it, find your Teddy," etc.
- **Make a cozy place in your home.** Just like adults, children sometimes need time alone to calm down. Give your child a space to do this by piling up some soft cushions and blankets, and adding a few stuffed animals and favorite stories. You can even get a large moving box, cut a door, and create a toddler-size "cozy room." Encourage your child to use this place when he is feeling overwhelmed or just wants some quiet time.
- **Suggest ways to manage strong emotions.** We often tell toddlers what not to do (e.g., "No screaming" or "Stop hitting"). Telling toddlers what they can do to express big feelings is even more important. When your child is really angry, suggest that she jump up and down, hit the sofa cushions, rip paper, cuddle up in a cozy area for alone time, paint an angry picture, or some other strategy that you feel is appropriate. The goal is to teach your child that any emotion is okay to feel and that she can learn to express feelings in healthy, non-hurtful ways.
- **Empathize with your child's feelings.** Sometimes the choices your child is being offered are not the ones he wants. Because your reaction gives him a cue of how to respond, it's best to stay matter-of-fact when you explain: "I know that

Pow! Bam! Take That! And That!

As you watch your child playact a battle between two action figures, your impulse might be to stop this aggressive play. But this is very typical for the toddler years. Play is the perfect time for children to work out strong feelings, even difficult ones like anger, frustration, or fear. Watching children as they play, and playing with them, helps you understand what they are thinking about or struggling with. You can also get insight into where they need a little support and how you can help them make sense of the world around them. If an upsetting play theme continues for a while or you are worried about your child's play, talk with your child's health care provider, teacher or caregiver, or a child development specialist.

you do not want the doctor to give you a shot. You are feeling really worried. But the shot keeps you healthy. It will hurt a little, but not too much. And it will be over with very quickly." This helps your child cope and, hopefully, move on.

- **Help your child understand her feelings and behavior.** When you can make connections between your child's temperament and her feelings, it helps her learn about herself. For example, you might say to a child who has a hard time moving between activities, "It's hard for you to get ready for nap right after we finish lunch. Your body needs time to relax after playing and eating. I will help you settle down and start to feel sleepy. Let's choose a story and get cozy." Over time this helps your child learn to manage situations that are challenging for her.

Teaching Feeling Words

 We often think only of teaching words for common emotions like happy, sad, mad, etc. But there are many, many other feeling words that we can use to describe the range of complex emotions each of us (and our children) experience every day. Children benefit when they develop a "feelings vocabulary" that they can use to communicate what they are feeling and experiencing. While babies and toddlers won't understand these words right away, over time and with practice they will grasp their meaning and begin to use these words themselves. Here are some ideas:

Brave	Frustrated	Embarrassed	Safe
Cheerful	Curious	Jealous	Relieved
Worried	Friendly	Angry	Peaceful
Joyful	Shy	Bored	Overwhelmed
Frightened	Ignored	Surprised	Loving
Calm	Lonely	Silly	Cranky
Excited	Interested	Uncomfortable	
Confused	Proud	Stubborn	

- **Plan for tantrums.** Tantrums are very common in the toddler years because children are still learning—and sometimes really struggling—with managing and expressing their feelings. Tantrums are their way of saying, "I am out of control and need your help to calm down." Rather than getting angry, too (which is easy to do, but can be scary for your child), help your child recover. Here's what you can try:
  1. Put into words how you think your child is feeling: "You are really mad. You are so frustrated!"
  2. Give him a way to show his strong feelings: "Do you want to throw some pillows?"
  3. Give him the support he needs (hugs, time alone, his teddy, etc.) to recover.
  4. Suggest another activity to shift his energy to something positive: "Let's play with blocks."
  5. And, as hard as it is sometimes, try to stay calm during your child's tantrums. You teach your child self-control by staying calm when he has "lost it." This helps him feel safe and lets him know that you'll always be there to support him—even during the tough times.
- **Offer choices.** Choices give toddlers a sense of control and can help them cope with disappointment. You might say, "It is bedtime. But you can choose whether you put pajamas on first or whether you brush teeth first." Choices can also help children deal with angry feelings and move on. For example, during a tantrum, you might say, "I can see you need to cry right now. Would you like me to hold you or do you want to be alone?"

Putting It All Together

Understanding feelings is an important part of a child's social-emotional development. Babies and toddlers experience feelings just like you do, and know when you are feeling happy or down as well. When you use words to describe emotions, share in their good feelings, and comfort them when they feel sad or overwhelmed, young children are learning important social-emotional skills. This learning takes a lot of practice on their part, and a lot of patience on yours. But the time and effort are worth it. The social-emotional skills children develop in the first two years are ones they will use and build on for the rest of their lives.

Reference: *Greenspan, S. (with Breslau Lewis, N.). (1999). Building healthy minds: The six experiences that create intelligence and emotional growth in babies and young children. Cambridge: Perseus Books.*

The Center on the Social and Emotional
Foundations for Early Learning

Child Care
Bureau

Office of
Head Start

Recommended Toy List for PCIT-Toddlers

Pretend Play

Puppets

Farm sets

Chunky train sets

Little People play sets

Kitchen / House sets

Baby dolls & items (doll bed, clothes, stroller)

Large wood / plastic toy vehicles with wheels

Stacking, Drop & Dump Play

Plastic bowls

Nesting toys / stacking rings

Large beads (non-choking hazard)

Soft blocks & cubes

Large Duplo blocks

Shape sorters

Relaxing Play

Board books

Bead Maze

Peg boards

Wooden peg puzzles

Motor Movement Play

Learning tables

Learning walkers

Push & pull toys

Crawl tunnels

Ride on / scoot vehicles

Toys with cause and effect/pop-up

(turn dials, switches, knobs, lids)

Creative Play

Jumbo/Palm crayons & large paper

Large empty cardboard boxes

Music / songs to dance

Simple sturdy musical instruments

PCIT-Toddlers Home Therapy Practice

Child's Name:_____   Date:_____

☐ Mom   ☐ Dad   ☐ Other Caregiver: _____

Your In Session 5-minute PRIDE Skills

| | Labeled Praise | Reflection | Behavior Description | Question/Command/Criticism |

Use your CDI "Do Skills / PRIDE" & play with your child 5 minutes daily.
Use CARES steps when signals of big emotions are present and your child needs your help.

	Did you engage in **Relaxation** before Special Time?		Did you spend 5 minutes in **Special Time** today?		Activity or Toys Played	List any signals of big emotions your child showed. Was CARES used?	PRIDE Skills used today… Any problems or questions during Special Time?
	Yes	No	Yes	No			
Monday							
Tuesday							
Wednesday							
Thursday							
Friday							
Saturday							
Sunday							

Write a time during the week when you felt an intense emotion and what impact did it have on your child?

_____

_____

Adapted from Eyberg and Funderburk (2011) CDI Homework sheet, pg 28.

Relationship Enhancement Tracker of
CDI-Toddlers Skills

Session #	Baseline CLP								
Date									
Home Therapy Practice									
7	X								
6	X								
5	X								
4	X								
3	X								
2	X								
1	X								
0	X								
Labeled Praise									
10+									
9									
8									
7									
6									
5									
4									
3									
2									
1									
0									
Reflection									
10+									
9									
8									
7									
6									
5									
4									
3									
2									
1									
0									
Behavior Description									
10+									
9									
8									
7									
6									
5									
4									
3									
2									
1									
0									

Relationship Enhancement Tracker of CDI-Toddlers Skills

Session #	Baseline CLP								
Date									

Emotion Labeling

10+									
9									
8									
7									
6									
5									
4									
3									
2									
1									
0									

Question/Command/Critical Statement

10+									
9									
8									
7									
6									
5									
4									
3									
2									
1									
0									

CARES

Satis-factory									
N/A									
Needs Improv.									

Other Positive Skills
(Imitate, Enjoy, Affection, Eye Contact, Animation, etc.)

Satis-factory									
N/A									
Needs Improv.									

Redirection and Under-Reaction

Satis-factory									
N/A									
Needs Improv.									

Limit-Setting "No Hurting"

Satis-factory									
N/A									
Needs Improv.									

PCIT-Toddlers
Check-In Sheet

Have any major stressors occurred since your last session that your therapist should be aware of?

_____

_____

_____

_____

If so, have these major stressors impacted your mood, behavior, and ability to deliver the therapy to your child for five minutes each day?

_____

_____

_____

_____

How have you noticed the impact of your expression of your emotions and behavior on your child's expression of his or her emotions and behavior?

_____

_____

_____

_____

Please note one time during the previous week where you felt connected to your child or you noticed a strength in your child.

_____

_____

_____

_____

References

Eisenstadt, T. H., Eyberg, S., McNeil, C. B., Newcomb, K., & Funderburk, B. W. (1993). Parent-Child Interaction Therapy with behavior problem children: Relative effectiveness of two stages and overall treatment outcome. *Journal of Clinical Child Psychology, 22*, 42–51.

Eyberg, S., & Funderburk, B. W. (2011). Parent-child interaction therapy protocol. Gainesville, FL: PCIT International.

Lieneman, C. C., Brabson, L. A., Highlander, A., Wallace, N. M., & McNeil, C. B. (2017). Parent–Child Interaction Therapy: current perspectives. *Psychology Research and Behavior Management, 10*, 239–256.

Slade, A. (2005). Parental reflective functioning: An introduction. *Attachment & Human Development, 7*(3), 269–281.

Vanderbilt University Center on the Social and Emotional Foundations for Early Learning. (1999). Teaching Your Child About Feelings Does This from Birth to Age 2. Retrieved from http://csefel.vanderbilt.edu/documents/teaching_your_child-feeling.pdf

1998 Cooper, Hoffman, Marvin, & Powell circleofsecurity.org

Chapter 14
Child-Directed Interaction Toddler Coach Session

The purpose of the child-directed interaction-toddler (CDI-T) coaching sessions is to help parents increase their use of the previously discussed PRIDE skills along with specific strategies to manage more difficult emotions and behavior (i.e., the CARES model, under-reaction, and redirection). Sessions will begin with the presentation of a clear visual stimulus presented to the child in the waiting area. Given the importance of consistency and predictability in the lives of toddlers, it is important that the patterns of each session remain as clear and similar as possible. Given the developmentally limited attention span of toddlers, it is not expected that sessions occur for the typical 45–60 minutes. Instead, therapists may consider a briefer 30–45-minutes session to aide in self-regulation and decrease the chances of managing high-level emotions in this phase of treatment. Most of the session will be spent on coaching the parent and child in the use of child-directed skills using in vivo bug-in-the-ear equipment. If two parents are present, therapists may consider splitting the coaching session in half, having one brief session per week with each parent or alternating between parents from week to week in order to allow each parent adequate coaching time. Finally, it remains important that the initial session check-in remain as brief as possible given the attention needs of the toddler age group. Therapists may consider completing this check-in at the conclusion of the session on the way to the car, if possible. In some cases, the therapist may decide to speak with the parent via phone more frequently between sessions in order to minimize long check-in and check-out durations.

Note Developmental tip of the day cards are provided in Appendix H at the conclusion of this manual. Clinicians may use their clinical judgment to determine if the parent is able to take in and utilize selected cards at the beginning or conclusion of each session.

© Springer Nature Switzerland AG 2018
E. I. Girard et al., *Parent-Child Interaction Therapy with Toddlers*,
https://doi.org/10.1007/978-3-319-93251-4_14

Session Preparation Items

1. Bug-in-the-ear equipment
2. Selected toys
3. DPICS-T coding sheets
4. Transition visual cards

CDI-T Coaching Tips

1. Working with toddlers and their parents is hard, particularly when working at an emotional level. It's important for coaches to be aware of their own feelings and exercise good emotion regulation skills themselves so that they may effectively support parents throughout the therapy process.
2. It is essential that the therapist specifically praise the child while coaching the parent, thereby teaching the parent to notice the child's strengths and positive qualities.
3. Coaching, particularly during the first few sessions, should be highly positive, focused on each instance in which the parent utilizes a PRIDE or positive skill (e.g., "good reflection," "nice labeled praise," "excellent behavioral description," "great imitation").
4. Coaches should become **more directive** (i.e., telling the parent exactly what to say and do) in implementation of the CARES model and response to aggression steps should dysregulation occur, particularly until the parent feels confident in accurately using the CARES model.
5. Coaching statements should remain short – between two and seven words each.
6. Coaching statements should occur often, after approximately each statement made by the parent.
7. A coach's ratio of positive comments to constructive suggestions should be about 5:1 throughout all CDI-T coaching sessions.
8. The coach's voice should always reflect the manner in which the parent should be speaking to the child.

    (a) During CDI-T, this should primarily be calm, gentle, and consistent.
    (b) Coaches should model and point out their exaggerated use of animated voices and facial expressions during any interactions with the parent (e.g., peek-a-boo game, expressive facial emotions, accompanying hand gestures). The use of such expressions may cause the parent or coach to feel as if he or she is behaving like an animated character, and this is developmentally appropriate.

9. The coach should infuse developmental knowledge whenever possible following coaching statements (e.g., "your reflection statements seem to have increased the clarity of his speech").

10. The coach should point out changes in the attachment behaviors of the parent-child relationship when they are observed (e.g., child visually referencing the parent, child seeking physical comfort when upset, moments of shared joy).
11. Coaching requires careful observation to identify cues in behavior. It is important for parents and therapists to understand that toddlers' behaviors are often outward expressions of children's internal emotions. Given toddlers' lack of ability to verbally communicate, it is critical that the coach assist the parent in trying to prevent the escalation of extreme emotions and behaviors by tuning in to the child's needs and responding to their early signs of distress.
12. Although children at this age may not have a lot of words, it is critical for language development that the coach prompt the parent to reflect any noises or approximations to words that occur.
13. Toddlers have a difficult time with change and transitions (e.g., going from the waiting room to the therapy room, when two parents are switching roles, when the therapist enters the room at the end of the session).

    (a) It is important that coaches help parents be sensitive to children's needs during transitions by using the CARES model. Additionally, teaching parents to maintain developmentally appropriate expectations for children helps parents to feel more confident managing the toddler's behavior.
    (b) Infusing playfulness, creativity, silliness, and imagination throughout the treatment helps parents and children to connect with one another while also helping to diffuse battles and increase mutual enjoyment.
    Examples:

    Parents and clinicians model walking out of the room while acting like soldiers, ballerinas, animals, and choo-choo trains or other movements that are fun for the child to enhance the rewarding value of the transition.

14. Coaches should point out changes that they notice in the parent's ability to remain calm during stressful emotional situations.
15. Coaches should teach and encourage parents to develop and implement novel play approaches with a variety of toys (e.g., filling a box with blocks and dumping them out versus building with the blocks).

Session Goals

1. Improve the parent's awareness of the direct impact of his or her expression of emotions and behavior upon the child's expression of emotions and behavior.
2. Increase the parent's use of the child-directed skills via direct coaching of the parent-child dyad during play with the child.
3. Increase the parent and child's familiarity with the session routine (e.g., transition to the room using visual aids, brief check-in, Home Therapy Practice submission and brief discussion, coaching, Home Therapy Practice assignment, check-out, transition out of the room using visual aids).

Session Outline

1. **Greet the parent and child in the waiting room.**

   (a) Provide the parent with the check-in sheet (included at the conclusion of this session) if not provided by front office.

   (b) Collect the parent's current Home Therapy Practice sheet, and place the information on the Relationship Enhancement Tracker of CDI-T Skills. Use a highlighter to graph those weeks where the parent completed four or more of the daily therapy sessions. For three or fewer, use a black pen or pencil to mark the number of days completed on the progress sheet.

   (c) Allow the parent to complete the check-in sheet for approximately 5 minutes if not completed in the waiting room.

   NOTE: Depending upon the setup of the waiting area at a given agency and/or the parent's difficulties managing the child's behavior, therapists may consider transitioning the parent-child dyad to a therapy room and playing with the child to allow the parent time to complete such procedures. If a parent has problems completing the form because of reading difficulty or because the child is too demanding, the therapist has the option of reading the sheet to the parent and recording the answers during the check-in. If the aforementioned transition occurs during this step, the therapist should utilize visual aids (described in the following step) when initially approaching the dyad in the waiting area.

2. **After the check-in sheet is completed, approach the parent and child prepared with the transitional cue cards/visual aids provided in the handouts of Chapter 14. Review the visual aide with the child while also prompting the parent to take the child's hand while walking to the therapy room.**

   (a) Given the parent's lack of familiarity with the PRIDE skills at this point in treatment, tell the parent that today you will model the use of the PRIDE skills while walking with the child and parent to the therapy room. However, the parent can contribute using any skills that he or she feels comfortable using. Praise the child and describe his or her behavior while walking. Praise the parent for any correct use of the skills used.

   Note: As CDI-T sessions progress and the parent's CDI-T skills improve, the therapist should transition to coaching the parent in his or her use of the CDI-T skills during this transition period.

3. **Review the completed check-in sheet. While reviewing the check-in sheet, the therapist should simultaneously interact with the child and model the use of CARES for the child if necessary.**

   (a) Briefly note any major changes that may have occurred since the previous session.

(b) Remind the parent of the parallel process. Select one parallel process question from the following examples:

  (i) Was there a time when you felt a lot of frustration or anger and you kept it in check because you wanted to be a good role model for your child?

  (ii) When was a time when you had to work hard to keep yourself calm in front of child? How did you do it?

  (iii) Did your interactions with your child bring up any thoughts of your own childhood or the impact of your parents' parenting on you?

  (iv) During the past week, did you notice the impact of someone else's emotions or behavior on your child's emotions or behavior?

  (v) Were there any moments that you felt proud of yourself for managing your emotions or behavior while around or interacting with your child differently than you may have in the past?

  (vi) Has anybody else commented on or noticed changes in your ability to regulate your emotions and behavior or your child's ability to regulate his or her emotions and behavior? If so, how?

  (vii) What did you do to take care of yourself during the past week? How does your self-care indirectly impact your child? In other words, what do you notice about your ability to be emotionally available for your child when you have taken time to care for your own needs?

4. **Praise the parent's ability to reflect on, and share thoughts about emotions and behavior, and explain how such insight contributes to the therapy process.**

(a) If in the course of the conversation it is clear that the parent needs additional support, the therapist may consider offering the parent an additional, individual session at another time to discuss the parent's thoughts and feelings.

5. **Remark on the parent's example of a time during the previous week when he/she felt connected to his/her child or noticed a strength in his/her child.**

(a) If the parent was unable to independently generate an example, prompt him or her to do so using one of the following scripts.
    Sample scripts:
    "Tell me about a time that you really enjoyed your child, felt connected to your child, you and your child were 'in sync,' when you laughed, or experienced a special bonding time where you felt like you 'clicked.'"
    Or
    "Tell me about a positive quality or a strength that you noticed in your child this week. How do you feel that your behavior impacts his or her ability to maximize this strength?"

6. **Review Home Therapy Practice.**

(a) Praise the parent for his or her effort in completing and returning the practice sheet.

(b) Briefly discuss the nature of the Home Therapy Practice session while problem-solving any difficulties that arose. Review the nature of the toys used, time practiced (given the child's developmental needs), and space in which the practice occurred.

(c) Provide confident reassurance to the parent following any expressions of uncertainty with the use of the skills or management of any child behavior during the practice session.

(d) If Home Therapy Practice was not returned, have the parent complete a new Home Therapy Practice sheet in session. If Home Therapy Practice was not conducted, problem-solve barriers to practice and reiterate the importance of "Home Therapy Practice" for the success of the current treatment. Problem-solve ways in which to help the parent remember to complete and return the Home Therapy Practice sheet (e.g., reminder in his or her phone, placing the sheet on the refrigerator). Explain to the parent that the real therapy happens at home during the 5-minute daily practice. The clinic sessions are designed to teach the parent to be a play therapist to provide the intervention at home.

7. **Check in on the parent's current emotion regulation, mood, and emotional ability to be a therapeutic parent for his or her child, while emphasizing the pivotal impact of the parent's emotions and behavior on the child's emotions and behavior. Guide the parent through cognitive check-in questions.**
    Cognitive Check-In Questions:

    (a) How am I feeling?
    (b) Am I in the right place to interact with my baby?

8. **Explain that the parent should be asking himself or herself such check-in questions prior to engaging his or her child in special playtime at home.**

9. **Briefly guide the parent through each of the four steps listed below in a brief diaphragmatic breathing relaxation exercise.**
    Step 1: Move to a comfortable position, either seated in a chair or on the floor.
    Step 2: Place one hand on your stomach. Take a slow, deep breath in.
    Step 3: Exhale slowly while pushing your stomach outward.
    Step 4: Repeat the process 2–3 times.

10. **Ask the parent about the impact of such procedures on his or her emotional and cognitive state. Emphasize the importance of engaging in the exercise to help the parent prepare for therapeutic play with the child in the home environment.**

11. **Transition to CDI-T coaching by presenting the coaching transition visual to the child. Provide the parent with the necessary bug-in-the-ear device.**
    Sample script: "It's time for mommy/daddy/caregiver to play with you! I'm going to go into my room [point to corresponding picture on visual] while you play with mommy/daddy/caregiver in here with these toys [point to corresponding picture on visual]."
    NOTE: When it is clear that the child understands the transition to coaching and the visual prompt is no longer needed, the visual cue may be discontinued.

12. **Direct parent to indicate to the child that it is time for the parent and child to play together with the toys.**

    "It's time for [child's name] and mommy/daddy/caregiver to play together!"

    (a) **Let the parent know that you will be quiet for the first 5 minutes, while the parent uses the child-directed skills with the child. Let the parent know that you will observe the parent and child play and specifically note all of the child-directed skills that the parent uses during the interaction.**

    Sample script: "I'm going to watch while you and [child's name] play together for five minutes. I want you to use as many child-directed skills that you can while you play. Should [child's name] become dysregulated during these 5 minutes, remember to use the CARES steps and I will be right here to assist in coaching CARES if needed. Follow your child's lead and have fun."

    Note: Should the child become extremely dysregulated during this 5-minute period, the therapist should pause coding and begin to coach the parent in the procedure most appropriate to the behavior.

13. **Following the 5-minute coded interaction, immediately put the data on the summary sheet before providing the parent with a feedback sandwich in which a labeled praise is given, followed by an area in which the parent may improve and goals for the day, followed by another labeled praise (a feedback sandwich).**

    Sample script: "You did a really nice job praising [child's name] for his gentle play. I can tell that you have been practicing! Today, we'll work on reducing your questions so that [child's name] can really direct the play. I love how closely you sit near [child's name], it seems like it makes him feel really safe."

14. **Coach the parent and child in the child-directed skills for approximately 15–25 minutes (one caregiver present). Attempt to conclude coaching when the child is in a positive mood.**

    (a) Provide the parent with high levels of positive reinforcement for any positive skills used, particularly those in contrast to any identified areas of weakness.
    (b) Avoid corrective statements.
    (c) Be aware of the parent's ability to regulate his or her emotions and behavior. Help the parent recognize signals that they are stressed or upset. If needed, coach the parent in the use of diaphragmatic breathing during the session. Therapists may also choose to prompt the parent to intentionally tense and hold select muscles (e.g., shoulders, hands, legs) for 3–4 seconds before releasing such tension. The contrast between such tensing and relaxing exercises function to assist selected muscle groups in relaxation.

        (i) Particularly following moments of a child's emotion dysregulation, therapists should coach the parent in the implementation of the CARES model for themselves.

C: Check cognitions, clue into yourself – before beginning special time with your toddler.

A: Assist self – if not emotionally ready for play, implement relaxation techniques to help refocus.

R: Reassure self – parenting presents challenges, and no one technique works for all children.

E: Emotional awareness – special time allows for fun and connection to be experienced.

S: Sensitive and soothing – be kind and sensitive to yourself in how you reassure yourself.

*NOTE: Steps are interchangeable and can be used in any order. The therapist can choose how many of these steps are needed for a particular parent at any given time.

(d) Therapists should highlight moments in which the parent's emotions (e.g., tone of voice, words) and behavior (e.g., engagement with the child, gentle touch) positively impact the child's emotions and behavior.

(e) When approximately 3 minutes remain in the session, prompt the caregiver to indicate the upcoming conclusion of the session to the child.

(f) Have the caregiver generate two praise statements in relation to the child's positive behavior during the session.

(g) Prompt the caregiver to begin to sing a "cleanup" song while cleaning up to aid child in transition. Therapists may search online for a suggested song if one is not known.

The Clean Up Song
by Barney
Clean up clean up everybody everywhere.
Clean up clean up everybody do your share.
Clean up clean up everybody everywhere.
Clean up clean up everybody do your share.
Clean up clean up everybody everywhere.
Clean up clean up everybody do your share
Lyrics © EMI Music Publishing, Sony/ATV Music Publishing LLC
Written by: JOSEPH K PHILLIPS, TRAD
Lyrics Licensed & Provided by LyricFind

15. **If two caregivers present: Coach the first parent and child in the child-directed skills for approximately 10 minutes. Then provide transition coaching to switch to the second parent:**

(a) Have the currently coached parent come in close to the toddler, within touching distance and perhaps rubbing their back while stating, "Now [Daddy] is coming to play with you."

(b) The "new" parent enters the room bringing with them upon entry a different toy to serve as a technique to decrease separation problems by using the toy as a distraction.

(c) The "new" parent then gives a transitional statement, "[Daddy] is here to play with you," while showing the new toy as a distraction.

(d) Both the "new" parent and "old" parent remain in close proximity with a gentle hand placed on the toddler and then fade the "old" parent out of the room, while the "new" parent begins to play with the toddler.

16. **After the toddler has successfully transitioned to the second parent, follow the same steps listed on Item 14, and coach the second parent and child in the child-directed skills for approximately 10 minutes.**

17. **Conduct the session wrap-up.**

(a) Enter the therapy room with the end-of-session transition visual.

(b) Present the Relationship Enhancement Tracker of CDI-Toddlers Skills.

(c) Provide the parent with brief feedback and praise related to initially coded CDI-T skills with emphasis on any improvements made throughout the session.

(d) Prompt the parent to comment on his or her ability to regulate his or her emotions throughout the session. Praise the parent for any positive changes or growth noted between the current session and previous sessions.

(e) Frame such discussion around the impact of the parent's emotion regulation on the child's emotion regulation. Remark on any skills that the parent used throughout the session (e.g., cognitive awareness, diaphragmatic breathing) that assisted the dyad in achieving positive results.

(f) If any difficulties with emotion regulation arose for the parent throughout the session, discuss relaxation and calming techniques that the parent may use should similar instances arise in the future.

18. **Provide the parent with the Home Therapy Practice sheet.**

19. **Present the transition visual to the child specifically indicating each picture related to leaving the therapy room and walking to the car.**

"Now it's time to go 'bye bye' [points to picture of child leaving therapy room] and walk to the car [point to picture of child in car]."

Important Notes

The current session should be repeated until parental mastery of the CDI-T skills is achieved within a 5-minute coded sequence conducted at the initial outset of the session. CDI-T mastery includes the following. In addition, no more than three (3) questions, commands, and critical comments can be provided during the 5-minute coded sequence in which CDI-T mastery is achieved, see Table 14.1, (Eyberg and Funderburk, 2011).

Table 14.1 Mastery criteria requirements for CDI-T

Parent skill	Mastery level to be achieved
Labeled praise	10 statements
Behavior description	10 statements
Reflection	10 statements
Emotion labeling	Satisfactory status
Positive skills (imitation, enjoyment, physical affection, redirection, animated tone of voice, animated facial expressions, play style at the child's developmental level)	Satisfactory status
CARES steps in response to emotion dysregulation	Satisfactory status

20. Complete Integrity Checklist: CDI-T Coach Session

Integrity Checklist: CDI-T Coach Session

 As you view the session, place a checkmark under the appropriate column, Yes (Y), Not Applicable (NA) or No (N). List these totals in the appropriate blanks below the table. See expanded session outlines for more information on each item. (Integrity checklist and directions are based on Eyberg & Funderburk, 2011).

Integrity Checklist: PCIT-Toddlers CDI Coach Session		
Client & Caregiver:		
Therapist Conducting Session:		
Checklist Completed By:	**Date:**	

	ITEMS	Y	NA	N
1	Greets the parent and child in the waiting area: Provides check-in sheet and collects Home Therapy Practice sheet			
2	Introduces session with visual transition prompt to the child and models PRIDE skills while supporting the caregiver/s to enter the therapy room safely			
3	Reviews check-in sheet and reviews major changes and reminds caregiver of the parallel process			
4	Praises caregiver for reflectiveness on the dyadic relationship			
5	Discusses a time in the previous week that the dyad felt connected			
6	Reviews Home Therapy Practice sheet			
7	Checks in with caregiver's emotional status and guides through cognitive check-in questions			
8	Educates caregiver on use of cognitive check-in and relaxation techniques prior to daily special play/ Home Therapy Practice			
9	Guides caregiver through relaxation breathing technique, if needed			
10	Introduces the visual prompt to the child for CDI-T			

11	Directs caregiver to introduce CDI-T to the child			
	With one caregiver in treatment			
12a	Codes DPICS-T with caregiver and child in CDI-T for 5 minutes			
13a	Gives caregiver feedback on skills and set goals for coaching			
14a	Coaches caregiver with child for about 10-20 minutes			
	With two caregivers in treatment			
12b	Codes DPICS-T with first caregiver and child CDI-T for 5 minutes			
13b	Gives first caregiver feedback in skills and set goals for coaching			
14b	Coaches first caregiver for about 5-10 minutes			
14c	Codes DPICS-T with second caregiver and child in CDI-T for 5 minutes			
14d	Gives second caregiver feedback on skills and sets goals for coaching			
14e	Coaches second caregiver with child for about 5 minutes			
	Wrap up Session Enter Treatment Room			
15	Debriefs session, discusses key points and use of CARES with caregivers			
16	Reviews Relationship Enhancement Tracker of CDI-Toddlers Skills with caregivers			
17	Provides Home Therapy Practice sheet to caregivers			
18	Presents transitional visual prompt to child specifically indicating the picture of leaving the therapy room and walking to the car			
	TOTALS			

Therapist comments about session

_____
_____
_____

Integrity checker comments about sessions:

_____
_____
_____

Integrity = $\dfrac{\text{Yes Total}}{\text{Yes Total + No Total}}$ = _____ %

Length of session = _____ minutes

Handouts and Forms

PCIT-Toddlers
Check-In Sheet

Have any major stressors occurred since your last session that your therapist should be aware of?

_____

_____

_____

_____

If so, have these major stressors impacted your mood, behavior, and ability to deliver the therapy to your child for five minutes each day?

_____

_____

_____

_____

How have you noticed the impact of your expression of your emotions and behavior on your child's expression of his or her emotions and behavior?

_____

_____

_____

_____

Please note one time during the previous week where you felt connected to your child or you noticed a strength in your child.

_____

_____

_____

_____

Transitional Visual Cue Card: Office to Playroom

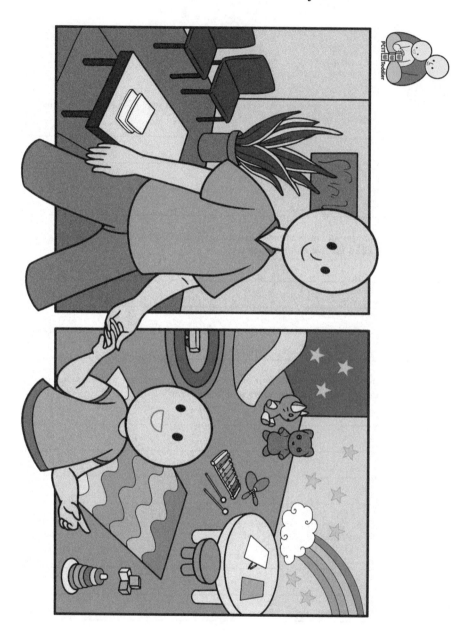

Transitional Visual Cue Card: Playroom to Leaving Office

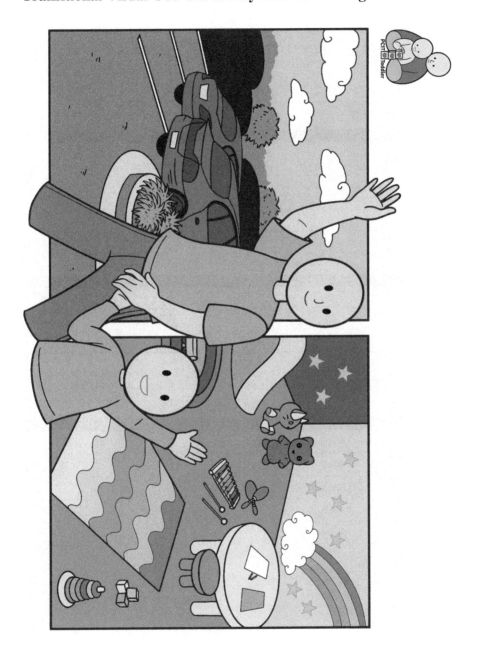

DPICS-T Coding Sheet for Therapist
Adapted from Eyberg and Funderburk (2011)

Child Name/ ID _____Date:_____

Parent: □ Mother   □ Father   □ Other _____

Coder:_____   Start Time:_____ End Time:_____

| o CDI Coach # _____ | o PDI Coach # _____ | o PDI LE # _____ |

Number of Days Homework Completed?   □ 0   □ 1   □ 2   □ 3   □ 4   □ 5   □ 6   □ 7

Do Skills	Tally Count	TOTAL	Mastery
Neutral Talk			--
Emotion Labeling			--
Behavioral Description			10
Reflection			10
Labeled Praise			10
Unlabeled Praise			--
Don't Skills	Tally Count	TOTAL	
Question			
Commands			0 ≤ 3
Negative Talk			

Coach caregiver through any missed CARES step (if needed) in the moment,
INCLUDING getting on the microphone during the 5 minutes of DPCIS Coding.

Big Emotion Present?	YES	NO	# Tally	
CARES Skills Used	CIRCLE ONE			NOTES
Come in Calm & Close	Satisfactory	Needs Practice	N/A	
Assist Child	Satisfactory	Needs Practice	N/A	
Reassure Child	Satisfactory	Needs Practice	N/A	
Emotional Validation	Satisfactory	Needs Practice	N/A	
Soothe	Satisfactory	Needs Practice	N/A	

(Continues onto next page)

DPICS-T Coding Sheet for Therapist
Adapted from Eyberg and Funderburk (2011)

PCIT Toddler

Child Name/ ID _____Date:_____

Parent: □ Mother   □ Father   □ Other _____

Coder:_____   Start Time:_____ End Time:_____

Positive Skills		Circle One		NOTES
Imitate	Satisfactory	Needs Practice		
Show Enjoyment	Satisfactory	Needs Practice		
Physical Affection	Satisfactory	Needs Practice		
Mutual Eye Contact	Satisfactory	Needs Practice		
Animated Tone of Voice	Satisfactory	Needs Practice		
Animated Facial Expressions	Satisfactory	Needs Practice		
Play Style at Developmental Level	Satisfactory	Needs Practice		
Bx Management Skills		Circle One		NOTES
Skill of Redirection	Satisfactory	Needs Practice	N/A	
Skill of Under Reaction	Satisfactory	Needs Practice	N/A	
Limit Setting - 'No Hurting'	Satisfactory	Needs Practice	N/A	

General Notes & Observations:

_____
_____
_____
_____
_____
_____
_____

Relationship Enhancement Tracker of CDI-Toddlers Skills

Session #	Baseline CLP								
Date									
Home Therapy Practice									
7	X								
6	X								
5	X								
4	X								
3	X								
2	X								
1	X								
0	X								
Labeled Praise									
10+									
9									
8									
7									
6									
5									
4									
3									
2									
1									
0									
Reflection									
10+									
9									
8									
7									
6									
5									
4									
3									
2									
1									
0									
Behavior Description									
10+									
9									
8									
7									
6									
5									
4									
3									
2									
1									
0									

Relationship Enhancement Tracker of CDI-Toddlers Skills

Session #	Baseline **CLP**								
Date									

Emotion Labeling

10+									
9									
8									
7									
6									
5									
4									
3									
2									
1									
0									

Question/Command/Critical Statement

10+									
9									
8									
7									
6									
5									
4									
3									
2									
1									
0									

CARES

Satis-factory									
N/A Needs Improv.									

Other Positive Skills
(Imitate, Enjoy, Affection, Eye Contact, Animation, etc.)

Satis-factory									
N/A Needs Improv.									

Redirection and Under-Reaction

Satis-factory									
N/A Needs Improv.									

Limit-Setting "No Hurting"

Satis-factory									
N/A Needs Improv.									

PCIT-Toddlers Home Therapy Practice

Child's Name:_____   Date:_____

□ Mom   □ Dad   □ Other Caregiver:_____

Your In Session 5-minute PRIDE Skills

| | Labeled Praise | Reflection | Behavior Description | Question/Command/Criticism |

Use your CDI "Do Skills / PRIDE" & play with your child 5 minutes daily.
Use CARES steps when signals of big emotions are present and your child needs your help.

	Did you engage in **Relaxation** before Special Time?		Did you spend 5 minutes in **Special Time** today?		Activity or Toys Played	List any signals of big emotions your child showed. Was CARES used?	PRIDE Skills used today… Any problems or questions during Special Time?
	Yes	No	Yes	No			
Monday							
Tuesday							
Wednesday							
Thursday							
Friday							
Saturday							
Sunday							

Write a time during the week when you felt an intense emotion and what impact did it have on your child?

_____

_____

Adapted from Eyberg and Funderburk (2011) CDI Homework sheet, pg 28.

Reference

Eyberg, S., & Funderburk, B. W. (2011). Parent-child interaction therapy protocol. Gainesville, FL: PCIT International.

Chapter 15
Parent-Directed Interaction-Toddler Teach Session

Previous research has supported the notion that authoritative parenting in which the caregiver exhibits a balance of both warmth and control is related to positive child outcomes (Vanderbilt University Center on the Social and Emotional Foundations for Early Learning, 1999). The implementation of such principles must be applied within a developmental framework unique to the infant and early toddler years. Therefore, procedures typically used to modify child compliance in preschoolers (i.e., time-out in a chair) are not considered to be developmentally appropriate for the toddler age group. However, given past research indicating increases in infant compliance following positive, parenting-focused intervention (Bagner et al., 2016), additional toddler-based compliance procedures may serve a preventative role to protect against future compliance difficulties. The goals of the parent-directed interaction phase of PCIT-T, therefore, are to teach and improve child compliance utilizing evidence-based principles that are likely to persist into the toddler and preschool years. Only a single session is dedicated to teaching caregivers the PDI-T skills. Given the volume of material covered in this session, it is strongly advised that the parent attend this session without the child (or bring another caregiver to assist with the child during the didactics). Although PDI-T is covered in a single teach session, ongoing practice and discussion of such skills are provided throughout subsequent coaching sessions. Accompanying handouts for the current session are included.

Note Developmental tip of the day cards are provided in Appendix H at the conclusion of this manual. Clinicians may use their clinical judgment to determine if the parent is able to take in and utilize selected cards at the beginning or conclusion of each session.

© Springer Nature Switzerland AG 2018

E. I. Girard et al., *Parent-Child Interaction Therapy with Toddlers*,

https://doi.org/10.1007/978-3-319-93251-4_15

Session Preparation Items

1. Necessary handouts:

    (a) PCIT-T check-in sheet
    (b) CDI-T Home Therapy Practice sheet
    (c) Relationship Enhancement Tracker of CDI-Toddlers Skills
    (d) Rules of effective commands
    (e) PDI-T guided compliance flow chart
    (f) Mid-treatment assessment measures (DECA and/or BITSEA) in addition to any other supplemental agency measures

Session Goals

1. Congratulate parents on their achievement of CDI-T mastery. Note any anecdotal changes observed in the child's behavior, emotion regulation abilities, child-parent relationship, or parent behavior since beginning treatment.
2. Provide parents with a brief understanding of PDI-T. Include the expected setup of treatment sessions.
3. Inform parents of the goals of the parent-directed interaction-toddler skills as well as the rationale behind and importance of teaching such skills.
4. Increase children's opportunities to develop language acquisition and production via directive language stimulation and coaching procedures.
5. Teach parents the steps involved in providing an effective instruction.
6. Emphasize the rationale behind limiting the types of commands provided to toddlers given their developmental level.
7. Teach parents the steps involved in the guided compliance technique.
8. Discuss the ongoing importance of Home Therapy Practice to the success of this new phase of the intervention.
9. Conclude with an opportunity for the parents to reflect on the potential impact of such skills for their child/family and ask remaining questions.

Session Outline

1. **Greet the parent in the waiting room.**

    (a) Provide the parent with the check-in sheet if not provided by front office personnel.
    (b) Provide the parent with a second administration of mid-treatment assessment measures if not provided by front office personnel. Specifically, if the DECA or BITSEA was initially administered, they are readministered for the mid-treatment assessment point. If any additional measures were

administered (e.g., the Ages and Stages Questionnaire, the Parenting Stress Index – Short Form, the Edinburgh Postnatal Depression Scale, the Child Behavior Checklist), they should also be readministered at this mid-treatment assessment point.

(c) Collect the parent's current Home Therapy Practice sheet, and place the information on the Relationship Enhancement Tracker of CDI-T Skills. Use a highlighter to graph those weeks where the parent completed four or more of the daily therapy sessions. For three or fewer, use a black pen or pencil to mark the number of days completed on the progress sheet.

2. **Review the completed check-in sheet. While reviewing the check-in sheet, the therapist should simultaneously interact with the child and model the use of CARES for the child if necessary.**

(a) Briefly note any major changes that may have occurred since the previous session.

(b) Remind the parent of the parallel process. Select one parallel process question from the following examples:

(i) Was there a time when you felt a lot of frustration or anger and you kept it in check because you wanted to be a good role model for your child?

(ii) When was a time when you had to work hard to keep yourself calm in front of your child? How did you do it?

(iii) Did your interactions with your child bring up any thoughts of your own childhood or the impact of your parents' parenting on you?

(iv) During the past week, did you notice the impact of someone else's emotions or behavior on your child's emotions or behavior?

(v) Were there any moments that you felt proud of yourself for managing your emotions or behavior while around or interacting with your child differently than you may have in the past?

(vi) Has anybody else commented on or noticed changes in your ability to regulate your emotions and behavior or your child's ability to regulate his or her emotions and behavior? If so, how?

(vii) What did you do to take care of yourself during the past week? How does your self-care indirectly impact your child? In other words, what do you notice about your ability to be emotionally available for your child when you have taken time to care for your own needs?

- Praise the parent's ability to reflect on and share such thoughts in relationship to her or her commitment to his or her child. If, in the course of the conversation, it is clear that the parent needs additional support, the therapist may consider offering the parent an additional, individual session to discuss the parent's thoughts and feelings.

- Remark on the parent's example of a time during the previous week when he/she felt connected to his/her child or noticed a strength in his/her child. If the parent was unable to independently generate an example, prompt him or her to do so using one of the following scripts.

Sample scripts:

"Tell me about a time that you really enjoyed your child, felt connected to your child, you and your child were 'in sync,' when you laughed, or experienced a special bonding time where you felt like you 'clicked'."

Or

"Tell me about a positive quality or a strength that you noticed in your child this week. How do you feel that your behavior impacts his or her ability to maximize this strength?"

3. **Review Home Therapy Practice.**

   (a) Praise the parent for his or her effort in completing and returning the practice sheet.
   (b) Briefly discuss the nature of the Home Therapy Practice session while problem-solving any difficulties that arose. Review the nature of the toys used, time practiced (given the child's developmental needs), and space in which the practice occurred.
   (c) Provide confident reassurance to the parent following any expressions of uncertainty with the use of the skills or management of any child behavior during the practice session.
   (d) If Home Therapy Practice was not returned, have the parent complete a new Home Therapy Practice sheet in session. If Home Therapy Practice was not conducted, problem-solve barriers to practice and reiterate the importance of such practice for the success of the current treatment. Problem-solve ways in which to help the parent remember to complete and return the Home Therapy Practice sheet (e.g., reminder in his or her phone, placing the sheet on the refrigerator).

4. **Congratulate the parent on his or her mastery of CDI-T skills. Discuss individual parent, child, or parent-child relationship-based changes that have occurred since beginning treatment with the parent. Review any remaining behavioral concerns that the parent may have.**

   Sample script: "Congratulations again on mastering, CDI-T. I'm really impressed by the hard work you put into practicing and achieving this challenging step in this treatment process. I've noticed that [child's name] is better able to calm himself down when he is upset. You've really helped support him through some difficult situations in this process, and as a result, it seems like your bond with him is even closer. How do you feel things have changed since you've begun treatment? What do you still feel you'd like to change with regard to [child's name]'s behavior?"

5. **Check in on any major changes that may have occurred since the previous session. Ask the parent to think of an example of one time during the previous week where he/she felt connected to his/her child or noticed a strength in his/her child.**

(a) If the parent exhibits difficulty finding a time when he/she felt connected to his/her child, ask the parent to think of a moment when he/she noticed a strength of the child (e.g., physically strong, smart, funny, compassionate).

Sample Script: "Tell me about a time that you really enjoyed your child, felt connected to your child, you and your child were 'in sync,' when you laughed, or experienced a special bonding time where you felt like you 'clicked'."

6. **Collect the parent's CDI-T Home Therapy Practice sheet, and add data to the Relationship Enhancement Tracker of CDI-Toddler Skills. Use a highlighter to graph those weeks where the parent completed four or more of the daily therapy sessions. For three or fewer, use a black pen or pencil to mark the number of days completed on the progress sheet. Praise the parent for his or her ongoing commitment to CDI-T, as such skills will continue to form the foundation of the PDI-T phase.**

   Sample script: "Great job completing your home therapy practice and bringing the sheet in today. This work is going to continue to be a critical piece of our work with [child's name] in this next phase of treatment."

7. **Discuss the primary objectives of PDI-T and the goals of the current teach session. Discuss the structure of ongoing treatment sessions. Review ongoing expectations for treatment attendance and importance of Home Therapy Practice completion.**

Primary objectives of PDI-T

   (a) Increase child compliance to parental directives.
   (b) Increase children's appropriate/functional language production via directive language stimulation and coaching. Improve parents' developmentally informed understanding of age-appropriate demands to be placed on toddlers.
   (c) Improve parents' ability to deliver effective instructions to their toddler-aged children.
   (e) Apply the PDI-T skills to real-life situations relevant to the family's needs.

Goals of the current teach session

   (a) Teach parents the PDI-T skills.
   (b) Practice the PDI-T skills in role-play situations with the therapist.

Sample script: "Today, we will focus on learning and practicing the PDI-T skills that you will use with [child's name] during the next session. The goals of PDI-T are different from CDI-T but CDI-T skills will continue to be used during our future PDI-T sessions. The major goal of PDI-T is to increase your child's compliance to developmentally appropriate demands targeted for his/her age. In this process, we expect that your ability to support [child's name] in his/her ability to listen will improve as you will provide him/her with the types of instructions that we know are most effective in helping children to listen. We will also help [child's name] learn to use his or her language to access things that he/she wants. This will help him/her to increase his/her vocabulary and use his/her language to get his/her needs met. Finally, we will use these skills to help improve any real-life challenges that you have with [child's name]'s behaviors during activities such as going out in public and meal times. The structure of our PDI-T sessions will be similar to our CDI-T sessions. I will begin by coding you and [child's name] in CDI-T. I will then code your PDI-T skills. You will continue to play with [child's name] using CDI-T but you will intermittently include commands, following PDI-T rules during your play. You will then practice both CDI-T and PDI-T skills at home with [child's name]. Of course, your ongoing treatment attendance and consistent Home Therapy Practice of the skills with [child's name] remain critical to treatment success."

8. **Emphasize the overriding principles of PDI-T: consistency, predictability, and following through.**

   (a) These principles help children feel safe and learn to trust the relationship between a parent's words and actions.

9. **Note that the PDI-T procedure always begins with an effective command. Teach parents the rules of effective instruction delivery based on Eyberg and Funderburk (2011).**

   Sample script: "Now, we will talk about the rules that we will follow when we tell [child's name] what to do. These rules have been shown to increase the chances that [child's name] will learn to follow directions quickly."

   Rule 1: Commands should be directly, rather than indirectly, stated.

   (a) Direct commands are provided in the form of a statement, rather than a question to clearly communicate that the child is independently expected to complete the task.

   Rule 2: Commands should be given one at a time.

   (a) Increases the chances that the child can process and execute the provided task, particularly given toddler's developmental level
   (b) Improves the parent's ability to determine if compliance has occurred

   Rule 3: Commands should be limited to simple concepts and phrases appropriate to toddler's developmental level.

   (a) Increases the child's ability to understand the provided task.
   (b) Given the population specific focus of this treatment, only the commands listed in Table 15.1 will be provided and practiced. The following commands represent the limited, toddler-directed commands that should be provided to and expected from this age group.
   (c) **Have the parent rank-order the following commands from most to least likely in which the child will comply.**

Table 15.1 List of developmentally appropriate toddler-directed commands

Developmentally appropriate, toddler-directed commands
"Please hand me_____" "Please give me_____"
"Please hand me the dinosaur"
"Please give me the dinosaur"
"Please put the _____ in the box"
"Please put the doll in the box"
"Please put the _____ in _____ (location)"
"Please put the truck in the basket"
"Please put the cup on the chair"
"Please hold my hand" (*only to be used when parent is close and child is calm)
"Please sit down"

Rule 4: Commands should always be specific, rather than stated in general terms.

(a) Improves children's understanding of what is expected

(b) Improves congruence between parent's and children's expectation for what is to be completed

Rule 5: A positive touch (e.g., touching the child's back) and clear, physical gestures (e.g., pointing) must accompany the provision of an effective command.

(a) Increases toddlers' chance of compliance by gaining their attention and allowing them to use their visual skills to orient toward the desired stimuli

Rule 6: Commands should be provided in a typical, speaking tone of voice.

(a) Limits the intensity of the emotional feedback the child receives prior to compliance

(b) Improves parent's ability to remain calm throughout the compliance sequence

Rule 7: Explanations should remain brief and provided prior to the command or following child compliance.

(a) Decreases the chances that the child will become distracted by an explanation provided in between the command and child compliance

(b) Increases the likelihood of compliance by providing context to demands

Rule 8: The parent must be in close proximity to the child prior to giving a command. When possible, the parent should physically position themselves on the child's level (e.g., crouch down on the floor next to the child).

(a) Increases the child's likelihood that he or she will comprehend that he or she must independently complete the task.

(b) Increases the likelihood of child compliance by assisting in orienting the child's attention toward the task.

10. **Reiterate the overriding rule that commands should be used sparingly and only when the child is emotionally able to practice listening.**

    (a) Given the natural fluctuation of toddler's moods depending upon the state of their biological needs (e.g., sleep, hunger, thirst), parents must be mindful of the likelihood that the toddler will be successful in compliance practice procedures. As much as possible, compliance procedures should not occur during times in which a biological need should be met (e.g., just prior to nap time, meal time). Discuss the application of this critical principle with the parent. Determine times in which listening practice should and should not occur.
    (b) An approximate ratio of five positive statements to every one corrective or command statement should be maintained throughout the day.

    Procedures Following an Effective Instruction
    A Summary of the Compliance Steps: An applied behavior analysis-based procedure, often referred to as "guided compliance," will be used to teach listening skills to toddlers. Modifications have been made to increase the toddler's likelihood of success by adding a "try again step" to the sequence. Therefore, the sequence includes "Tell-Show-Try Again-Guide." This procedure prevents escape from compliance while teaching toddlers, in a developmentally appropriate manner, the compliance skills that they will need to be successful. Steps 11–17 summarize and provide examples of each step related to the "Tell-Show-Try Again-Guide" procedure.

11. **Discuss the need to balance listening skill practice with the child's need to develop autonomy.**

    (a) Gaining independence is an important developmental process in this age range.
    (b) Teaching listening skills must be balanced with supporting the child's natural need to assert independence and develop a sense of control in the world.
    (c) During most of the day, indirect commands and choices are preferred whenever possible to foster toddler independence.
    (d) PDI-T is largely focused on the 5 minute per day listening practice sessions.
    (e) PDI-T procedures are used in ways that set the child up for success.
    (f) Listening practice sessions are conducted only when the child is in a positive mood
    (g) Listening practice is structured as an upbeat teaching tool to celebrate the child's emerging ability to follow directions and is limited in practice to a maximum of three commands.

12. **Discuss the 5-second waiting + physical gesture (e.g., point) rule along with provision of labeled praise for compliance. This step constitutes the "TELL" portion of the procedure.**

    (a) Young children need 5 seconds to comprehend and process an effective instruction.
    (b) Parents should be completely silent, while continuing to point to between the items necessary for compliance (e.g., pointing back and forth between the truck and the basket).

(c) The visual prompting helps the toddler associate words/vocabulary to objects and provides clarity about what the parent is expecting and where object is to be placed. The calm and silent repetition of the pointing gesture demonstrates patience and promotes a calm learning environment.

Example:

(a) Parent: "Please put the truck in the basket" (parent continuously points back and forth between the truck and the basket, while remaining verbally silent).

13. **Following compliance, an immediate, enthusiastic labeled praise and physical touch should be provided, and the parent should then return to following the child's lead with the PRIDE skills.**

(a) Immediate, clear, enthusiastic reinforcement is critical to reinforcing compliance.
(b) The inclusion of physical touch provides an additional layer of reinforcement while improving the positive connection between the parent and child.

Example:

(a) Parent: "Good listening to Mommy!" [parent rubs child's back]. "Now you are pushing the car. You picked up a truck…"
(b) **Practice Situation:** The therapist should role-play the parent, while the parent role-plays the child. The therapist should begin using CDI-T skills for 5 seconds. An effective instruction should be given. The parent should comply following the initial command.

14. **If compliance does not occur within a 5-second window following instruction delivery, the parent should physically demonstrate to the child how to complete the instruction. This step constitutes the "Show" portion of the procedure.**

Example:

(a) Parent: "Put the truck in the basket like this" [parent physically puts truck in basket and then immediately removes it, placing it back in its original position on the floor].

15. **If compliance occurs, an immediate, enthusiastic labeled praise should be provided, along with a positive, physical touch. The parent should then return to following the child's lead with the PRIDE skills.**

(a) Immediate, clear, enthusiastic reinforcement is critical to reinforcing compliance.
(b) An animated tone of voice is particularly important when reinforcing toddler's positive behavior.
(c) The inclusion of physical touch provides an additional layer of reinforcement while improving the positive connection between the parent and child.

Example:

(a) Parent: "Good listening to Mommy!" [parent rubs child's back].
(b) **Practice Situation:** The therapist should role-play the parent, while the parent role-plays the child. The therapist should begin using CDI-T skills for 5 seconds. An effective instruction should be given. The parent should comply **following the "Show" step of the procedure.**

16. **If compliance does not occur within a 5-second window following the demonstration, the parent should point to the child and say, "Your turn" and subsequently repeat the original command.**

    (a) This step helps to reiterate and clarify expectations while providing the child with an additional opportunity to practice independent compliance.

Example:

(a) Parent: "Your turn [parent points to child]. Put the truck in the basket" [parent points between the truck and the basket and waits 5 seconds].

17. **If compliance occurs, an immediate, enthusiastic labeled praise should be provided, along with a positive, physical touch. The parent should then return to following the child's lead with the PRIDE skills.**

    (a) Immediate, clear, enthusiastic reinforcement is critical to reinforcing compliance.
    (b) An animated tone of voice is particularly important when reinforcing a toddler's positive behavior.
    (c) The inclusion of physical touch provides an additional layer of reinforcement while improving the positive connection between the parent and child.

Example:

(a) Parent: "Good listening to Mommy!" [parent rubs child's back].
(b) **Practice Situation:** The therapist should role-play the parent, while the parent role-plays the child. The therapist should begin using CDI-T skills for 5 seconds. An effective instruction should be given. The parent should comply **following the "Try Again" step of the procedure.**

18. **If compliance does not occur within a 5-second window following the demonstration, the parent should say, "[Caregiver's relationship to child] will help you [original command]" [parent should gently, physically guide the child's hand and help him/her complete the original command]. As always, such words should be spoken in a neutral tone of voice. This step constitutes the "Guide" portion of the procedure. The Guide portion is completed by finishing the sequence with a behavioral description of the task.**

Example:

(a) Parent: "Mommy will help you put the truck in the box" [parent guides the child's hand to pick up the truck and place it in the box].
(b) Parent: "That's putting the truck in the box" [behavior description given to end GUIDE sequence]

(c) **Practice Situation:** The therapist should role-play the parent, while the parent role-plays the child. The therapist should begin stating five PRIDE skills before an effective instruction should be given. The parent should allow the therapist to physically guide the final step of the procedure.

19. **Practice the entire sequence using effective commands in two role-play situations with the therapist.**

   (a) **Practice Situation One:** The parent should role-play themselves, while the therapist role-plays the child. The parent should begin by using CDI-T skills for 10–20 seconds. An effective instruction should be given. The therapist should comply prior to the "GUIDE" step.

   (b) **Practice Situation Two:** The parent should role-play themselves, while the therapist role-plays the child. The parent should begin by using CDI-T skills for 10–20 seconds. An effective instruction should be given. The therapist should not comply throughout the sequence and allow the parent to progress through the entire sequence with completion at GUIDE procedure.

20. **Following the sequence, parent and child should resume CDI-T skills or implement the CARES model should emotion dysregulation be present.**

21. **Discuss the use of language encouragement** (Hansen & Shillingsburg, 2016; Tempel, Wagner, & McNeil, 2009). *This should never be punitive only motivational. If a child does not have language, this step of the protocol should not be conducted. This should not be used when children are cranky, hungry or desiring affection. Meeting children's primary needs is always paramount*

   (a) Toddlerhood is an ideal time, developmentally, to help children learn appropriate, functional ways to get their needs met.

   (b) Previous behavioral intervention with young children has demonstrated improvements in children's language acquisition and production abilities.

   (c) Verbal prompts should only be used when the child is naturally reaching for/desires an object.

   (d) Enthusiastic labeled praise along with desired object should be provided to child upon any approximation toward desired verbalization.

   (e) Following a 5-second delay, object should be handed to the child regardless of verbalization.

   (f) Purpose of the delay: gives them time to process and use their words and teaches them that access to the desired object occurs more quickly following language production.

   Sample script: "Toddlerhood is a key time for language stimulation and development. Helping [child's name] to increase his/her language will help him/her learn better ways to manage his/her big emotions while also getting his/her needs met. During PDI-T, we will help [child's name] develop his/her language skills by prompting him/her to use his/her words when he/she wants something. If after your prompt to him/her, no words are spoken, wait for five seconds before handing him/her the object. Therefore, this procedure isn't meant to frustrate him/her but provide him/her with opportunities to use his/her language to get his/her needs met. We will only use these verbal prompts when [child's name] is calm and seems emotionally ready to attempt them."

Example 1:

Child: [pointing toward toy truck that parent is holding] "Ah, ah."
Parent: "truck please."
Child: "Tuck pea."
Parent: "Good job saying truck please!" [parent claps and hands child the truck].

Example 2:

Child: [walking toward light-up toy that parent is playing with, arms outstretched].
Parent: [picks up the toy] "Say toy please."
Child: [no attempt at verbalization present, 5 seconds has passed].
Parent: [hands child the toy] "T – T – Toy. Here's the toy."

22. **Discuss PDI-T mastery criteria.**

    PDI-T mastery criteria is a 5-minute coded sequence at the initial outset of a PDI-T session:

    (a) 75% effective commands
    (b) 75% effective follow-through
    (c) Satisfactory implementation of:

        (i)   Language encouragement and coaching procedures
        (ii) CARES model
        (iii) Response to dangerous behaviors

    Sample script: "Just like CDI-T, we will continue to practice these procedures until mastery of PDI-T is achieved. We will continue to practice CDI-T steps during PDI-T but sessions will also include PDI-T procedures. You will also practice PDI-T procedures during Home Therapy Practice with [child's name]. PDI-T mastery will be met when you are able to provide [child's name] with 75% effective commands, 75% effective follow through in a five-minute coded sequence at the initial outset of a PDI-T session and are able to satisfactorily utilize directive language stimulation procedures, the CARES model, and use the steps that we talked about in response to [child's name] dangerous behaviors."

23. **Provide the parent with the CDI-T Home Therapy Practice sheet and the compliance sentence stems guide to review at home. Provide the rationale for waiting until the next session to practice PDI-T procedures.**

    Sample script: "This week, I'd like you to continue to practice CDI-T with [child's name]. I want to be sure that everything goes well the first time we introduce [child's name] to PDI-T so we'll practice the PDI-T steps for the first time here during our next session."

24. **Complete Integrity Checklist: PDI-T Teach Session**

Integrity Checklist: PDI-T Teach Session

 As you view the session, place a checkmark under the appropriate column, Yes (Y), Not Applicable (NA) or No (N). List these totals in the appropriate blanks below the table. See expanded session outlines for more information on each item. (Integrity checklist and directions are based on Eyberg & Funderburk, 2011).

Integrity Checklist: PCIT-Toddlers PDI Teach Session			
Client & Caregiver:			
Therapist Conducting Session:			
Checklist Completed By:		**Date:**	

	ITEMS	Y	NA	N
1	Congratulates caregiver/s mastery CDI-T skills			
2	Checks-in on any major changes and ask the caregiver/s a time in the past week that they have felt connected to their child or have noticed a strength in their child			
3	Reviews CDI-T Home Therapy Practice sheet			
4	Discusses CDI-T as the foundation of treatment			
5	Presents overview of PDI-T and introducing concept of developing listening skills			
6	Discusses the expectations of attendance and Home Therapy Practice			
7	Emphasizes the overriding principles of PDI-T: Consistency, Predictability, Follow through			
8	Rule 1: Commands should be direct rather than indirect			
9	Rule 2: Commands should be given one at a time			
10	Rule 3: Commands should be limited to simple concepts and phrases appropriate to toddler's developmental level			
11	Rule 4: Commands should be specific, rather than in general terms			
12	Rule 5: A positive touch and clear, physical gesture must accompany the provision of an effective command			
13	Rule 6: Commands should be provided in a typical, speaking tone of voice			
14	Rule 7: Explanations should remain brief and provided prior to the command or following child compliance			
15	Rule 8: Caregiver/s close proximity to the child prior to giving the command is required			
16	Asks caregiver to rank-order commands			
17	Reiterates the overriding rule that commands should be used sparingly and when the child has the emotional capacity to listen and practiced a maximum of three times per day			

18	Summarizes the compliance steps: Tell, Show, Try again, Guide			
19	TELL: Discusses 5 second waiting and gesturing			
20	Following compliance an enthusiastic label praise and physical touch is given			
21	Practices Situation: Role plays demonstrating CDI-T for 5 seconds, effective command and praising compliance			
22	SHOW: Discusses if compliance does not occur within 5 seconds the caregiver will physically demonstrate how to complete the instruction. Praise compliance with enthusiastic label praise and physical touch			
23	Practice Situation: Role plays demonstrating CDI-T for 5 seconds, effective command and compliance following the SHOW step			
24	TRY AGAIN: Discusses if compliance does not occur within 5 seconds following the demonstration the caregiver should point and say: "Your turn" and subsequently repeats the original command and caregiver points repeatedly to task. If compliance occurs caregiver gives an enthusiastic label praise and physical touch			
25	Practice Situation: Role plays demonstrating CDI-T for 5 seconds, effective command and Try Again step			
26	GUIDE: Discusses if compliance does not occur within 5 seconds following the demonstration the caregiver says: "I will help you...(restates the original command)" while physically guiding the child's hand to complete the command and using a behavioral description to label completion of the task. A label praise may be provided after the behavior description			
27	Practice Situation: Role plays demonstrating CDI-T 5 seconds and Guide procedure			
28	Practice Situation One: CDI-T skills for 10-20 seconds and effective command up the Try Again step			
29	Practice Situation Two: CDI-T for 10-20 seconds and effective command up to the completion of the Guide step			
30	Discusses language encouragement			
31	Discusses PDT-T mastery criteria			
32	Provides CDI-T Home Therapy Practice sheet and emphasizes importance of CDI-T this week			
33	Discusses rationale for not practicing PDI-T this week			
	TOTALS			

Therapist comments about session

_____

_____

_____

Integrity checker comments about sessions:

_____

_____

_____

Integrity =   Yes Total _____   = _____ %
                 Yes Total + No Total

Length of session = _____minutes

Handouts and Forms

PCIT-Toddlers
Check-In Sheet

Have any major stressors occurred since your last session that your therapist should be aware of ?

_____

_____

_____

_____

If so, have these major stressors impacted your mood, behavior, and ability to deliver the therapy to your child for five minutes each day?

_____

_____

_____

_____

How have you noticed the impact of your expression of your emotions and behavior on your child's expression of his or her emotions and behavior?

_____

_____

_____

_____

Please note one time during the previous week where you felt connected to your child or you noticed a strength in your child.

_____

_____

_____

_____

PCIT-Toddlers 8 Rules of Effective Commands* (PDI-T phase)

Adapted from Eyberg and Funderburk (2011), Eight Rules of Effective Commands, pgs 72-73

*Over-riding rule that commands are used sparingly and only when the child is emotionally able to practice listening with a maximum of three commands practiced during session and during PDI-T Home Therapy Practice.

RULE	REASON	EXAMPLES
1. Commands should be **DIRECTLY,** rather than indirectly stated.	• Direct commands are provided in the form of a statement, rather than a question to clearly communicate that the child is independently expected to complete the task.	• **Please hand me the block.** • **Put the train in the box please.** • **Sit by Mommy.** Instead of: Will you hand me the block? Let's put the train in the box. Come sit by me, ok.

2. Commands should be given **ONE AT A TIME**.	• Increases the chances that the child can process and execute the provided task, particularly given toddler's developmental level.
	• Improves the parent's ability to determine if compliance has occurred.
		• **Please put the doll in the basket.**
		    Instead of:
		
		Put the doll, play clothes and wipes up on the counter.
		
		• **Hold my hand.**
		    Instead of:
		
		Let's go home. (gathering items & holding hands)

3. Commands should be limited to **SIMPLE CONCEPTS & PHRASES** appropriate to toddler's developmental level.	• Increases the child's ability to understand the provided task. • Only the commands listed on your handout will be provided and practiced as they represent the limited, toddler-directed commands that should be provided to and expected from this age group.	• **Sit by Daddy.** *Instead of:* *Stop running and calm down.*

4. Commands should always be **SPECIFIC,** rather than stated in general terms.	• Improves children's understanding of what is expected.
	• Improves congruence between parent's and children's expectation for what is to be completed.
		• **Sit by Mommy.**
		    Instead of:
		
		Behave!
		
		• **Hold my hand.**
		    Instead of:
		
		Stop touching everything!

5. A **POSTIVE TOUCH** (touching the child's back) **& CLEAR PHYSICAL GESTURES** (e.g., pointing to objects) must accompany an effective command.	• Increase toddlers' chance of compliance by gaining their attention and allowing them to use their visual skills to orient toward the desired task.	• **Parent: (place hand softly on child's back and holds out opposite hand) Please hold Daddy's hand.** *Instead of:* *Parent: (from across the room)* *Come hold my hand!*
6. Commands should be provided in a **TYPICAL, SPEAKING TONE OF VOICE**.	• Limits the intensity of the emotional feedback the child receives prior to compliance. • Improves parent's ability to remain calm throughout the compliance sequence.	• **Parent: (at eye level of child and with typical tone of voice) Please give Mommy the train.** *Instead of:* *Parent: (from across the room)* *Give me the train!*
7. **EXPLANATIONS** should remain **BRIEF** and **PROVIDED PRIOR** to the command **OR FOLLOWING** toddler **COMPLIANCE**.	• Decreases the chances that the child will become distracted by an explanation provided in between the command and child compliance. • Increases the likelihood of compliance by providing context to demands. • Method for teaching rationale and sequencing.	• **Parent: Uh-oh, time to go home. Hold Daddy's hand please. Child: (complies)** **Parent: Good listening! (while providing facial expressions and enthusiastic tone of voice).** *Instead of:* *Parent: Hold my hand. - Child: Why?* *Parent: Clean up. –* *Child: Me play.*
8. Parent must be in **CLOSE PROXIMITY** to the child **PRIOR TO** issuing a **COMMAND.**	• When possible, parent should physically position themselves on the child's level (e.g., crouch down on the floor next to the child). • Increases likelihood child will comprehend and independently complete the task. • Increases the likelihood of child compliance by assisting in orienting the child's attention toward the task.	• **Child: (running around room) Parent: (gets near child closing off their running path and down to eye level) Wow, story time! (holding out book) Please sit with Mommy.** *Instead of:* *Parent: (chasing child around room) Sit down with me so we can read a story.*

PDI-Toddlers Identified Commands Worksheet

*Over-riding rule that commands are used sparingly and only when the child is emotionally able to practice listening.

**Please rank-order the following commands
from the most (#1) to least likely (#5) your child will comply.**

Rank #	Developmentally Appropriate, Toddler-Directed Commands
	"Please hand me_____" "Please give me_____" *"Please hand me the dinosaur"* *"Please give me the dinosaur"*
	"Please put the _____ in the box" *"Please put the doll in the box"*
	"Please hold my hand" (*only to be used when parent is close and child is calm)
	"Please sit down"

**Please list any other commands you would like to have your child comply with
in order to review with your therapist:**

1. _____

2. _____

3. _____

4. _____

5. _____

PDI-T: Teaching Compliance Skills
TELL-SHOW-TRY AGAIN-GUIDE FLOW CHART

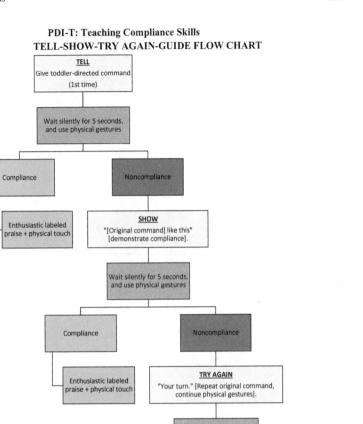

PCIT-Toddlers Home Therapy Practice

Child's Name:_____   Date:_____

☐ Mom   ☐ Dad   ☐ Other Caregiver: _____

Your In Session 5-minute PRIDE Skills

10			
5			
0			
Labeled Praise	Reflection	Behavior Description	Question/Command/Criticism

<u>Use your CDI "Do Skills / PRIDE"</u> & play with your child 5 minutes daily.
<u>Use CARES steps</u> when signals of big emotions are present and your child needs your help.

	Did you engage in **Relaxation** before Special Time?		Did you spend 5 minutes in **Special Time** today?		Activity or Toys Played	List any signals of big emotions your child showed. Was CARES used?	PRIDE Skills used today... Any problems or questions during Special Time?
	Yes	No	Yes	No			
Monday							
Tuesday							
Wednesday							
Thursday							
Friday							
Saturday							
Sunday							

Write a time during the week when you felt an intense emotion and what impact did it have on your child?

_____

_____

Adapted from Eyberg and Funderburk (2011) CDI Homework sheet, pg 28.

References

Bagner, D. M., Coxe, S., Hungerford, G. M., Garcia, D., Barroso, N. E., Hernandez, J., & Rosa-Olivares, J. (2016). Behavioral parent training in infancy: A window of opportunity for high-risk families. *Journal of Abnormal Child Psychology, 44*(5), 901–912.

Eyberg, S., & Funderburk, B. W. (2011). Parent-child interaction therapy protocol. Gainesville, FL: PCIT International.

Hansen, B., & Shillingsburg, A. M. (2016). Using a modified parent-child interaction therapy to increase vocalizations in children with autism. *Child & Family Behavior Therapy, 38*(4), 318–330.

Tempel, A. B., Wagner, S. M., & McNeil, C. B. (2009). Parent-child interaction therapy and language facilitation: The role of parent-training on language development. *The Journal of Speech and Language Pathology – Applied Behavior Analysis, 3*(2–3), 216–232.

Vanderbilt University Center on the Social and Emotional Foundations for Early Learning. (1999). Teaching your child about feelings does his from birth to age 2. Retrieved from http://csefel. vanderbilt.edu/documents/teaching_your_child-feeling.pdf

Chapter 16
Parent-Directed Interaction-Toddler Coach Session

The purpose of the parent-directed interaction coaching sessions is to help parents build upon the use of their previously mastered CDI-T skills (e.g., PRIDE skills, CARES steps, under-reaction, redirection) by increasing children's opportunities to develop functional language and consistent, high levels of child compliance while elevating parents' abilities to manage behaviors. Finally, PDI-T skills are applied to typical life situations, such as diapering and nap time. The ongoing importance of Home Therapy Practice is critical to the success of this new phase of the intervention. Sessions will continue to begin with the presentation of a clear visual stimulus to the child in the waiting area indicating the "when-then" steps of holding the parents hand and then walking to the playroom. The principles of consistency and predictability continue to underlie the foundations of this phase of the intervention. Again, therapists may consider a 30–45-minute session to aide in children's self-regulation. Additionally, such constraints model the importance of maintaining developmentally appropriate time limitations in order to help young children better regulate their emotions and behavior. Similar to CDI-T, the majority of PDI-T sessions will be spent coaching the parent and child in the use of parent-directed skills using in vivo bug-in-the-ear equipment. Compliance practice will occur in graduated steps such that commands with a higher chance of compliance will be practiced prior to commands with a lower chance of compliance.

Note Developmental tip of the day cards are provided in Appendix H at the conclusion of this manual. Clinicians may use their clinical judgment to determine if the parent is able to take in and utilize selected cards at the beginning or conclusion of each session.

Session Preparation Items

1. Bug-in-the-ear equipment
2. Visual transition aide card

© Springer Nature Switzerland AG 2018
E. I. Girard et al., *Parent-Child Interaction Therapy with Toddlers*,
https://doi.org/10.1007/978-3-319-93251-4_16

3. Necessary handouts:

    (a) CDI-T Home Therapy Practice sheet
    (b) PDI-T Home Therapy Practice sheet
    (c) DPICS-T Coding sheet
    (d) PDI-T Coding compliance sheet (for PDI-T coach 3 and greater)
    (e) Relationship Enhancement Tracker for CDI-Toddlers Skills
    (f) Listening/Compliance Tracker for PDI-Toddlers Skills

PDI-T Coaching Tips

1. In this age group, we are teaching listening skills versus discipline, and therefore, an overall feeling of fun, lighthearted compliance interactions that often include "game-like" listening activities should be present.
2. During the PDI-T phase, the CDI-T skills continue to be the foundation of the treatment. Therefore, inclusion of all of the CDI-T coaching tips should continue.
3. The coach's voice should always reflect the manner in which the parent should be speaking to the child.

    (a) When coaching parents through the guided compliance procedure in the PDI-T phase, this should primarily be clear, calm, and consistent.
    (b) Coaches may be more directive during the first few sessions of the PDI-T phase as parents learn the guided compliance steps. As sessions continue, coaches should allow parents to become increasingly more independent in their use of the skills.

4. Children in this age group often take extra time to comprehend and comply with effective commands, and therefore some children may need more than 5 seconds to complete the given task.
5. It is essential that coaches help parents observe children's cues, including approximations toward compliance (e.g., searching for the desired object, attempts to complete the request) prior to moving to the next step in the compliance sequence.
6. Coaches should model enthusiasm while prompting parents to issue a labeled praise and positive touch in response to child compliance.
7. Despite the circumscribed steps in the PDI command sequence, motivating parents to be enthusiastic and playful while implementing the steps helps children maintain focus while keeping the interaction warm and enjoyable.
8. The number of attempts at compliance practice throughout the session should be guided by the parent's and child's moods (e.g., a happy and well-rested dyad provides more opportunities to teach and learn listening skills; a tired and irritable dyad provides limited, if any, opportunity to teach and practice listing skills) and limited to a maximum of three attempts per coaching session and during PDI-T Home Therapy Practice.

Session Goals

1. Increase the parent's use of the parent-directed skills via direct coaching of the parent-child dyad during play with the child.
2. Maintain the parent's ability to utilize previously mastered CDI-T skills.

Session Outline

1. **Greet the parent and child in the waiting room.**

   (a) Provide the parent with the check-in sheet if not provided by front office personnel, and allow the parent to complete the sheet for approximately 5 minutes.

   (b) Collect the parent's current Home Therapy Practice sheet, and place the information on the Relationship Enhancement Tracker of CDI-T Skills in front of the parent. Use a highlighter to graph the weeks where the parent completed four or more of the daily therapy sessions. When 3 days, or fewer, of Home Therapy Practice is completed, use a black pen or pencil to mark the number of days completed on the Relationship Enhancement Tracker of CDI-T Skills.

   NOTE: Depending upon the set-up of the waiting area at a given agency and/or the parent's difficulties managing the child's behavior, therapists may consider transitioning the parent-child dyad to a therapy room and playing with the child to allow the parent time to complete such procedures. If the aforementioned transition occurs during this step, the therapist should utilize visual aids (described in the following step) when initially approaching the dyad in the waiting area.

2. **After the check-in sheet is completed, approach the parent and child prepared with the transitional cue cards/visual aids provided in the hand-outs section of this chapter. Review the visual aide with the child while also prompting the parent to take the child's hand while walking to the therapy room.**

   (a) Given the parent's previous mastery of the PRIDE skills, the therapist should prompt the parent to use such skills walking with the child and parent to the therapy room, thereby reinforcing skill use.

   Note: As CDI-T sessions progress and the parent's CDI-T skills improve, the therapist should transition to coaching the parent in his or her use of the CDI-T skills during this transition period.

3. **Review the completed check-in sheet. While reviewing the check-in sheet, the therapist should simultaneously interact with the child and model the use of CARES for the child if necessary.**

(a) Briefly note any major changes that may have occurred since the previous session.

(b) Remind the parent of the parallel process. Select one parallel process question from the following examples:

   (i) Was there a time when you felt a lot of frustration or anger and you kept it in check because you wanted to be a good role model for your child?

   (ii) When was a time when you had to work hard to keep yourself calm in front of child? How did you do it?

   (iii) Did your interactions with your child bring up any thoughts of your own childhood or the impact of your parents parenting on you?

   (iv) During the past week, did you notice the impact of someone else's emotions or behavior on your child's emotions or behavior?

   (v) Were there any moments that you felt proud of yourself for managing your emotions or behavior while around or interacting with your child differently than you may have in the past?

   (vi) Has anybody else commented on or noticed changes in your ability to regulate your emotions and behavior or your child's ability to regulate his or her emotions and behavior? If so, how?

   (vii) What did you do to take care of yourself during the past week? How does your self-care indirectly impact your child? In other words, what do you notice about your ability to be emotionally available for your child when you have taken time to care for your own needs?

   - Praise the parent's ability to reflect on, and share such thoughts in relationship to her or her commitment to his or her child. If, in the course of the conversation, it is clear that the parent needs addition support, the therapist may consider offering the parent an additional, individual session to discuss the parent's thoughts and feelings.

   - Remark on the parent's example of a time during the previous week when he/she felt connected to his/her child or noticed a strength in his/her child. If the parent was unable to independently generate an example, prompt him or her to do so using one of the following scripts.

Sample scripts:
"Tell me about a time that you really enjoyed your child, felt connected to your child, you and your child were 'in sync,' when you laughed, or experienced a special bonding time where you felt like you 'clicked'."
   or
   "Tell me about a positive quality or a strength that you noticed in your child this week. How do you feel that your behavior impacts his or her ability to maximize this strength?"

(a) **Review Home Therapy Practice.**

   (i) Praise the parent for his or her effort in completing and returning the practice sheet.
   (ii) Briefly discuss the nature of the Home Therapy Practice session while problem-solving any difficulties that arose. Review the nature of the toys used, time practiced (given the child's developmental needs), and space in which the practice occurred.
   (iii) Provide confident reassurance to the parent following any expressions of uncertainty with the use of the skills or management of any child behavior during the practice session.
   (iv) If Home Therapy Practice was not returned, have the parent complete a new Home Therapy Practice sheet in session. If Home Therapy Practice was not conducted, problem-solve barriers to practice and reiterate the importance of such practice for the success of the current treatment. Problem-solve ways in which to help the parent remember to complete and return the Home Therapy Practice sheet (e.g., reminder in his or her phone, placing the sheet on the refrigerator).

4. **Check in on the parent's current emotion regulation, mood, and emotional ability to be a therapeutic parent for his or her child while emphasizing the pivotal impact of the parent's emotions and behavior on the child's emotions and behavior. Guide the parent through cognitive check-in questions. Cognitive Check-In Questions:**

   (a) How am I feeling?
   (b) Am I in the right place to interact with my baby?

5. **Explain that the parent should be asking him or herself such check-in questions prior to engaging his or her child in special playtime at home.**
6. **Briefly guide the parent through each of the four steps listed below in a brief diaphragmatic breathing relaxation exercise.**

   Step 1: Move to a comfortable position, either seated in a chair or on the floor.
   Step 2: Place one hand on your stomach. Take a slow, deep breath in.
   Step 3: Exhale slowly while pushing your stomach outward.
   Step 4: Repeat the process 2–3 times.

7. **Ask the parent about the impact of such procedures on his or her emotional and cognitive state. Emphasize the importance of engaging in the aforementioned exercise to help the parent prepare for therapeutic play with the child in the home environment.**
8. **Transition to PDI-T coaching by presenting the coaching transition visual (if needed) to the child. Provide the parent with the necessary bug-in-the-ear device.**

Sample script: "It's time for mommy/daddy/caregiver to play with you! I'm going to go into my room [point to corresponding picture on visual] while you play with mommy/daddy/caregiver in here with these toys [point to corresponding picture on visual]."

9. **Direct parent to indicate to the child that it is time for the parent and child to play together with the toys.**

   "It's time for [child's name] and mommy/daddy/caregiver to play together!"

10. **[First PDI-T coaching session] – Begin with CDI-T coaching for 5 minutes, omit DPICS Coding in this session to allow for more coaching time to be spent on PDI-T sequence, and skip to Step 15.**

11. **[Second PDI-T coaching session] – Let the parent know that you will be quiet for the first 5 minutes, while the parent uses the child-directed skills with the child. Let the parent know that you will observe the parent and child play and specifically note all of the child-directed skills that the parent uses during the interaction.**

    Sample script: "I'm going to watch while you and [child's name] play together for five minutes. I want you to use as many child-directed skills that you can while you play. Should [child's name] become dysregulated during these 5 minutes, remember to use the CARES steps. Follow your child's lead and have fun."

    Note: Should the child become extremely dysregulated during this five-minute period, the therapist should pause coding and begin to coach the parent in the procedure most appropriate to the behavior.

12. **Following the 5-minute coded interaction, allow the caregiver to play for an extra minute after coding. Put the data on the Relationship Enhancement Tracker for CDI-Toddler Skills before providing the parent with a feedback sandwich in which a labeled praise is provided, followed by an area in which the parent may improve and goals for the day, and followed by another labeled praise.**

    Sample script: "You did a really nice job praising [child's name] for his gentle play. I can tell that you have been practicing! Today, we'll work on reducing your questions so that [child's name] can really direct the play. I love how closely you sit near [child's name], it seems like it makes him feel really safe."

13. **Once the caregiver has reached their third PDI-T coach session, let the parent know that you will be quiet, while the parent uses the parent-directed toddler skills with the child. Let the parent know that you will observe the parent and child play and specifically note all of the parent-directed skills that the parent uses during the interaction including use of commands and the Tell-Show-Try Again-Guide procedure.**

Sample script: "I'm going to watch while you and [child's name] play together for five minutes. I want you to aim to use 4 commands during this five-minute period and as many child-directed (PRIDE) skills that you can while you play. Should [child's name] become dysregulated during these 5 minutes, remember to use the CARES steps."

14. **Following the five-minute coded interaction, provide the parent with a feedback sandwich in which a labeled praise is provided, followed by an area in which the parent may improve and goals for the day, and followed by another labeled praise.**

    Sample script: "You did a really nice job using developmentally appropriate commands with [child's name]. I can tell that you have been practicing! Today, we'll work on changing some of your indirect commands into direct commands. I love how all of the positive touches you give [child's name] while you play are helping to build your relationship."

15. **Coach the parent and child in the parent-directed toddler skills for approximately 15–25 minutes (one caregiver). Attempt to conclude coaching when the child is in a positive mood. (See Chapter 9 "Coaching Considerations During PDI-T," e.g., vignette)**

    (a) Initially focus on commands ranked high on the caregiver's rating of the child's likelihood of compliance. Once compliance to such commands is achieved within the "tell" or "show" step, move on to the next command on the rank-order hierarchy (PDI diagram follows).

    (b) Coach the parent to implement the directive language stimulation procedures when the child naturally desires a toy throughout the session.

    (c) Be aware of the parent's ability to regulate his or her emotions and behavior. Help the parent recognize signals that they are stressed or upset. If needed, coach the parent in the use of diaphragmatic breathing during the session. Therapists may also choose to prompt the parent to intentionally tense and hold select muscles (e.g., shoulders, hands, legs) for 3–4 seconds before releasing such tension. The contrast between such tensing and relaxing exercises function to assist selected muscle groups in relaxation.

    (d) Particularly following moments of a child's emotion dysregulation, therapists should coach the parent in the implementation of the CARES model for themselves.

    C: Check cognitions – clue into yourself, before beginning special time with your toddler.

    A: Assist self – if not emotionally ready for play, implement relaxation techniques to help refocus.

    R: Reassure self – parenting presents challenges and no one technique works for all children.

    E: Emotional awareness – special time allows for fun and connection to be experienced.

S: Sensitive and soothing – be kind and sensitive to yourself in how you reassure yourself.

*NOTE: Steps are interchangeable and can be used in any order.

(a) Therapists should highlight moments in which the parent's emotions (e.g., tone of voice, words) and behavior (e.g., engagement with the child, gentle touch) positively impact the child's emotions and behavior.

(b) When approximately 3 minutes remains in the session, prompt the caregiver to indicate the upcoming conclusion of the session to the child (i.e., provide a transition statement to assist the child in preparing for the end of play).

(c) Have the caregiver generate two praise statements in relation to the child's positive behavior during the session.

(d) Prompt the caregiver to begin to sing a "clean-up" song while cleaning up to aid child in transition. Therapists may search online for a suggested song if one is not known.

16. **If two caregivers present: Coach the first parent and child in the parent-directed toddler skills for approximately 10 minutes. Then provide transition coaching to switch to the second parent:**

(a) Have the currently coached parent come in close to the toddler, within touching distance and perhaps rubbing their back while stating, "Now [Daddy] is coming to play with you."

(b) The "new" parent enters the room bringing with them upon entry a different toy to serve as a technique to decrease separation problems by using the toy as a distraction.

(c) The "new" parent then gives a transitional statement, "[Daddy] is here to play with you." While showing the new toy as a distraction.

(d) Both the "new" parent and "old" parent remain in close proximity with a gentle hand placed on the toddler and then fade the "old" parent out of the room, while the "new" parent begins to play with the toddler.

17. **After the toddler has successfully transitioned to the second parent, follow the same steps listed on Item 15 and coach the second parent and child in the parent-directed toddler skills for approximately 10 minutes**

18. **Enter the therapy room with the end-of-session transition visual. Present the Relationship Enhancement Tracker for CDI-T Skills, and if third or greater PDI-T coaching sessions, present the Listening/Compliance Tracker for PDI-T Skills. Provide parent with brief feedback related to initially coded CDI-T and PDI-T skills with emphasis on any improvements made throughout the session.**

19. **Provide the parent with CDI-T and PDI-T Home Therapy Practice sheets.**

20. **Present the transition visual to the child specifically indicating each picture related to leaving the therapy room and walking to the car.**

Sample script: "Now it's time to go 'bye bye' [points to picture of child leaving therapy room] and walk to the car [point to picture of child in car]."

Table 16.1 Mastery criteria requirements for PDI-T

Parent skill	Mastery level to be achieved
Effective delivery of the PDI-T guided compliance sequence	75% effective commands during a five-minute sequence mastered at the outset of the session 75% effective follow-through to effective commands
Effective use of the directive language stimulation and coaching procedures	Satisfactory implementation
Effective use of the physical aggression response procedures (if applicable)	Satisfactory implementation
Effective use of the self-injurious behavior response procedures (if applicable)	Satisfactory implementation

Important Notes:

The current session should be repeated until parental mastery of the PDI-T skills is achieved within a five-minute coded sequence conducted at the initial outset of the session. PDI-T mastery includes the following (Table 16.1):

21. When PDI-T mastery is achieved, the therapist should provide the parent with post-treatment assessment measures to be completed immediately, prior to advancement to the life-enhancement situation session.
22. Complete Integrity Checklist: PDI-T Coach Session

Integrity Checklist: PDI-T Coach Session

 As you view the session, place a checkmark under the appropriate column, Yes (Y), Not Applicable (NA) or No (N). List these totals in the appropriate blanks below the table. See expanded session outlines for more information on each item. (Integrity checklist and directions are based on Eyberg & Funderburk, 2011).

Integrity Checklist: PCIT-Toddlers PDI Coach Session			
Client & Caregiver:			
Therapist Conducting Session:			
Checklist Completed By:		Date:	

	ITEMS	Y	NA	N
1	Approaches the dyad in the waiting room with prepared visual aid. Reviews visual aid with the child and prompting the caregiver to use CDI-T skills and coach models PCIT-T skills			
2	Checks-in on any major changes and asks the caregiver/s a time in the past week that they have felt connected to their child or have noticed a strength in their child			
3	Reviews CDI-T & PDI-T Home Therapy Practice sheets and reinforces their importance and problem solves any challenges			
4	Tells the caregiver that even if you have memorized the Tell-Show-Try Again-Guide procedure completely, you will coach them on every step			
5	Introduces CDI-T Statement and DPICS Code for the first 5 minutes CDI-T Skills, provides feedback			
6	Codes PDI-T Listening/Compliance for first caregiver for 5 minutes if 3rd PDI-T coaching session or greater and transfers data to Listening/Compliance Tracker			
7	Coaches the caregiver and the child in the PDI-T skills for 15-20 minutes			
8	Caregiver prepares child for clinician entering the room			
9	Reviews Relationship Enhancement Tracker for CDI-T, & Listening/Compliance Tracker for PDI-T if 3rd PDI-T coaching session or greater			
10	Provides CDI-T & PDI-T Home Therapy Practice sheets			
11	Instructs parent to call if they have any problems			
12	Prepares child for transition to leaving with transition visual aid			
13	Supports dyad as required during exit of session and clinician models CDI-T skills			
	TOTALS			

Therapist comments about session

_____

_____

_____

Integrity checker comments about sessions:

_____

_____

_____

Integrity = $\dfrac{\text{Yes Total}}{\text{Yes Total + No Total}}$ = _____ %

Length of session = _____minutes

Handouts and Forms

PCIT-Toddlers
Check-In Sheet

Have any major stressors occurred since your last session that your therapist should be aware of?

_____

_____

_____

_____

If so, have these major stressors impacted your mood, behavior, and ability to deliver the therapy to your child for five minutes each day?

_____

_____

_____

_____

How have you noticed the impact of your expression of your emotions and behavior on your child's expression of his or her emotions and behavior?

_____

_____

_____

_____

Please note one time during the previous week where you felt connected to your child or you noticed a strength in your child.

_____

_____

_____

_____

Transitional Visual Cue Card – Office to Play Room

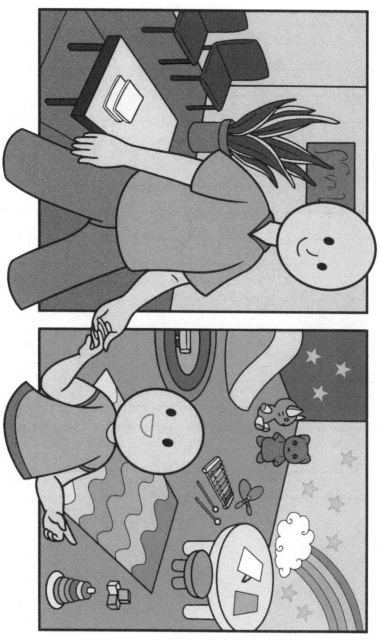

Transitional Visual Cue Card – Play Room to Leaving Office

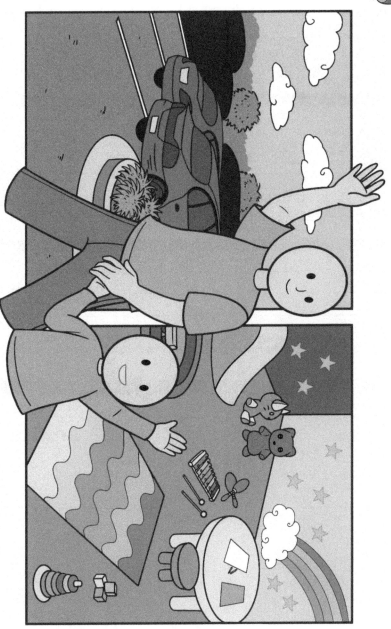

DPICS-T Coding Sheet for Therapist
Adapted from Eyberg and Funderburk (2011)

Child Name/ ID _____ Date: _____

Parent: □ Mother   □ Father   □ Other _____

Coder: _____   Start Time: _____ End Time: _____

| o CDI Coach # _____ | o PDI Coach # _____ | o PDI LE # _____ |

Number of Days Homework Completed?   □ 0   □ 1   □ 2   □ 3   □ 4   □ 5   □ 6   □ 7

Do Skills	Tally Count	TOTAL	Mastery
Neutral Talk			--
Emotion Labeling			--
Behavioral Description			10
Reflection			10
Labeled Praise			10
Unlabeled Praise			--
Don't Skills	Tally Count	TOTAL	
Question			
Commands			$0 \leq 3$
Negative Talk			

Coach caregiver through any missed CARES step (if needed) in the moment,
__INCLUDING__ getting on the microphone during the 5 minutes of DPCIS Coding.

Big Emotion Present?	YES	NO	# Tally	
CARES Skills Used	CIRCLE ONE			NOTES
Come in Calm & Close	Satisfactory	Needs Practice	N/A	
Assist Child	Satisfactory	Needs Practice	N/A	
Reassure Child	Satisfactory	Needs Practice	N/A	
Emotional Validation	Satisfactory	Needs Practice	N/A	
Soothe	Satisfactory	Needs Practice	N/A	

(Continues onto next page)

DPICS-T Coding Sheet for Therapist
Adapted from Eyberg and Funderburk (2011)

Child Name/ ID _____ Date:_____

Parent: □ Mother   □ Father   □ Other _____

Coder:_____ Start Time:_____ End Time:_____

Positive Skills	Circle One		NOTES
Imitate	Satisfactory	Needs Practice	
Show Enjoyment	Satisfactory	Needs Practice	
Physical Affection	Satisfactory	Needs Practice	
Mutual Eye Contact	Satisfactory	Needs Practice	
Animated Tone of Voice	Satisfactory	Needs Practice	
Animated Facial Expressions	Satisfactory	Needs Practice	
Play Style at Developmental Level	Satisfactory	Needs Practice	
Bx Management Skills	**Circle One**		**NOTES**
Skill of Redirection	Satisfactory	Needs Practice	N/A
Skill of Under Reaction	Satisfactory	Needs Practice	N/A
Limit Setting - 'No Hurting'	Satisfactory	Needs Practice	N/A

General Notes & Observations:

_____
_____
_____
_____
_____
_____
_____

Relationship Enhancement Tracker of
CDI-Toddlers Skills

Session #	Baseline CLP								
Date									

Home Therapy Practice

7	X								
6	X								
5	X								
4	X								
3	X								
2	X								
1	X								
0	X								

Labeled Praise

10+									
9									
8									
7									
6									
5									
4									
3									
2									
1									
0									

Reflection

10+									
9									
8									
7									
6									
5									
4									
3									
2									
1									
0									

Behavior Description

10+									
9									
8									
7									
6									
5									
4									
3									
2									
1									
0									

Relationship Enhancement Tracker of CDI-Toddlers Skills

Session #	Baseline CLP								
Date									

Emotion Labeling

10+									
9									
8									
7									
6									
5									
4									
3									
2									
1									
0									

Question/Command/Critical Statement

10+									
9									
8									
7									
6									
5									
4									
3									
2									
1									
0									

CARES

Satis-factory									
N/A									
Needs Improv.									

Other Positive Skills
(Imitate, Enjoy, Affection, Eye Contact, Animation, etc.)

Satis-factory									
N/A									
Needs Improv.									

Redirection and Under-Reaction

Satis-factory									
N/A									
Needs Improv.									

Limit-Setting "No Hurting"

Satis-factory									
N/A									
Needs Improv.									

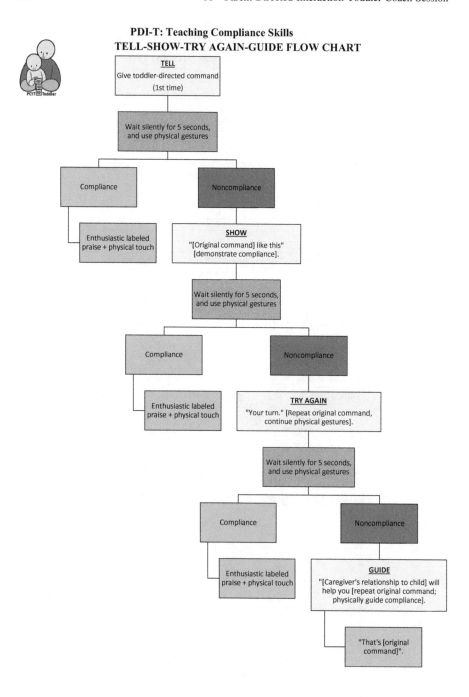

PDI-T: Teaching Compliance Skills
TELL-SHOW-TRY AGAIN-GUIDE FLOW CHART

PCIT-T PDI-T Coding Sheet for Therapists

Child's Name _____   ☐ Mother ☐ Father ☐ Other _____   Coder: _____

Start Time: _____   End Time: _____   PDI Session #: _____

TELL						SHOW						TRY AGAIN				GUIDE		
Command DC or IC?	Gesture Given?	NOC	CO	NC	Praise LP or UP or NP?	Praise w/ Animation - And or - + touch	5 sec	demo task repeats DC + Like This	CO	NC	Praise LP or UP or NP?	Praise w/ Animation - And or - + touch	5 sec	State, "Your Turn" + DC	CO	NC	5 sec	"… will help you." Hand-over-hand	BD to end task	Correct FT?
1																				
2																				
3																				
4																				
5																				
6																				
7																				
8																				
9																				
10																				
Total																				

A. # NOC _____   % Effective DC (C÷D) _____   ☐ 75% Effective DC

B. # IC _____

C. # effective DC _____   % CO to DC (E÷C) _____   ☐ % Child Compliance Skills

D. Total Commands _____   (Complete task at "Tell", "Show" or "Try Again" Step)

E. # CO to DC _____

F. # FT to DC _____   % FT to DC (F÷C) _____   ☐ 75% Correct FT

Adapted from Eyberg and Funderburk (2011) pg. 105

Listening/ Compliance Tracker of PDI-Toddlers Skills

Session #	Baseline PLP	Baseline CU						
Date								

PDI-T Home Therapy Listening Practice

7	X	X						
6	X	X						
5	X	X						
4	X	X						
3	X	X						
2	X	X						
1	X	X						
0	X	X						

Effective Direct Commands

100%								
90%								
80%								
70%								
75%								
60%								
50%								
40%								
30%								
20%								
10%								
0%								

Consistent Follow Through

100%								
90%								
80%								
75%								
70%								
60%								
50%								
40%								
30%								
20%								
10%								
0%								

Child Compliance Behavior*

100%								
90%								
80%								
75%								
70%								
60%								
50%								
40%								
30%								
20%								
10%								
0%								

*Compliance Behavior is calculated by task completion during the PDI-T sequence of "Tell", "Show" or "Try Again."

PCIT-Toddlers Home Therapy Practice

Child's Name:_____   Date:_____

☐ Mom   ☐ Dad   ☐ Other Caregiver: _____

Your In Session 5-minute PRIDE Skills

Labeled Praise   Reflection   Behavior Description   Question/Command/Criticism

Use your CDI "Do Skills / PRIDE" & play with your child 5 minutes daily.
Use CARES steps when signals of big emotions are present and your child needs your help.

	Did you engage in **Relaxation** before Special Time?		Did you spend 5 minutes in **Special Time** today?		Activity or Toys Played	List any signals of big emotions your child showed. Was CARES used?	PRIDE Skills used today… Any problems or questions during Special Time?
	Yes	**No**	**Yes**	**No**			
Monday							
Tuesday							
Wednesday							
Thursday							
Friday							
Saturday							
Sunday							

Write a time during the week when you felt an intense emotion and what impact did it have on your child?

_____

_____

Adapted from Eyberg and Funderburk (2011) CDI Homework sheet, pg 28.

PCIT-Toddlers Home Therapy Listening Practice
Identified Commands
Adapted from Eyberg and Funderburk (2011) pg. 105

Child's Name:_____ Date:_____

□ Mom   □ Dad   □ Other Caregiver: _____

Use the 8 Rules for Effective Commands & follow-up with a labeled praise every time your child complies.

USE CARES when needed before starting PDI-T, be sure your toddler is well rested to learn, 3 commands maximum.

Prompting Direct Command ✚ Compliance Tell, Show or Try Again ＝ Animated Labeled Praise

Date	Did you practice PDI for 5 min. in a play situation after CDI today? Yes	No	Place mark for each success after: **Tell**	Place mark for each success after: **Show**	Place mark for each success after: **Try Again**	Place mark for each task after: **Guide**	**Comments** Write the play command(s) you gave that required the "GUIDE" technique. Was CARES needed after GUIDE? Other Comments?
Monday							
Tuesday							
Wednesday							
Thursday							
Friday							
Saturday							
Sunday							

Call your PCIT-Toddler Coach IMMEDIATELY if you are struggling with Teaching Compliance Sequence

Example Identified Commands (fill in the blank):

Please pass me _____.

Please give me _____.

Please put _____ here.

Labeled Praises:

Great following directions!

You're good at listening!

Awesome job minding me!

Reference

Eyberg, S., & Funderburk, B. W. (2011). Parent-child interaction therapy protocol. Gainesville, FL: PCIT International.

Chapter 17
Life-Enhancement Situations Coach Session

The purpose of the life-enhancement situations coaching session is to help parents generalize and apply their previously mastered CDI-T and PDI-T skills (e.g., PRIDE skills, CARES steps, under-reaction, redirection, guided compliance, directive language stimulation coaching) to everyday, real-life situations that arise in the lives of toddlers and their families. It is critical that therapists empower parents by guiding them to apply previously learned developmental knowledge and mastered skills to such situations. Additionally, the ongoing importance of CDI-T and PDI-T skills during Home Therapy Practice provides the foundation of this phase of the intervention. Sessions will continue to begin with the presentation of a clear visual stimulus presented to the child in the waiting area indicating the "when-then" steps of holding the parent's hand and then walking to the playroom. The principles of consistency and predictability continue to underlie this phase of the intervention. Again, therapists may continue to consider a 30–45-minute session to aide in self-regulation. Additionally, such constraints model the importance of maintaining developmentally appropriate time limitations on helping children this age regulate their emotions and behavior. Similar to CDI-T and PDI-T sessions, the majority of the life-enhancement situations will be spent on coaching the parent and child in the use of parent-directed skills using in vivo bug-in-the-ear equipment.

Note Developmental tip of the day cards are provided in Appendix H at the conclusion of this manual. Clinicians may use their clinical judgment to determine if the parent is able to take in and utilize selected cards at the beginning or conclusion of each session.

Session Preparation Items

1. Bug-in-the-ear equipment
2. Visual transition aide cards

© Springer Nature Switzerland AG 2018
E. I. Girard et al., *Parent-Child Interaction Therapy with Toddlers*,
https://doi.org/10.1007/978-3-319-93251-4_17

3. DPICS-T Coding sheet
4. Listening/Compliance PDI-T Coding sheet
5. Necessary handouts:

  (a) CDI-T Home Therapy Practice sheet
  (b) PDI-T Home Therapy Practice sheet
  (c) Life-enhancement handouts as needed from Appendices

6. Appropriate toys
7. Life-enhancement scenario-focused items (e.g., pillows, books, snack)
8. Relationship Enhancement Tracker for CDI-T skills
9. Listening/Compliance Tracker for PDI-T skills

Session Goals

1. Increase the parent's use of the parent-directed skills via direct coaching of the parent-child dyad during play with the child
2. Maintain the parent's ability to utilize previously mastered CDI-T skills

Session Outline

1. **Greet the parent and child in the waiting room.**

  (a) Provide the parent with the check-in sheet if not provided by front office personnel.
  (b) Collect the parent's current CDI-T and PDI-T Home Therapy Practice sheet, and place the information on the Relationship Enhancement Tracker for CDI-T skills and Listening/Compliance Tracker for PDI-T skills sheets. Use a highlighter to graph those weeks where the parent completed four or more of the daily therapy sessions. For three or fewer, use a black pen or pencil to mark the number of days completed on the progress sheet.
  (c) Allow the parent to complete the check-in sheet for approximately 5 minutes if not completed in the waiting room.

  NOTE: Depending upon the setup of the waiting area at a given agency and/or the parent's difficulties managing the child's behavior, therapists may consider transitioning the parent-child dyad to a therapy room and playing with the child to allow the parent time to complete such procedures. If the aforementioned transition occurs during this step, the therapist should utilize visual aids (described in the following step) when initially approaching the dyad in the waiting area.

2. **After the check-in sheet is completed, approach the parent and child prepared with the transitional cue cards/visual aids provided in this Chapter. Review the visual aide with the child while also prompting the parent to take the child's hand while walking to the therapy room.**
3. **Review the completed check-in sheet. While reviewing the check-in sheet, the therapist should simultaneously interact with the child and model the use of CARES for the child if necessary.**

(a) Briefly note any major changes that may have occurred since the previous session.

(b) Remind the parent of the parallel process. Select one parallel process question from the following examples:

(i) Was there a time when you felt a lot of frustration or anger and you kept it in check because you wanted to be a good role model for your child?

(ii) When was a time when you had to work hard to keep yourself calm in front of child? How did you do it?

(iii) Did your interactions with your child bring up any thoughts of your own childhood or the impact of your parents parenting on you?

(iv) During the past week, did you notice the impact of someone else's emotions or behavior on your child's emotions or behavior?

(v) Were there any moments that you felt proud of yourself for managing your emotions or behavior while around or interacting with your child differently than you may have in the past?

(vi) Has anybody else commented on or noticed changes in your ability to regulate your emotions and behavior or your child's ability to regulate his or her emotions and behavior? If so, how?

(vii) What did you do to take care of yourself during the past week? How does your self-care indirectly impact your child? In other words, what do you notice about your ability to be emotionally available for your child when you have taken time to care for your own needs?

- Praise the parent's ability to reflect on and share such thoughts in relationship to her or her commitment to his or her child.
- Remark on the parent's example of a time during the previous week when he/she felt connected to his/her child or noticed a strength in his/her child. If the parent was unable to independently generate an example, prompt him or her to do so using one of the following scripts.

Sample scripts:
"Tell me about a time that you really enjoyed your child, felt connected to your child, you and your child were 'in sync', when you laughed, or experienced a special bonding time where you felt like you 'clicked'."
       or

"Tell me about a positive quality or a strength that you noticed in your child this week. How do you feel that your behavior impacts his or her ability to maximize this strength?"

4. **Review Home Therapy Practice.**

   (a) Praise the parent for his or her effort in completing and returning the practice sheet.
   (b) Briefly discuss the nature of the Home Therapy Practice session while problem-solving any difficulties that arose. Review the nature of the toys used, time practiced (given the child's developmental needs), and space in which the practice occurred.
   (c) Provide confident reassurance to the parent following any expressions of uncertainty with the use of the skills or management of any child behavior during the practice session.
   (d) If Home Therapy Practice was not returned, have the parent complete a new Home Therapy Practice sheet in session. If Home Therapy Practice was not conducted, problem-solve barriers to practice and reiterate the importance of such practice for the success of the current treatment. Problem-solve ways in which to help the parent remember to complete and return the Home Therapy Practice sheet (e.g., reminder in his or her phone, placing the sheet on the refrigerator).

5. **Check in on the parent's current emotion regulation, mood, and emotional ability to be a therapeutic parent for his or her child while emphasizing the pivotal impact of the parent's emotions and behavior on the child's emotions and behavior. Guide the parent through cognitive check-in questions.**

   Cognitive Check-In Questions:

   (a) How am I feeling?
   (b) Am I in the right place to interact with my toddler?

6. **Explain that the parent should be asking himself or herself such check-in questions prior to engaging his or her child in special playtime at home.**
7. **Briefly guide the parent through each of the four steps listed below in a brief diaphragmatic breathing relaxation exercise.**

   Step 1: Move to a comfortable position, either seated in a chair or on the floor.
   Step 2: Place one hand on your stomach. Take a slow, deep breath in.
   Step 3: Exhale slowly while pushing your stomach outwards.
   Step 4: Repeat the process 2–3 times.

8. **Ask the parent about the impact of such procedures on his or her emotional and cognitive state. Emphasize the importance of engaging in the aforementioned exercise to help the parent prepare for therapeutic play with the child in the home environment.**

9. **Briefly present the parent with the following life-enhancement scenarios.**

   (a) Feeding time
   (b) Diaper changing
   (c) Transitioning into the car seat
   (d) Reading time
   (e) Nap time
   (f) Public behavior

   Sample script: "Now that you've mastered by the child-directed and parent-directed phases of PCIT-T, I'm wondering if there are any other 'real-life' scenarios that continue to pose some challenges with [child's name]. Some of the common situations that we generally work on include areas such as feeding time, diaper changing, transitioning in the car seat, reading time, and nap time. Does managing [child's name]'s behavior become particularly difficult during any of these scenarios? Is this an area that you would like to work on?"

10. **Ask the parent if any of the previously mentioned areas remain an area of concern.**

11. **Determine if the scenario is appropriate to practice in session after accounting for the rules and policies of the individual clinic.**

12. **Option A: If it is determined that the scenario is *not approriate* to practice in the clinic, discuss the application of CDI-T and PDI-T skills to the scenario, as well as developmental guidance and overriding principles to be considered. Provide typical PDI-T coaching session.**

    Option B: If it is determined that a given scenario *may be practiced* in the clinic, discuss applicable CDI-T and PDI-T skills listed in the scenarios below. Following such discussion, *continue to Steps 13-18*.

    (a) Assist the parent in individualizing such skills to the specific needs of the child and family.

13. **Let the parent know that you will be quiet for the first 5 minutes, while the parent uses the child-directed skills with the child. Let the parent know that you will observe the parent and child play and specifically note all of the child-directed skills that the parent uses during the interaction.**

    Sample script: "I'm going to watch while you and [child's name] play together for 5 minutes. I want you to use as many child-directed skills that you can while you play. Should [child's name] become dysregulated during these 5 minutes, remember to use the CARES steps. Follow your child's lead and have fun."

    Note: Should the child become extremely dysregulated during this 5-minute period, the therapist should pause coding and begin to coach the parent in the procedure most appropriate to the behavior.

14. **Following the 5-minute coded interaction, provide the parent with a feedback sandwich in which a labeled praise is provided, followed by an area in which the parent may improve the goals for the day, and followed by another labeled praise.**

    Sample script: "You did a really nice job praising [child's name] for his gentle play. I can tell that you have been practicing! Today, we'll work on reducing your questions so that [child's name] can really direct the play. I love how closely you sit near [child's name]; it seems like it makes him feel really safe."

15. **Set up the scenario by providing the parent with appropriate materials to prepare the space.**

    (a) For example, provide the parent with pillows and age-appropriate books to practice reading time.
    (b) Prompt the parent to retrieve a snack from his or her diaper bag or provide the parent with an age-appropriate snack to practice feeding time.

16. **Coach the parent through the scenario set-up process.**

    (a) Prompt the parent to verbally prepare the child for the scenario.
    (b) PRIDE skills should be used during scenario setup.

       (i) Praise for assisting with setup
       (ii) Behavior descriptions for set-up behaviors

    Sample reading scenario set-up script: "Now it's time to set up the room for our practice reading scenario. I'd like you to take the pillows and books that I've placed in the room and tell [child's name] that it is time to read. Go ahead and use the PRIDE skills with [child's name] while you set up the space."

17. **Coach the parent in practice of the chosen scenario for 10–15 minutes using applicable CDI-T and PDI-T skills.**
18. **To end the session, enter the therapy room with the end-of-session transition visual. If a life-enhancement scenario was practiced in session, provide parent with brief feedback related to the selected life-enhancement situation. Otherwise, reinforce the importance of practicing the chosen scenario in the home environment during the coming week.**
19. **Provide the parent with the CDI-T Home Practice and PDI-T Home Therapy Listening Practice sheet.**
20. **Present the transition visual to the child specifically indicating each picture related to leaving the therapy room and walking to the car.**

    Sample script: "Now it's time to go 'bye bye' [points to picture of child leaving therapy room] and walk to the car [point to picture of child in car]."

Sleep and Settling

Important Note: Sleep and settling toddlers can be a complex and multifaceted area. Although this section is informed by recommendations by the Karitane Organization in Sydney, Australia, it is meant to be an overview of general sleeping and settling guidelines. Should sleep and settling difficulties persist beyond these recommendations, therapists should assist parents in seeking individualized consultation with a sleep expert.

Summary of Helpful Strategies for Sleep and Settling

A young child's sleep plays a critical role in his or her ability to regulate his or her emotions and behavior. While a successful sleep experience may come easily for some toddlers and their families, many young children with behavior difficulties also struggle to initiate and maintain healthy sleep, causing increased stress for them and their parents (reference). A child's successful sleep experience begins far before sleep initiation. Following are a list of strategies often recommended by sleep professionals that may help to improve the quality and quantity of a child's sleep.

- A consistent bedtime routine should be used including calming activities such as a warm bath, story, calming music, and/or cuddle time with parents.
- Parents may consider creating a visual schedule to increase predictability in the toddler's life. The schedule may include pictures of each activity. The parent may consider guiding the toddler through the routine each evening while simultaneously pointing to each picture as it occurs.
- A relaxing atmosphere should be created, whereby extraneous noises in the atmosphere are minimized, the parent speaks in a calming tone of voice, and/or calming background music is played.
- A child should sleep in a consistent location. A familiar comfort object may help children self-soothe and, when consistently paired with bedtime, help induce sleep.
- Parents should take steps to ensure their own calm emotional demeanor throughout the sleep routine. Should difficult-to-manage emotions arise for the parent or child, parents may consider taking a break to help themselves regain a calm composure, while another caregiver supervises the child.

  - When possible, caregivers may consider dividing toddler's bedtime responsibilities or trading places when difficult to manage emotions manifest. The caregiver's ability to remain calm and consistent throughout the bedtime process is paramount to the toddler's sleep success.
  - Relaxation strategies such as positive self-talk, diaphragmatic breathing, or progressive muscle relaxation may be used.

Table 17.1 Recommended hours of sleep per day by chronological age

Age	Recommended sleep per day (hours, including naps)
Newborn (0–3 months)	14–17 hours
Infant (4–12 months)	12–16 hours
Toddler (1–2 years)	11–14 hours
Preschool (3–5 years)	10–13 hours

- Parents should keep in mind that even minor changes to the bedtime routine may take time for young children to adjust to, particularly given young children have limited emotional resources during this time. Persistence, along with consistency and predictability, is critical to helping reestablish new, successful habits and patterns.
- See Appendix C for Karitane Sleep and Settling Resources (Karitane, 2018).
- See the CDC website for information regarding recommended hours of sleep per day by chronological age (Centers for Disease Control and Prevention, 2017) (Table 17.1).

Summary of Strategies to Avoid for Sleep and Settling

- The use of electronic devices including televisions, phones, and tablets should not be used to help induce sleep. Such devices should be discontinued prior to bedtime.
- Children should not be allowed to use a bottle filled with milk or other sugar-rich drinks during or just prior to sleep initiation as such substances have been found to increase children's risk for dental disease.
- Whenever possible, parents should avoid the use of the car, swing, or stroller to help induce sleep as children may become dependent upon such environments for sleep initiation.

Applicable CDI-T Skills for Sleep and Settling

- Verbally prepare children prior to initiation of the activity (such warning should not be given more than 2–3 minutes in advance).
- PRIDE skills
  - Praise for steps toward nap initiation (e.g., staying in crib, lying down, holding comfort object)
  - Describe behaviors, particularly those that relate to sleep (e.g., yawning, rubbing eyes, sitting in crib).
- CARES model in response to emotion dysregulation.

Applicable PDI-T Skills for Sleep and Settling

- Simple commands such as "sit down," "hold your [comfort object]," and "hold your bottle" may be practiced.
- Parents may choose to avoid commands if the child is unlikely to be successful due to high levels of emotion dysregulation.

Developmental Guidance/Overriding Principles for Sleep and Settling

- Development of and adherence to a clear, simple, predictable schedule and routine.
- As often as possible, allow the child to sleep in the same place each day, thereby increasing consistency and predictability.
- Engage in calming activities shortly before the routine begins (e.g., avoid high-energy activities).
- A calming tone and soothing voice should be used to help children associate such cues with sleep.
- Create a quiet, calm, dark environment free from distraction (e.g., television) to motivate sleep initiation.

Feeding Time

Applicable CDI-T Skills for Feeding Time

- Verbally prepare children prior to initiation of the activity (such warning should not be given more than 2–3 minutes in advance).
- PRIDE skills
  - Praise for approximations toward feeding behavior (e.g., picking up the spoon, sitting in the chair, eating a bite).
- Enthusiasm should be enhanced when children take bites of food (e.g., singing, clapping, enjoyable sounds)
  - Games can be used to enhance the rewarding value of eating (e.g., "open the tunnel, here comes the choo choo!")
- Under-reaction for nonemotional games (e.g., repeatedly dropping a sippy cup on the floor and laughing).

Applicable PDI-T Skills for Feeding Time

- Parents may choose to avoid commands if the child is unlikely to be successful due to high levels of emotion dysregulation.
- Modeling eating behavior is encouraged (e.g., taking a bite from the child's plate, enthusiastic reaction such as rubbing belly, saying "yum, yum" following eating).
- Joint family meals are encouraged to model appropriate feeding behavior and encourage family interaction.
- Feeding commands should be limited to feeding support skills (e.g., "pick up your spoon," "hold your cup," "scoop the noodles like this").

**It is critical that the parent and child do not enter into control battles. Force feeding of any kind is not recommended.

Developmental Guidance/Overriding Principles for Feeding Time

- Avoid confrontations by carefully watching children's cues (e.g., pushing food away).
- When-then statements may be considered if the child is developmentally able to understand the concept (e.g., "if you sit in your seat, then I'll give you some pasta").
- Modeling can be a powerful tool to demonstrate proper feeding behaviors. Parents should eat alongside their children when possible.

Diaper Changing

Applicable CDI-T Skills for Diaper Changing

- Verbally prepare children prior to initiation of the activity (such warning should not be given more than 2–3 minutes in advance).
- PRIDE skills

  - Praise for lying down, looking at the parent, and playing with provided object.
  - Behavior descriptions for diaper-changing-related activities.

- Enthusiasm/silliness should be enhanced when children are engaging in desired behaviors.
- Parents are organized and quick with needed supplies
- Music and singing are encouraged. Diaper-changing songs can be found on YouTube (YouTube, 2018) (e.g., https://www.youtube.com/results?search_query=diaper+changing+songs)

Applicable PDI-T Skills for Diaper Changing

- Parents may choose to avoid commands if the child is unlikely to be successful due to high levels of emotion dysregulation.
- Diaper-changing-related commands may be practiced in a fun, "game-like" way (e.g., lying down, retrieving diaper, bringing wipes, pulling out wipes from dispenser, throwing dirty diaper into trash like a basketball).

Developmental Guidance/Overriding Principles for Diaper Changing

- Parents may consider engaging other desirable activities throughout the session.
- Parents may consider providing the child with a simple, highly desired item with which to play (and withhold this object until diaper changing occurs).
- Simple diaper-changing-related cues may be associated with diaper changing (e.g., a specific light-up toy, song).

Transitioning into the Car Seat

Applicable CDI-T Skills for Transitioning into the Car Seat

- Verbally prepare children prior to initiation of the activity (such warning should not be given more than 2–3 minutes in advance).
- PRIDE skills

  - Parents may consider distraction while placing the child in the seat, "You have your Thomas the Train shoes on today!"
  - Praise should be provided for any approximations toward car seat behaviors (e.g., sitting in the seat, allowing parent to put seatbelt on).

- Parents may provide children with desired objects in the car (if toy throwing is of concern, parents should avoid this suggestion).
- Therapists may consider practicing car seat behavior in the clinic using an additional car seat and large stuffed animal or doll. Car seat behaviors may be modeled and practiced using such items in a fun, game-like scenario (e.g., pretend to "drive" the stuffed animal to grandma's house; allow child to practice buckling himself/herself into seat after stuffed animal) to promote toddlers' comfort, security, and mastery with the activity.
- Parents model being calm throughout the process.

Applicable PDI-T Skills for Transitioning into the Car Seat

- Parents may choose to avoid commands if the child is unlikely to be successful due to high levels of emotion dysregulation.
- Car seat-related commands (e.g., sitting in the seat, holding provided toy/object).

Developmental Guidance/Overriding Principles for Transitioning into the Car Seat

- Parents should take the temperature of the car seat, buckle, and car itself into consideration prior to placing their child in the seat. Extreme temperatures can impact a child's reaction to transition.

Reading to Your Child

Applicable CDI-T Skills for Reading to Your Child

- PRIDE skills
  - Praise for sitting, looking at the book, and helping to turn pages
  - Description of appropriate behaviors (e.g., picking out book, sitting with parent)
- Particularly high levels of enthusiasm while reading

Applicable PDI-T Skills for Reading to Your Child

- PDI-T-guided compliance skills may be considered using commands such as "come here," "sit down," and "turn the page."

Developmental Guidance/Overriding Principles for Reading to Your Child

- Modifications may be considered based on the child's ability to attend to the entire story. The parent may choose to describe or simply label pictures.
- Books with engaging pictures/activities (e.g., lift the flap) and topics of interest to the child should be chosen.

- Parents should consider using sturdy, board books to avoid page tearing and to promote fine motor skills.
- Quality of a brief reading session, rather than length of session, should be prioritized.
- See Appendix G for Toddler Book Suggestions.

Public Outing

Applicable CDI-T Skills for Public Outing

- Verbally prepare children prior to initiation of the public outing (such warning should not be given more than 2–3 minutes in advance)
- PRIDE skills

  - Praise the child for listening while explaining expectations about the outing.
  - Think ahead about behaviors to give attention to, so praise the opposite, e.g., "Great job holding hands."
  - Give a running commentary about what is going to happen.
  - Use behavioral descriptions to keep the child focused.
  - Use enthusiasm to make the activity fun and engaging.
  - Use distraction and redirection to move the child along.

Applicable PDI-T for Public Outing

- Safety direct commands, e.g., "Please hold my hands."
- PDI-T-guided compliance skills may be considered such as "come here" or "sit down."

Developmental Guidance/Overriding Principle for Public Outing

- Need to assess the child's capacity to manage the public outing

  - Avoid public outings if the child is hungry, tired, or unwell.
  - Time may be shortened/limited due to the child's developmental level.

- Parents are educated on necessary preparation and items to bring during a public outing (i.e., Public Outing Checklist Handout).
- The first few practice outings should be kept to optimum learning situations, e.g., playing in the park

Table 17.2 Public outing toddler bag checklist

Public outing toddler bag checklist	✓
1. Appropriate change of clothes for weather	
2. Diaper-changing-related items, e.g., change mat, diaper, cleaning lotion	
3. Healthy snack and drink	
4. Desired toy to be used for distraction	
5. Wash cloth to be used to freshen child and parent	
6. Child's blanket/comforter	
7. Child's comfort item/toy	
8. Hat or beanie (weather dependent)	
9. Sun screen	

Public Behavior Bag Checklist (Table 17.2)

21. Complete Integrity Checklist: PCIT-T Life-Enhancement Session

Integrity Checklist: PCIT-T Life-Enhancement Session

 As you view the session, place a checkmark under the appropriate column, Yes (Y), Not Applicable (NA) or No (N). List these totals in the appropriate blanks below the table. See expanded session outlines for more information on each item. (Integrity checklist and directions are based on Eyberg & Funderburk, 2011).

Integrity Checklist: PCIT-Toddlers Life Enhancement Session		
Client & Caregiver:		
Therapist Conducting Session:		
Checklist Completed By:	**Date:**	

	ITEMS	Y	NA	N
1	Greets the parent and child in the waiting area: Provides check-in sheet and collect CDI-T & PDI-T Home Therapy Practice sheets			
2	Enters session with visual transition prompt to the child and models PRIDE skills while supporting the caregiver/s to enter the therapy room safely			
3	Reviews check-in sheet and reviews any major changes and reminds caregiver of the parallel process			
4	Discusses a time in the previous week that the dyad felt connected			
5	Reviews Home Therapy Practice and Home Listening Practice			
6	Discusses the use of cognitive check-in and relaxation techniques prior to daily special play			
7	Discusses life enhancing scenarios and prioritizes scenarios of concern for caregiver/s			
8	Reviews and provides handouts for appropriate scenarios			
9	Problem solves barriers			
10	Sets up Life Enhancement Scenario space with appropriate materials			
11	Coaches the caregiver/s through chosen Life Enhancement Scenario for 10-15 minutes using CDI-T and PDI-T skills as applicable			
12	Introduces the visual prompt to the child for CDI-T to begin special play, if time permits			

13	Directs the caregiver to begin CDI-T to the child, if time permits			
14	Observes CDI-T and CARES for 5 minutes, if time permits			
15	Gives CDI-T feedback sandwich and identifies goal for the session, if beyond goal obtained during Life Enhancement coaching and time permits			
16	Observes PDI-T and CARES FOR 5 minutes, if time permits			
17	Gives PDI-T feedback and identifies goal for the session, if time permits			
18	Coach PDI-T for 10-15 minutes, if time permits			
19	Provides warning for end of the session			
20	Enters room with end of session transitional aide			
21	Provides brief feedback with life enhancing skills, CDI-T, PDI-T and discuss CARES for the caregiver/s			
22	Gives CDI-T & PDI-T Home Therapy Practice sheets and discusses importance of practicing CDI-T, PDI-T and Life Enhancing Skills			
23	Introduces transitional visual prompt to child specifically indicating picture leaving the therapy room and walking to the car			
	TOTALS			

Therapist comments about session

_____

_____

_____

Integrity checker comments about sessions:

Integrity = $\dfrac{\text{Yes } (\checkmark\text{'s})}{\text{Yes } (\checkmark\text{'s}) + \text{No } (X\text{'s})}$ = _____ %

Length of session = _____ minutes

Handouts and Forms

**PCIT-Toddlers
Check-In Sheet**

Have any major stressors occurred since your last session that your therapist should be aware of?

_____

_____

_____

_____

If so, have these major stressors impacted your mood, behavior, and ability to deliver the therapy to your child for five minutes each day?

_____

_____

_____

_____

How have you noticed the impact of your expression of your emotions and behavior on your child's expression of his or her emotions and behavior?

_____

_____

_____

_____

Please note one time during the previous week where you felt connected to your child or you noticed a strength in your child.

_____

_____

_____

_____

Transitional Visual Cue Card – Office to Play Room

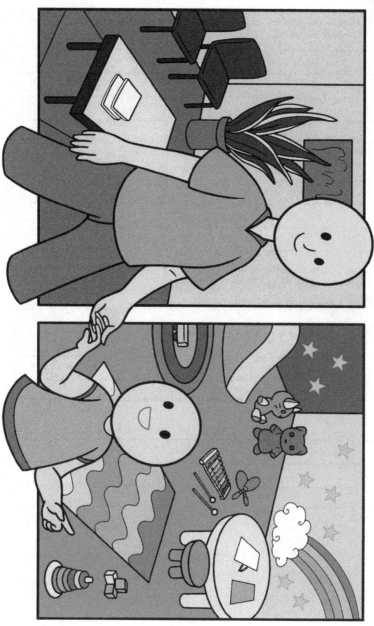

Transitional Visual Cue Card – Play Room to Leaving Office

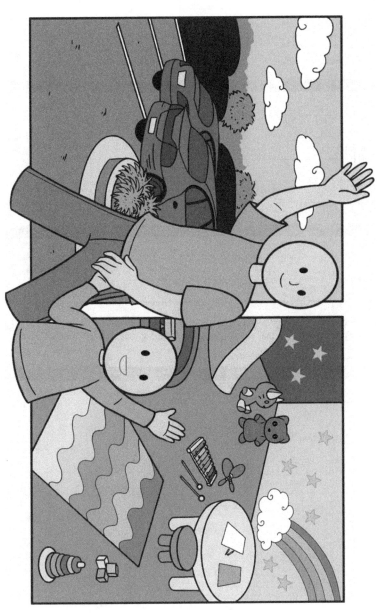

DPICS-T Coding Sheet for Therapist
Adapted from Eyberg and Funderburk (2011)

Child Name/ ID _____Date:_____

Parent: □ Mother   □ Father   □ Other _____

Coder:_____   Start Time:_____ End Time:_____

o CDI Coach # ____	o PDI Coach # ____	o PDI LE # ____

Number of Days Homework Completed?   □ 0   □ 1   □ 2   □ 3   □ 4   □ 5   □ 6   □ 7

Do Skills	Tally Count	TOTAL	Mastery
Neutral Talk			--
Emotion Labeling			--
Behavioral Description			10
Reflection			10
Labeled Praise			10
Unlabeled Praise			--
Don't Skills	Tally Count	TOTAL	
Question			
Commands			0 ≤ 3
Negative Talk			

Coach caregiver through any missed CARES step (if needed) in the moment,
INCLUDING getting on the microphone during the 5 minutes of DPCIS Coding.

Big Emotion Present?	YES	NO	# Tally	
CARES Skills Used	CIRCLE ONE			NOTES
Come in Calm & Close	Satisfactory	Needs Practice	N/A	
Assist Child	Satisfactory	Needs Practice	N/A	
Reassure Child	Satisfactory	Needs Practice	N/A	
Emotional Validation	Satisfactory	Needs Practice	N/A	
Soothe	Satisfactory	Needs Practice	N/A	

(Continues onto next page)

DPICS-T Coding Sheet for Therapist
Adapted from Eyberg and Funderburk (2011)

Child Name/ ID _____Date:_____

Parent: □ Mother   □ Father   □ Other _____

Coder:_____   Start Time:_____ End Time:_____

Positive Skills	Circle One		NOTES
Imitate	Satisfactory	Needs Practice	
Show Enjoyment	Satisfactory	Needs Practice	
Physical Affection	Satisfactory	Needs Practice	
Mutual Eye Contact	Satisfactory	Needs Practice	
Animated Tone of Voice	Satisfactory	Needs Practice	
Animated Facial Expressions	Satisfactory	Needs Practice	
Play Style at Developmental Level	Satisfactory	Needs Practice	
Bx Management Skills	Circle One		NOTES
Skill of Redirection	Satisfactory	Needs Practice	N/A
Skill of Under Reaction	Satisfactory	Needs Practice	N/A
Limit Setting - 'No Hurting'	Satisfactory	Needs Practice	N/A

General Notes & Observations:

_____
_____
_____
_____
_____
_____
_____

Relationship Enhancement Tracker of
CDI-Toddlers Skills

Session #	Baseline CLP								
Date									
Home Therapy Practice									
7	X								
6	X								
5	X								
4	X								
3	X								
2	X								
1	X								
0	X								
Labeled Praise									
10+									
9									
8									
7									
6									
5									
4									
3									
2									
1									
0									
Reflection									
10+									
9									
8									
7									
6									
5									
4									
3									
2									
1									
0									
Behavior Description									
10+									
9									
8									
7									
6									
5									
4									
3									
2									
1									
0									

Relationship Enhancement Tracker of CDI-Toddlers Skills

Session #	Baseline CLP							
Date								

Emotion Labeling

10+								
9								
8								
7								
6								
5								
4								
3								
2								
1								
0								

Question/Command/Critical Statement

10+								
9								
8								
7								
6								
5								
4								
3								
2								
1								
0								

CARES

Satis-factory								
N/A								
Needs Improv.								

Other Positive Skills
(Imitate, Enjoy, Affection, Eye Contact, Animation, etc.)

Satis-factory								
N/A								
Needs Improv.								

Redirection and Under-Reaction

Satis-factory								
N/A								
Needs Improv.								

Limit-Setting "No Hurting"

Satis-factory								
N/A								
Needs Improv.								

TELL-SHOW-TRY AGAIN-GUIDE FLOW CHART

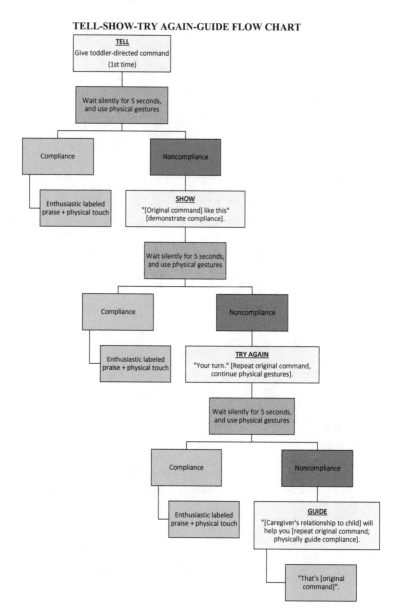

PCIT-T PDI-T Coding Sheet for Therapists

Child's Name _____ □ Mother □ Father □ Other _____ Coder: _____

Start Time: _____ End Time: _____ PDI Session #: _____

TELL								**SHOW**							**TRY AGAIN**					**GUIDE**		
Command DC or IC?	Gesture Given?	NOC	CO	NC	Praise LP or UP or NP?	Praise w/ Animation - And or - + touch		5 sec	demo task repeats DC + Like This	CO	NC	Praise LP or UP or NP?	Praise w/ Animation - And or - + touch		5 sec	State "Your Turn" + DC	CO	NC	5 sec	"…will help you." Hand-over-hand	BD to end task	Correct FT?
1																						
2																						
3																						
4																						
5																						
6																						
7																						
8																						
9																						
10																						
Total																						

A. # NOC _____   % Effective DC (C÷D) _____   □ 75% Effective DC

B. # IC _____

C. # effective DC _____   % CO to DC (E÷C) _____   □ % Child Compliance Skills

D. Total Commands _____   (Complete task at "Tell", "Show" or "Try Again" Step)

E. # CO to DC _____   % FT to DC (F÷C) _____   □ 75% Correct FT

F. # FT to DC _____

Adapted from Eyberg and Funderburk (2011) pg. 105

Listening/ Compliance Tracker of PDI-Toddlers Skills

Session #	Baseline **PLP**	Baseline **CU**						
Date								

PDI-T Home Therapy Listening Practice

7	X	X						
6	X	X						
5	X	X						
4	X	X						
3	X	X						
2	X	X						
1	X	X						
0	X	X						

Effective Direct Commands

100%								
90%								
80%								
70%								
75%								
60%								
50%								
40%								
30%								
20%								
10%								
0%								

Consistent Follow Through

100%								
90%								
80%								
75%								
70%								
60%								
50%								
40%								
30%								
20%								
10%								
0%								

Child Compliance Behavior*

100%								
90%								
80%								
75%								
70%								
60%								
50%								
40%								
30%								
20%								
10%								
0%								

*Compliance Behavior is calculated by task completion during the PDI-T
 sequence of "Tell", "Show" or "Try Again."

PCIT-Toddlers Home Therapy Practice

Child's Name:_____   Date:_____

☐ Mom   ☐ Dad   ☐ Other Caregiver: _____

Your In Session 5-minute PRIDE Skills

Use your CDI "Do Skills / PRIDE" & play with your child 5 minutes daily.
Use CARES steps when signals of big emotions are present and your child needs your help.

	Did you engage in **Relaxation** before Special Time?		Did you spend 5 minutes in **Special Time** today?		Activity or Toys Played	List any signals of big emotions your child showed. Was CARES used?	PRIDE Skills used today… Any problems or questions during Special Time?
	Yes	No	Yes	No			
Monday							
Tuesday							
Wednesday							
Thursday							
Friday							
Saturday							
Sunday							

Write a time during the week when you felt an intense emotion and what impact did it have on your child?

_____

_____

Adapted from Eyberg and Funderburk (2011) CDI Homework sheet, pg 28.

PCIT-Toddlers Home Therapy Listening Practice
Identified Commands
Adapted from Eyberg and Funderburk (2011) pg. 105

Child's Name:_____   Date:_____

□ Mom   □ Dad   □ Other Caregiver: _____

Use the 8 Rules for Effective Commands & follow-up with a
labeled praise every time your child complies.

USE CARES when needed before starting PDI-T, be sure
your toddler is well rested to learn, 3 commands maximum.

Date	Did you practice PDI for 5 min. in a play situation after CDI today? Yes	No	Place mark for each success after: **Tell**	Place mark for each success after: **Show**	Place mark for each success after: **Try Again**	Place mark for each task after: **Guide**	**Comments** Write the play command(s) you gave that required the "GUIDE" technique. Was CARES needed after GUIDE? Other Comments?
Monday							
Tuesday							
Wednesday							
Thursday							
Friday							
Saturday							
Sunday							

Call your PCIT-Toddler Coach IMMEDIATELY if you are struggling with Teaching Compliance Sequence

Example Identified Commands (fill in the blank):

Please pass me _____.

Please give me _____.

Please put _____ here.

Labeled Praises:

Great following directions!

You're good at listening!

Awesome job minding me!

PCIT-Toddlers **PUBLIC OUTING TODDELR BAG CHECKLIST**	✓
1. Diaper changing related items (e.g., change mat, diapers, wipes, cleaning lotion)	
2. Healthy snack and drink	
3. Appropriate change of clothes for weather	
4. Wash cloth to be used to freshen child and parent	
5. Desired toy to be used for distraction	
6. Child's comfort item/toy	
7. Child's blanket/comforter	
8. Hat or beanie (weather dependent)	
9. Sun screen	

Comments

_____

_____

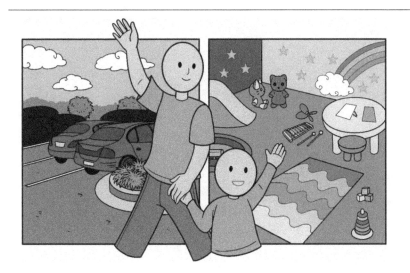

References

Centers for Disease Control and Prevention. (2017). How Much Sleep Do I Need? Retrieved from
    https://www.cdc.gov/sleep/about_sleep/how_much_sleep.html
Eyberg, S., & Funderburk, B. W. (2011). Parent-child interaction therapy protocol. Gainesville, FL:
    PCIT International.
Karitane. (2018). Resources. Retrieved from https://karitane.com.au/page/our-services/resources
YouTube. (2018). Retrieved from https://www.youtube.com

Chapter 18
Graduation Session

The purpose of the graduation session is to commemorate and reflect upon the journey and accompanying success that the parent and child have jointly achieved throughout their course of PCIT-T. While it is likely that many small successes have been noted, discussed, and celebrated as they occurred, a full session is dedicated to helping the parent process the meaning behind his or her completion of the full PCIT-T model. Although time for such reflection is built into the session, it is unlikely that the full extent of reflection will be appreciated for some families with the child present. As a result, clinicians may choose to ask the parent to come alone to the current session or to have a second graduation session with only the parent present. The current session provides closure to an often arduous and emotionally challenging treatment course while also serving to recognize any unacknowledged efforts of the parent who independently, recognized the need for early intervention and in turn, set his or her child on a promising developmental trajectory. A second focus of the current session is to allow the parent to show off his or her specialized parenting abilities to the treatment team, who in turn, help the parent to recognize the monumental impact of the parent's hard work on the child's behavior and emotions as well as the parent's behavior and emotions while relating such changes to the child and parent's future.

Note Developmental tip of the day cards are provided in Appendix H at the conclusion of this manual. Clinicians may use their clinical judgment to determine if the parent is able to take in and utilize selected cards at the beginning or conclusion of each session.

Session Preparation Items

1. Bug-in-the-ear equipment
2. Visual transition aide cards

© Springer Nature Switzerland AG 2018
E. I. Girard et al., *Parent-Child Interaction Therapy with Toddlers*,
https://doi.org/10.1007/978-3-319-93251-4_18

3. Pre−/post-assessment DPICS-T Coding sheets
4. Relationship Enhancement Tracker for CDI-T skills
5. Listening/Compliance Tracker for PDI-T skills
6. Appropriate toys
7. Necessary handouts:

   (a) Posttreatment measures
   (b) Graduation certificate

Session Goals

1. Commemorate and reflect upon the journey and accompanying success that the parent and child have jointly achieved throughout their course of PCIT-T.
2. Allow the parent to show off his or her specialized parenting abilities to the treatment team, who in turn, help the parent to recognize the monumental impact of the parent's hard work on the child's behavior and emotions as well as the parent's behavior and emotions while relating such changes to the child and parent's future.

Session Outline

1. **Greet the parent and child in the waiting room.**

   (a) Provide the parent with the check-in sheet if not provided by front office personnel and allow 5 minutes to complete.
   (b) Collect the parent's current CDI-T and PDI-T Home Therapy Practice sheet, and place the information on the Relationship Enhancement Tracker for CDI-T skills and Listening/Compliance Tracker for PDI-T skills sheets. Use a highlighter to graph those weeks where the parent completed four or more of the daily therapy sessions. For three or fewer, use a black pen or pencil to mark the number of days completed on the progress sheet.

   NOTE: Depending upon the set-up of the waiting area at a given agency and/or the parent's difficulties managing the child's behavior, therapists may consider transitioning the parent-child dyad to a therapy room and playing with the child to allow the parent time to complete such procedures. If the aforementioned transition occurs during this step, the therapist should utilize visual aids (described in the following step) when initially approaching the dyad in the waiting area.

2. **After the check-in sheet is completed, approach the parent and child prepared with the transitional cue cards/visual aids provided in this chapter. Review the visual aide with the child while also prompting the parent to take the child's hand while walking to the therapy room.**
3. **Review the completed check-in sheet. While reviewing the check-in sheet, the therapist should simultaneously interact with the child and model the use of CARES for the child if necessary.**
4. **Ask parent(s) to complete paper and pencil assessment measures if not provided prior to graduation session while clinician engages with toddler.** Assessment measures include:

   (a) The Devereux Early Childhood Assessment (DECA)

      (i) DECA-Infant (ages 12–18 months)
      (ii) DECA-Toddler (ages 18–36 months)

   (b) or The Brief Infant Toddler Social Emotional Assessment (BITSEA)

   Optional: The Ages and Stages Questionnaire (ASQ), the Modified Checklist for Autism in Toddlers, Revised, with Follow-Up ™, the Parenting Stress Index – Short Form (PSI-SF), the Child Behavior Checklist (CBCL), and the Edinburgh Postnatal Depression Scale (EPDS).

5. **Initiate three posttreatment DPICS observations (verbatim instructions are provided below).** Code all verbalizations according to DPICS coding rules. Additionally, determine the parent's skill with regard to positive skills and fulfillment of the CARES model during any moments of child emotion dysregulation.

   Important guidelines: If two parents or caregivers are present, each should complete his or her own behavior observations. Ideally, each parent should conduct the observations privately, without observation by the other parent. When possible, observations should be conducted on a small rug or blanket on the floor with selected developmentally appropriate toys to increase child safety. Guidelines for each situation may be given over a bug-in-the-ear walkie talkie device particularly when it is suspected that the therapist's guidance may otherwise affect the child's behavior (e.g., slightly older children). Guidelines may be provided in person for younger toddlers.

   Child-directed interaction script: "In this situation, tell [child's name] that he/she may play with whatever he/she chooses. Let him/her choose any activity he/she wishes. You just follow his/her lead and play along with him/her" (Eyberg & Funderburk, 2011, p.13). Begin to time a five-minute warm-up period prior to formally using the DPICS to code the five-minute situation.

Note: During the 5-minute warm-up prior to formally coding clinicians, score all posttreatment assessment measures, and prepare to review outcomes with caregiver.

Parent-directed interaction script: "That was fine. Now we'll switch to the second activity (Eyberg & Funderburk, 2011, p.13). Redirect [child's name] to play with a different toy in the room that you have chosen and see if you can get [child's name] to play with you." Begin to time and DPICS code the five-minute situation.

Cleanup script: "That was fine. Now please tell [child's name] that it is time to clean up the toys (Eyberg & Funderburk, 2011, p.13). Help him/her put all the toys in their containers and all the containers in the toy box [or designate location]." Begin to time and DPICS code the five-minute situation.

6. **Clinician completes Dyadic Parent-Child Interaction Coding System (DPICS) and records outcomes to corresponding skills tracking graphs**

   (a) Child-Led Play (CLP) graduation; Relationship Enhancement Tracker for CDI-T Skills
   (b) Parent-Led Play (PLP) graduation; Listening/Compliance Tracker for PDI-T Skills
   (c) Clean-Up (CU) graduation; Listening/Compliance Tracker for PDI-T Skills

7. **Debrief DPICS observation**

   (a) Discuss the parent's impression of changes from pre-treatment observation to post-treatment observation related to their child and their implementation of skills.
   (b) Review Relationship Enhancement Tracker for CDI-T Skills over the course of treatment
   (c) Review Listening/Compliance Tracker for PDI-T Skills over the course of treatment

8. **Review posttreatment assessment scores by comparing and contrasting scores to mid-treatment outcome measures and pretreatment outcome measures for the DECA and/or BITSEA in addition to any supplemental assessments provided prior.**

9. **Check in on the parent's current emotion and process meaning of graduation session.**

10. **Congratulate the parent on his or her ability to meet all the requirements necessary to graduate from PCIT-T. Introduce the purpose of the current, graduation session.**

    Sample Script: "Today is a really special day because it represents the conclusion of your formal journey through and graduation from PCIT-T. So, the purpose of today's session is two-fold – one, to recognize and commemorate your persistence and ability to meet all of the requirements necessary to complete PCIT-T and two, to reflect upon your path with [child's name] through this program. Your path and its accompanying changes represent an even greater accomplishment than any graduation certificate can ever describe – for you, for [child's name], for your relationship, and for your future together."

11. **Allow the parent to reflect upon his or her unique journey through PCIT-T. A list of questions to prompt the discussion are presented below:**

    (a) Tell me about what your journey through PCIT-T means to you.
    (b) What was a memorable moment through your course of PCIT-T?
    (c) What was the most challenging aspect of PCIT-T?
    (d) How do you feel your relationship with [child's name] has changed since beginning PCIT-T?
    (e) How do you feel that PCIT-T may impact [child's name]'s future?
    (f) How has PCIT-T impacted your life apart from parenting [child's name]?
    (g) What do you feel that you have learned from PCIT-T?
    (h) What do you wish you could have told yourself during week 1 of PCIT-T?
    (i) What changes have you noticed in yourself throughout the course of PCIT-T?
    (j) What changes have you noticed in [child's name] throughout the course of PCIT-T?
    (k) What do you wish you could tell other parents with situations similar to yours when you first began working with me?
    (l) How do you feel that you have impacted [child's name]'s development by dedicating yourself to PCIT-T?

12. **Discuss the concept of relapse prevention and indicators that the parent may need to seek help in the future.**
    Sample script: "There may come a time in [child's name]'s life that you may need to seek treatment again for his or her behavioral difficulties in the future. If this occurs, it does not mean that everything that you have done in this program has not worked. [Child's name]'s behavioral and emotional needs will continue to change as he/she develops and as a result, he/she may need specialized services to target the unique difficulties that he/she is experiencing at various points in development. This is similar to his or her medical needs, just because [child's name] may have been treated for the flu when she/he was 2, doesn't mean that he/she won't need treatment for the flu or something else later on. However, I want to do everything that we can to try to delay or prevent, [child's name] from needing treatment at any point in the near future. Let's talk about some of the key skills and concepts that will continue to be important in helping [child's name] to develop and regulate his or her emotions."

13. **Prompt the parent to brainstorm the skills that he/she believes will continue to be important to setting the child up for behavioral or emotional success. Praise the parent's efforts.**

14. **Expand upon the parent's ideas by summarizing the core concepts of this treatment. Such concepts should include positive reinforcement, emotion**

regulation, development of a warm, trusting relationship, age-appropriate limit setting, teaching listening skills, and providing consistency, predictability, and follow-through.

(a) These goals were achieved through therapeutic strategies of the PRIDE skills, CARES model, under-reaction, redirection, distraction, guided compliance, and daily skill practice.

15. **Present the parent with the graduation certificate and celebrate their success.**
16. **Present the transition visual to the child specifically indicating each picture related to leaving the therapy room and walking to the car.**
    Sample script: "Now it's time to go 'bye bye' [points to picture of child leaving therapy room] and walk to the car [point to picture of child in car]."

17. **Complete integrity checklist: PCIT-T graduation session**

Integrity Checklist: PCIT-T Graduation Session

 As you view the session, place a checkmark under the appropriate column, Yes (Y), Not Applicable (NA) or No (N). List these totals in the appropriate blanks below the table. See expanded session outlines for more information on each item. (Integrity checklist and directions are based on Eyberg & Funderburk, 2011).

Integrity Checklist: PCIT-Toddlers Graduation Session		
Client & Caregiver:		
Therapist Conducting Session:		
Checklist Completed By:	**Date:**	

	ITEMS	Y	NA	N
1	Greets the parent and child in the waiting area: Provides check-in sheet and collects CDI-T & PDI-T Home Practice sheets			
2	Uses visual transition prompt to the child and models PRIDE skills while supporting the caregiver/s to enter the therapy room safely			
3	Reviews check-in sheet and CDI-T/PDI-T Home Practice sheets and discusses any major changes			
4	Administers Post- treatment measures (score measure during 5-minute warm-up of CLP)			
5	Conducts Post-Treatment DPICS-T Observations, 3 scenarios (CLP, PLP, and CU) and transfers scores to appropriate Tracking sheets			
6	Debriefs caregiver on Post-Treatment DPICS-T			
7	Reviews Post-Treatment Assessment outcome scores, comparing to Pre-Treatment and Mid-Treatment measures			
8	Congratulates the caregiver/s on meeting mastery			
9	Allows caregiver/s to reflect on their PCIT-T journey			
10	Discusses the concept of relapse prevention and when to seek support			
11	Reviews skills mastered and summarizes core concepts, praises caregiver/s efforts			
12	Presents graduation certificates and celebrates			
13	Introduces the visual prompt transition to leave, end PCIT-T treatment			
	TOTALS			

Therapist comments about session

_____

_____

_____

Integrity checker comments about sessions:

_____

_____

_____

Integrity =   Yes Total _____   = _____ %
                    Yes Total + No Total

Length of session = _____ minutes

Handouts and Forms

PCIT-Toddlers
Check-In Sheet

Have any major stressors occurred since your last session that your therapist should be aware of?

_____

_____

_____

_____

If so, have these major stressors impacted your mood, behavior, and ability to deliver the therapy to your child for five minutes each day?

_____

_____

_____

_____

How have you noticed the impact of your expression of your emotions and behavior on your child's expression of his or her emotions and behavior?

_____

_____

_____

_____

Please note one time during the previous week where you felt connected to your child or you noticed a strength in your child.

_____

_____

_____

_____

Transitional Visual Cue Card – Office to Play Room

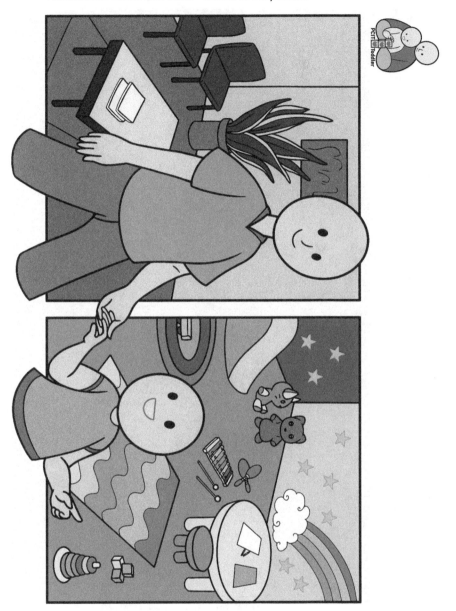

Transitional Visual Cue Card – Play Room to Leaving Office

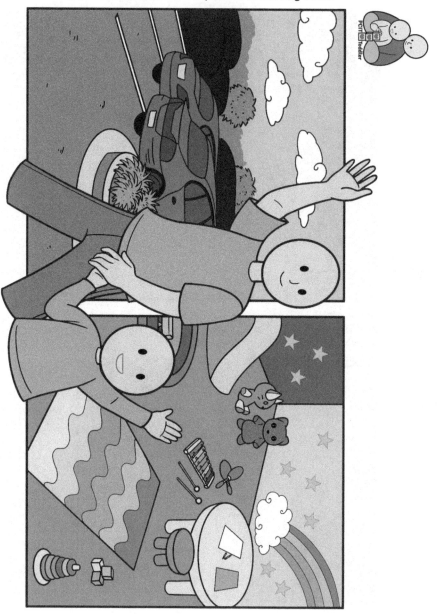

PCIT-T Pre/Post DPICS Assessment for Therapist
(Based on Eyberg & Funderburk, 2011)

Child Name/ ID _____Date:_____

Assessment:	□ **PRE**	□ **POST**	Coder:_____
Parent:	□ Mother	□ Father	□ Other _____
Situation:	□ **Child Led Play**	□ **Parent Led Play**	□ **Clean Up**

Start Time:_____   End Time:_____

Do Skills		Tally Count	TOTAL
Neutral Talk			
Emotion Labeling			
Behavioral Description			
Reflection			
Labeled Praise			
Unlabeled Praise			
Don't Skills		Tally Count	TOTAL
Question			
Direct	Comply (CO) Tell-Show-Try Again		
Command	Non-Comply (NC) Guide		
(DC)	No Opportunity (NOC)		
Indirect	Comply (CO) Tell-Show-Try Again		
Command	Non-Comply (NC) Guide		
(IC)	No Opportunity (NOC)		
Negative Talk			

PCIT-T Pre/Post DPICS Assessment for Therapist

Big Emotion Present?	YES	NO	# Tally	
CARES Skills Used	CIRCLE ONE			NOTES
Come In	Satisfactory	Needs Practice	N/A	
Assist Child	Satisfactory	Needs Practice	N/A	
Reassure Child	Satisfactory	Needs Practice	N/A	
Emotional Validation	Satisfactory	Needs Practice	N/A	
Soothe	Satisfactory	Needs Practice	N/A	

Coach caregiver through any missed step (if needed) in the moment,
INCLUDING getting on the microphone during the 5 minutes of DPCIS Coding.

Positive Skills	Circle One		NOTES
Imitate	Satisfactory	Needs Practice	
Show Enjoyment	Satisfactory	Needs Practice	
Physical Affection	Satisfactory	Needs Practice	
Mutual Eye Contact	Satisfactory	Needs Practice	
Animated Tone of Voice	Satisfactory	Needs Practice	
Animated Facial Expressions	Satisfactory	Needs Practice	
Play Style at Developmental Level	Satisfactory	Needs Practice	
Bx Management Skills	Circle One		NOTES
Skill of Redirection	Satisfactory	Needs Practice	N/A	
Skill of Under Reaction	Satisfactory	Needs Practice	N/A	
Limit Setting - 'No Hurting'	Satisfactory	Needs Practice	N/A	

Relationship Enhancement Tracker of CDI-Toddlers Skills

Session #	Baseline CLP							
Date								

Home Therapy Practice

7	X							
6	X							
5	X							
4	X							
3	X							
2	X							
1	X							
0	X							

Labeled Praise

10+								
9								
8								
7								
6								
5								
4								
3								
2								
1								
0								

Reflection

10+								
9								
8								
7								
6								
5								
4								
3								
2								
1								
0								

Behavior Description

10+								
9								
8								
7								
6								
5								
4								
3								
2								
1								
0								

Relationship Enhancement Tracker of
CDI-Toddlers Skills

Session #	Baseline CLP								
Date									

Emotion Labeling

10+									
9									
8									
7									
6									
5									
4									
3									
2									
1									
0									

Question/Command/Critical Statement

10+									
9									
8									
7									
6									
5									
4									
3									
2									
1									
0									

CARES

Satis-factory									
N/A									
Needs Improv.									

Other Positive Skills
(Imitate, Enjoy, Affection, Eye Contact, Animation, etc.)

Satis-factory									
N/A									
Needs Improv.									

Redirection and Under-Reaction

Satis-factory									
N/A									
Needs Improv.									

Limit-Setting "No Hurting"

Satis-factory									
N/A									
Needs Improv.									

Listening/ Compliance Tracker of PDI-Toddlers Skills

Session #	Baseline PLP	Baseline CU								
Date										
PDI-T Home Therapy Listening Practice										
7	X	X								
6	X	X								
5	X	X								
4	X	X								
3	X	X								
2	X	X								
1	X	X								
0	X	X								
Effective Direct Commands										
100%										
90%										
80%										
70%										
75%										
60%										
50%										
40%										
30%										
20%										
10%										
0%										
Consistent Follow Through										
100%										
90%										
80%										
75%										
70%										
60%										
50%										
40%										
30%										
20%										
10%										
0%										
Child Compliance Behavior*										
100%										
90%										
80%										
75%										
70%										
60%										
50%										
40%										
30%										
20%										
10%										
0%										

*Compliance Behavior is calculated by task completion during the PDI-T sequence of "Tell", "Show" or "Try Again."

Certificate of Accomplishment

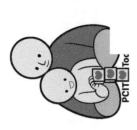

This Award is Hereby Presented to

_____

For Successful Completion of

Parent-Child Interaction Therapy with Toddlers (PCIT-T):

Improving Attachment and Emotion Regulation

_____

Clinician

_____

Date

Adapted from Eyberg and Funderburk (2011) pg. 170-171

Reference

Eyberg, S., & Funderburk, B. W. (2011). Parent-child interaction therapy protocol. Gainesville, FL: PCIT International.

Appendix A: Coaching Child Directed Interaction excerpt: McNeil, C.B., & Hembree-Kigin, T. (2010). Parent-Child Interaction Therapy: Second Edition (Chapter 5). New York: Springer

Reprinted by permission from Springer: McNeil, C.B., & Hembree-Kigin, T. (2010). *Parent-Child Interaction Therapy: Second Edition (Chapter 5)*. New York: Springer.

Chapter 5

Coaching Child-Directed Interaction

What to bring:

1. ECBI
2. DPICS-III Coding sheets
3. CDI Homework Sheets
4. PCIT Progress Sheet

When therapists coach CDI skills, we employ the same strategies and philosophies that parents are taught to use with their children during special playtime. Therapists provide labeled praises to parents to increase particular CDI skills. We also use strategic attention and selective ignoring to increase certain parent verbalizations while decreasing others. Just as a goal of special playtime is to improve the parent-child relationship, therapists use coaching strategies that enhance rapport with the parents. For example, therapists avoid criticism when coaching, particularly the words "no," "don't," "stop," "quit," and "not," in order to prevent parents from feeling judged or incompetent. These negative feelings damage our relationships with the parents and lead to treatment attrition. Rather than criticizing, we enthusiastically give attention to their positive behaviors by describing and praising. When correcting the parent, we use constructive feedback telling them what "to do" rather than what "not to do." Just as we teach parents to allow their children to lead the play, we allow parents to take the lead in their use of PRIDE skills. That is, we want parents to use their own words and develop a play style that is comfortable for them within the CDI guidelines. We only use constructive

© Springer Nature Switzerland AG 2018

E. I. Girard et al., *Parent-Child Interaction Therapy with Toddlers*,

https://doi.org/10.1007/978-3-319-93251-4

corrections when the parent is having difficulty with a particular skill. In fact, in the first CDI coaching session, Sheila Eyberg (1999) discourages the use of any correction at all, so as to make rapport a priority. When parents are using the CDI skills well, we follow their lead, using descriptions and praise to demonstrate acceptance. According to Dr. Eyberg (n.d.), the basic principles of client-centered therapy (empathy, genuineness, and positive regard) should guide our coaching. We want parents to leave coaching sessions feeling good about themselves, good about their child, and good about their progress in treatment.

Novice PCIT therapists can coach the basic child-directed interaction skills with little or no prior experience. However, coaching is an art that continuously develops as the therapist gains experience working with parents from diverse cultural groups, with various communication styles and disparate childrearing attitudes, and with children who present unique challenges. Although skillful coaching develops from experiences working with dysfunctional parent-child dyads, it is also grounded in an understanding of early childhood development and normative parent-child interactions. We feel it is particularly important for the PCIT therapist to develop and maintain an "internal barometer" for the wide range of interaction styles and communication patterns that characterize healthy, nurturing parent-child relationships. In this way, the therapist will broaden his or her repertoire of coaching strategies and will reduce the tendency to develop professional "myopia," in which similar interaction sequences are coached in all families, without regard to the family's unique communication strengths and style.

Overview of a Typical Coaching Session

Table 5.1 presents the steps involved in typical coaching sessions for families in which one or both parents are participating. Upon arrival to each PCIT session, parents complete the ECBI Intensity Scale in the waiting area. The therapist quickly

Table 5.1 Steps for conducting a child-directed interaction coaching session

One parent participating		
Step 1	Check-in and review of homework	10 min
Step 2	Coding of CDI skills	5 min
Step 3	Coaching of CDI skills	35 min
Step 4	Feedback on progress and homework assignment	10 min
Two parents participating		
Step 1	Check-in and review of homework	10 min
Step 2	Coding of first parent's CDI skills	5 min
Step 3	Coaching of first parent's CDI skills	15 min
Step 4	Coding of second parent's CDI skills	5 min
Step 5	Coaching of second parent's CDI skills	15 min
Step 6	Feedback on progress and homework assignment	10 min

tallies the score and records it on the PCIT Progress Sheet (see Appendix 5). The session begins with a review of the homework. After problem-solving issues that arise with the homework and inquiring about other familial stressors, we observe the parent conducting a five-minute play therapy session with the child, without doing any direct coaching. Parental use of CDI skills during these 5 min is recorded on a Dyadic Parent-Child Interaction Coding System-III (DPICS-III) recording sheet (see Appendix 1) and later transferred to the PCIT Progress Sheet (see Appendix 5) so that parents can view session-to-session changes. After this five-minute observation period, the parent is directly coached by the therapist while continuing to practice the PRIDE skills with the child. For two-parent families, the coaching session is divided in half so that each parent receives coaching. The parent who is not being coached learns through observation and is often taught to code from behind the mirror. The observing parent should be quiet so as not to interrupt the coaching. The last 10 min of the session is spent providing parents with feedback on their progress (see Appendix 5 for PCIT Progress Sheet) and identifying areas that should receive special focus during the next week's home practice. The therapist may choose to reserve an additional few minutes at the end of each coaching session for individual rapport-building as needed. This individual time can decrease resistance to therapy by encouraging children to view the therapist as an ally rather than as a conspirator with the parents. Although the number of CDI coaching sessions will vary based on how quickly parents master the skills, the basic steps outlined in this chapter are used in each coaching session.

Setting Up for the Coaching Session

The parent and child meet with the therapist in a childproofed playroom equipped with a table and chairs and three to five construction-oriented toys. Generally, the parent and child play on the floor during CDI, with the parent following the child around the room as the child plays with the toys that are available. However, it is up to the child to choose whether to play on the floor or at the table. For example, if the child chooses to color at the table, the parent should sit at the table as well. A few minutes later, the child may choose to drive cars on the carpet, and the parent should move to the floor to join in the play. Toys that are inappropriate for CDI should be removed from the room to avoid the unpleasantness that may occur if the child insists on playing with an inappropriate toy. Because parents will be asked to avoid limit-setting during CDI, the playroom should contain no items that may inspire the child to misbehave and require parental intervention. In our playroom, we do not include lamps, glass framed pictures, nicely upholstered furniture, sinks, boxes of tissues, or personal items such as handbags. Light switches are kept in the "on" position using lockable covers or tape.

If the therapist will be coaching via a bug-in-ear microphone device, the earpiece should be sterilized with an alcohol wipe and tested prior to the start of the therapy session. Additional materials that will be needed during each session are as follows: one DPICS-III coding sheet for each parent, one homework sheet for each parent, one PCIT Progress Sheet for each parent, and a clock or stopwatch.

Check-In and Homework Review

The session typically begins with the child playing independently nearby, while the parent and therapist review the child's home and school adjustment during the previous week, discuss familial stressors, and review the week's homework practice. We ask parents to bring in a homework sheet each week indicating whether or not they were able to practice each day and noting any questions, observations, or concerns they had during the course of the week. Because one of the goals for the CDI stage of PCIT is for parents to become more adept at recognizing and praising their child's positive qualities and behaviors, we are careful to prompt parents to note progress and accomplishments by the child, not just problems. We also use this check-in period as an opportunity to teach parents to shape independent play by giving their child intermittent labeled praises for playing quietly while the adults talk.

In order to maximize the amount of time spent in direct coaching of CDI, we restrict this initial "check in" to 5–10 min. Occasionally, the parents we work with have difficulty sticking to this time limit or bring in concerns about important marital or individual issues. If this occurs on a consistent basis, diverting focus away from the parent training intervention and slowing PCIT treatment progress, we recommend inviting parents to participate in adjunctive interventions such as individual treatment, support groups, or marital therapy. Thus, important concurrent issues may be addressed in a planful way often enhancing the effectiveness of PCIT. With some parents who tend to offer overly lengthy and detailed descriptions of their child's misbehavior, we choose to sequence the session so that this check-in period is saved for the last 10 min of the session. This limits nonproductive focus on child misbehavior both by decreasing the time available for it and by inviting parents to review child behavior only after they have been coached to focus on their child's positive attributes.

During the first CDI coaching session, the check-in period should include a brief review of the "do" and "avoid" skills. Most parents feel quite self-conscious about performing these new skills in front of the therapist. It is helpful to directly address this anxiety, letting parents know that it is a common experience that will quickly pass, and reminding them that the therapist does not expect them to be "masters" of play therapy after practicing it for only one week. Finally, the check-in period during the first CDI coaching session should be concluded with a developmentally appropriate explanation of the coaching process for the child. If the therapist-coach will be recording and coaching the skills from an observation room and the child is old enough to perceive that the parent is receiving instructions over the bug-in-ear, the following explanation might be given:

> It's time for me to leave now so you can have special playtime with your mom (dad). But, I'm going to watch you and your mom (dad) play. I'll be watching from behind that mirror. Do you want to see? [Allow child to enter observation room and briefly view the playroom]. I'm going to help your mom (dad) learn to play in a special way. Sometimes I might say things that she (he) will hear in that funny thing in her (his) ear. That thing is not a toy. You can look at it but you can't play with it. Your job is to just play along with your mom (dad) and have fun, OK?

If the therapist-coach will be recording and coaching from within the playroom, the child might be told something like:

> It's time for you to have special playtime with your mom (dad) now. I'm going to stay here and watch you and your mom (dad) play. My job is to help your mom (dad) learn to play with you in a very special way. Sometimes I will watch quietly and write things down, and sometimes I will say some things to your mom (dad). Your job is to keep playing and pretend like I'm not even here, like I'm invisible! That means you don't look at me or talk to me. You just play with your mom (dad) and pretend like I'm not here, OK?

Both of these explanations should be adapted to fit the cognitive and language development of the individual child, and some therapist-coaches may choose to have the parent repeat the explanation in their own words to enhance the child's understanding. If coaching from within the room, some children will have initial difficulty remembering not to interact with the therapist. The first time this occurs, the therapist should remind the child to pretend that the therapist is not there and subsequently the therapist should completely ignore any further overtures from the child. Most children will quickly learn to tune out the therapist's coaching and to attend to the play with the parent. If the therapist continues to respond to the child's overtures, the latter will become more frequent and coaching will be compromised.

Parental Noncompliance with CDI Homework

Although parents often leave the early CDI sessions with the best of intentions to complete their daily homework, we find that the majority of parents have great difficulty getting their homework done on a consistent basis. Therapists should expect homework noncompliance and be proactive about problem-solving homework issues. Because clinic improvements will not readily generalize to the home without practice, both therapists and parents must view homework as a critical element of the treatment. We recognize that it is rare for families to be able to complete 100% of the assigned homework. And, we find that many families can progress well through treatment if they are completing most of their homework. When parents complete homework fewer than 3 times per week, we become seriously concerned that treatment may not progress. In those cases, we analyze the possible reasons for the homework noncompliance and employ strategies to correct the problem. Table 5.2 provides four common functions of homework noncompliance and associated remedies.

Table 5.2 Functions of homework noncompliance solutions

1. Parent does not "buy in" to CDI	1. Put the issue on the table
	2. "Sell" CDI again (see Chapter 3)
	3. Introduce idea of an "experiment"
2. Parent is too stressed and disorganized to make homework a priority	1. Give them a folder
	2. Night-before reminder call
	3. Give them a physical reminder for refrigerator
	4. Midweek reminder call
	5. Incentives
	6. Help them develop a routine for CDI
3. Therapist has not sent a consistent message that homework should be a priority	1. Avoid inadvertently reinforcing noncompliance with supportive statements such as "It's okay. I can see it was a tough week."
	2. Consistently pick up homework sheet with ECBI, making homework sheet a "ticket" to the session
	3. Give labeled praises for remembering homework sheet
	4. Give labeled praises for completing most of the homework (e.g., 4 out of 7 days)
	5. Require parents to re-create the homework sheet if it is forgotten
	6. Repeatedly educate the parents about the importance of homework and attribute child changes to home practice (or lack thereof)
4. Parent practice is being sabotaged by others in the home	1. Attempt to engage the significant others in therapy
	2. Problem solve ways for parent to practice with privacy
	3. Empower the parent to be assertive with others
	4. Educate parent that others who have been criticized for CDI practice have found ways to complete homework
	5. Forecast that significant others will stop sabotaging when they see the treatment work

Parent Does Not "Buy In" to CDI Some families enter treatment more motivated for CDI than others. Our highly educated parents are typically convinced easily of the potential benefits of CDI. In contrast, our court-ordered, school-referred, and less educated families tend to be harder to persuade. Homework noncompliance may be an early indicator of treatment resistance in these families. We find it helpful to address the resistance directly. We might say, "I'm sensing that you don't really believe that special playtime is going to make any difference." This opens the door for parents to directly discuss skepticism and provides us with an opportunity to further "sell" CDI. As discussed in Chapter 3, five points to emphasize when "selling" CDI are (1) the parent must have a strong relationship with the child for the intensive discipline program to work, (2) daily practice leads to faster mastery of CDI so that the family progresses to the discipline program more quickly, (3) CDI is "therapy" not just play, (4) having a short daily connection with the child adds up and leads to the child wanting to please the parent, and (5) by practicing each day, the parent overlearns important behavior management skills that become habits that occur naturally throughout the day. For parents who remain resistant even after receiving the five "selling points" above, we encourage parents to think of CDI practice as an "experiment." As part of the experiment, we have the parent generate the number of CDI practices that they are willing to commit to for the upcoming week. We write the agreed upon number on the top of the homework sheet and introduce the experiment in the following way:

> So you think you can get in 4 times this week. Is that a realistic number? Are you able to commit to that for this week only? Great. Then, when I see you next week, the first thing that I will ask you is whether you were able to do *your* part of the experiment. I will ask you whether you did special playtime 4 times during the week. It is important for you to get in all 4 practices so that we give the play therapy a chance to work. Together we will look at whether the practice time led to any good changes in your child's behavior, your relationship with your child, or your own skills as a play therapist.

We use this "experiment" as a way of shaping homework behavior. If we get the parent to do one week of homework, then we have a foot in the door. We can praise the parent for the accomplishment and make observations about how it is helping.

Parent Is Too Stressed and Disorganized to Make Homework a Priority We find that many of our multi-stressed, disorganized families are sufficiently sold on the merits of CDI but have just been unsuccessful at making it happen at home. These families lack routine, are often just trying to get through their days, are responding to crises, and feel overwhelmed by the addition of one more task. When we recognize a family as disorganized and stressed, we often give them a folder at the beginning of treatment. We tell them to put all of their handouts and homework sheets in this folder. We also help them pick one place in the home to keep the folder, and we emphasize that they need to bring this folder to every session. When possible, we instruct our staff to provide the family with a reminder call the day before their next session. In the call, the family is reminded about the time of the session, who should come to the session, and the need to bring the folder. Sometimes these families benefit from posting a visual reminder to practice special playtime at home. Instead of expecting them to generate the reminder, we may hand them a sign to post on a wall, the door, or the refrigerator. Some therapists may choose to give the family a reminder call midway through the week to get them going on the homework and make them feel more accountable. Finally, therapists and/or agencies may choose to implement an incentive program for homework practice. Examples include the following: (1) collecting a deposit early in treatment that is refunded as parents practice homework, (2) allowing the child to select something from the "homework treat box" whenever a sufficient amount of homework was completed, and (3) awarding raffle tickets for larger prizes based on successful homework practice.

Therapist Has Not Sent a Consistent Message that Homework Should Be a Priority When training to be mental health professionals, we are taught to be supportive and client-centered with an emphasis on following the client's lead in sessions. We have found that this supportive approach can sometimes undermine our message that homework is critical for treatment progress. When our multi-stressed families present with crises, we can be easily derailed by focusing our efforts on providing support. It is not uncommon for therapists to use active listening, empathic responding, and questioning to encourage parents to talk more about the weekly crises. We often respond by saying, "You've had a really rough week," "You've got a lot on your plate," "What did you do when your ex-husband did not return her on time?" and "What did you say to the teacher when she called you?" Although it is our job to be supportive, we must be careful not to inadvertently send a message to parents that homework is not very important. For example, in the midst of providing supportive statements and inquiries about crises, we can easily find ourselves half way through the session before we ever ask about homework. And, sometimes we get so caught up in the crises that we forget to ask for homework at all. At other times, parents report to us that they were unable to do their homework because of stressful life events (e.g., death of a grandparent, a child protective services report, overtime at work, a sick child, out-of-town visitors). Our training in supportive therapy leads us to respond by saying, "That's okay. It was a tough week." Yet, with multiproblem families, *every* week is tough. If PCIT is to progress, we have to avoid giving these families permission to not do their homework because of stressful life events. As good clinicians, we work hard every session to maintain balance between providing support and making it clear to families that we expect them to do their daily homework.

To ensure that we communicate to parents that homework is a priority, we can employ several strategies. First, just as we collect an ECBI from the parents before they enter the session, we can also collect their homework sheet up front. In this way, we can make the homework sheet a sort of "ticket" to the session. Consistently asking for the homework sheet prior to the session has two benefits: (1) it increases the chance that the therapist will remember to ask for the homework, and (2) it sends a message to the client that daily practice is so important that we do not even begin the session without examining the homework sheet. If the parents turn in their homework, they should receive labeled praise for remembering the sheet, regardless of how many times they actually practiced at home. If the parents forget to bring the homework paper, the therapist should require them to re-create the homework sheet in the waiting area prior to the beginning of the session. Completing the homework sheet in the waiting area is aversive to parents because it postpones their access to the therapist and the supportive aspects of the treatment. During sessions, we repeatedly educate parents about the importance of daily practice. We teach them that the 5 min per day of special playtime is critical for (1) the development of their parenting skills, (2) improvement in the parent-child relationship, and (3) generalization of child behavior improvements from the clinic to the home setting. To help parents perceive the link between homework practice and treatment progress, we review ECBI and

DPICS results. Behavioral improvements reported on the ECBI and skill improvements coded on the DPICS are directly attributed to how well parents have followed through on their homework. When progress is slow, parents are educated about the need for them to increase homework completion in order to speed up treatment gains. Finally, in those cases in which parents actually succeed in completing all or most of their homework, we make it a point to provide labeled praise for their efforts.

Parent Practice Is Being Sabotaged Many parents tell us that it is hard to complete homework because significant others in the home observe and interfere. These significant others usually include spouses and extended family members, like grandparents, who are not participating in PCIT. Examples of interference include interrupting, showing nonverbal disapproval (e.g., shaking head, rolling eyes), inducing guilt ("Why are you wasting time playing instead of making dinner?"), and using blatant criticism ("You're stupid if you think this is going to do any good."). If we do not give parents specific strategies for dealing with interference from family members, there is a good chance that the participating parent will discontinue homework, hampering treatment progress. Our efforts to deal with sabotage include the following: (1) attempt to engage the significant others in therapy, (2) problem-solve ways for parent to practice with privacy, (3) empower the parent to be assertive with others, (4) educate the parent that other clients have encountered the same types of interference and still have found ways to complete their homework, and (5) forecast that significant others will stop sabotaging when they see the treatment work.

Observing and Recording Child-Directed Interaction Skills

As mentioned earlier, we devote a brief period of time at the beginning of each session to recording parental skills progress. This allows us to closely monitor the effectiveness of our previous coaching, provides us with objective information that can be charted and shared with interested parents, and supplies us with information about what skills should receive particular focus during the subsequent coaching.

We get the most accurate picture of how parents are performing their skills at home when we conduct our recording period early in the session, before doing any coaching. If recording is done at the end of the session, after several minutes of skills coaching, nearly all parents are able to perform at a high skill level. However, this performance is artificially enhanced by short-term retention and typically is uncharacteristic of how parents perform independently in home play therapy sessions throughout the week.

We begin the recording period by telling parents:

> I would like for you to go ahead and begin special playtime now. I'll just watch you for five minutes and make some notes to myself before I jump in and begin coaching, OK? Show me your best CDI skills.

We then allow a minute or so to go by so that the parents may warm up and let any initial nervousness subside as they devote their full attention to their child. We begin timing for 5 min and record tally marks in the appropriate boxes on the DPICS-III recording form. At the end of the 5 min, we take a minute or so to make notes about qualitative aspects of the interaction that we would like to address in the coaching or discuss with the parent at the end of the session. We then quickly transfer the data from the recording sheet to the parent's PCIT Progress Sheet. This form makes it easy for the therapist to track the family's week-to-week progress.

Immediately after the five-minute coding, we find it helpful to provide the parent with a "constructive feedback sandwich." The feedback sandwich consists of a hefty slice of labeled praise, followed by a delicately sliced suggestion regarding what the parent could do even better, and finished with another substantial slice of labeled praise. For example, the therapist might say, "You did a great job of increasing your reflections this week. You went from three to eight. And congratulations, you met mastery on behavioral descriptions with 12 of those. The one thing that you might want to focus on is increasing your labeled praises. I counted four and you need 10 for mastery. But overall, I thought that your play was warm and fun, and you did a good job of letting Sasha lead the play."

The skill progress information we collect also helps us to determine how close the family has come to meeting a pre-determined set of criteria for mastery of CDI skills and progressing to the discipline portion of PCIT. The "gold standard" for mastery of CDI skills established by Eyberg (www.pcit.org) is presented in Table 5.3. Because the mastery criteria involve using ten each of the labeled praises, reflections, and behavioral descriptions, when talking with parents, we often refer to the mastery criteria as the "ten-ten-ten." It should be noted that the criteria presented in Table 5.3 were established based on the concept of "over-learning." We know that after treatment is concluded and parents no longer receive weekly coaching, their CDI skills will backslide. However, if they have over-learned the skills, we expect that their skills will still be sufficient to maintain the child's positive behavior over time, even if some backsliding occurs. Over-learning also is important because it enhances generalization outside of the playtime. A goal is for the positive parenting skills to become over-learned habits that occur effortlessly throughout the day. For example, when the child tells an elaborate story in the car on the way home from school, we hope that the parent will automatically provide a reflection of the content. Or, when

Table 5.3 Criteria for mastery of child-directed interaction skills during a 5-min play session

10 labeled praises
10 reflections
10 behavioral descriptions
3 or fewer commands + questions + negative talk (criticism and sarcasm)
Ignore all negative attention-seeking behaviors
Imitate the child's play
Be enthusiastic

the two children in the family are playing amiably together in the living room, our goal is for the parent to reflexively provide a labeled praise. It is the over-practicing and over-learning of skills during playtime sessions that lead to the spontaneous use of these skills throughout the day.

Coaching the "Do" and "Avoid" Skills: Tips for Therapists

Skillful coaching of the parent-child interactions requires that the therapist-coach provide frequent, specific feedback to parents while not disrupting the natural flow of the interaction. That is a tall order for novice therapists who feel awkward sandwiching their comments between parent and child verbalizations. The following general principles are important for effective skills coaching.

Make Coaching Brief, Fast, and Precise The best coaching statements contain few words. Full sentences and lengthy explanations interrupt the flow of the interaction and may cause parents to become flustered as they attempt to divide their attention between the therapist-coach and their child. Not only should the coaching statement contain few words; it should be fast in that it should be delivered immediately after the parent's verbalization. Because every word must count, the language used should be precise rather than general or vague. Occasionally, a situation will arise in which the therapist-coach needs to provide a longer explanation or observation. In those rare situations, the coach could ask the parent to allow the child to play independently for a moment, while the coach provides feedback. Situations in which we have done this include times when a parent is not responding to our coaching (e.g., remains flat for 10 min despite intensive coaching on enthusiasm) and when we are providing instructions for a special exercise (e.g., praise exercise). Another situation in which we have taken a moment to talk to a parent in more detail is one in which a parent becomes emotional during the coaching. For example, we worked with a mother who was so touched by a picture her child drew that she became tearful. Her son, who had seldom seen her cry, became worried that she was hurt or that something bad had happened. The mother became flustered and did not know how to proceed with the special playtime. We talked with her for just a moment while the child played, giving her suggestions for how to explain "happy tears" to her son. Yet, the overwhelming majority of coaching should be brief so that it promotes rather than interferes with rapid skill acquisition. The coaching statements may take the form of labeled praises, gentle corrections, directives, and observations. Table 5.4 presents examples of commonly used coaching statements in each of these four categories.

Coach After Nearly Every Parent Verbalization Every verbalization the parent makes provides the therapist-coach with an opportunity to teach, and the more input the parent receives, the faster and better the skills will be learned. Also, by providing feedback after each verbalization, parents learn to pause and wait for therapist input. Coaching will proceed more smoothly when the therapist and parent

Table 5.4 Common child-directed interaction coaching statements

Labeled praises	
Good imitation	Nice physical praise
I like how you're ignoring now	Good description
Great job of following his lead	Good answering his question
Good encouraging his creativity	Great teaching!
Nice timing on giving him back your attention	Terrific enthusiasm!
Nice eye contact	Nice labeled praise
Gentle Corrections	
Oops, a question!	Sounds a little critical
Looks like a frown	Was that a command?
A little leading	Might be better to say…
You're getting a little ahead of her now	
Directives	
Try to label it	Can you reflect that?
Say "Nice manners!"	More enthusiasm!
Say it again, but drop your voice at the end	Let's ignore until he does something neutral or positive
Say "I like it when you use your big girl voice."	Say "It's so much fun to play with you when you're careful with the toys"
Praise her for sharing	How about a hug with that praise?
What can you praise now?	
Observations	
He's enjoying this	Sounds very genuine
He's sitting nicely now	Now he's imitating you
She wants to please you	He loves that praise
He's talking more now because you're reflecting	She's handling frustration a little better now
She's staying with it longer because of your descriptions	There's a big self-esteem smile!
	You see, anything you praise will increase
That praise is good for her self-esteem	By saying "I'm sorry," you just set a good example for polite manners
That's good practice for fine motor skills	

develop this type of pacing. Providing intensive feedback requires that the therapist think quickly and react with an appropriate labeled praise, gentle correction, observation, or direction. For novice therapists (and even very experienced ones!), this requires intense concentration and sustained effort which can be exhausting. Therapists must resist the inclination to reduce the frequency of their feedback or to coach in a mechanical fashion.

Give More Praise Than Correction Many parents begin therapy feeling incompetent in their parenting roles. It is critical for good outcome in PCIT that parents feel supported and successful from the outset. For that reason, the therapist-coach must stay in tune with the proportion of praise to correction being provided.

Most parents correctly perform many of the skills from the beginning, providing natural opportunities for the therapist-coach to provide a preponderance of labeled praises. If parents are not producing descriptions, reflections, and praises on their own, the therapist should use directives to get the parent to make particular statements, followed by labeled praises after the statements are made, and observations concerning the child's responses. For example:

Parent: (watches child build but does not speak)
Therapist: (gives directive) "Say, 'Good idea to make a zoo!'"
Parent: "I like that zoo you're building!"
Therapist: (gives labeled praise) "Nice labeled praise. (makes two observations) She really lights up when you praise her. She's working even harder now"

Although it is important to provide feedback as frequently as possible, it is not wise to correct every mistake the parent makes, particularly early in treatment when errors are frequent. Correcting every mistake, even if done in a gentle way, can tip the scale in the negative direction, causing a parent to feel criticized, inept, and discouraged. We recommend that therapist-coaches strive for a ratio of at least five supportive statements for every correction. An alternative to corrections is the use of selective ignoring for incorrect skill use, followed by strategic attention when the skill is used properly. The following is an example:

Parent: "What do you want to do now?"
Therapist: (selectively ignores question)
Parent: "Are you pretending to take the dog for a walk?"
Therapist: (selectively ignores question)
Parent: "Your dog is going for a walk."
Therapist: (provides strategic attention) "Terrific description! You said it as a statement. Good job reducing those questions."

After the first coaching session, most parents are performing so many skills correctly that most of the errors can be gently corrected while still maintaining the overall positive tone of the coaching.

Coach Easier Skills Before Harder Ones Some of the "do" and "avoid" skills are generally easier to learn than others, and parents are more likely to feel immediate success if more focus is placed on the easier skills initially. In our experience, describing is typically the easiest of the CDI skills, followed by imitating, reflecting, avoiding criticism, and avoiding commands. The skills that appear to be most difficult for parents to master are avoiding questions and giving praise. We believe that eliminating questions is particularly difficult because of the very high rate of questions most parents give young children at baseline. Asking questions is a difficult habit to break. For some parents, praising is difficult because they are not comfortable expressing affection verbally. Others may believe that too much praise will spoil their child or cause him or her to become boastful. Many parents resist praising because they are caught up in a coercive cycle in which they do not want to praise during special playtime if the child has displayed disruptive behavior earlier in the day. Still other parents simply have difficulty identifying their child's positive and praiseworthy qualities and behaviors. Most parents find that praise comes more easily and naturally after they have been practicing play therapy for a couple of weeks and have been coached on praise for one or two sessions. If the parent continues to experience difficulty generating praise, we recommend processing this issue with the parent in detail.

Use Special Exercises for Difficult Skills When the parent is performing many skills at the desired rate but one skill appears to be lagging well behind, we may interrupt the CDI to conduct special exercises in which the parent is encouraged to concentrate on the particular skill. For example, we may tell the parent, "I want to try a little experiment. I want to see how many times in the next minute you can praise Katie, OK? Are you ready? Now begin." During that minute, we stop coaching other skills and count aloud for the parent the number of praises given. For example:

> Good, there's one…that's two…three… now you're really going…think of another one…four…time is up. That was fantastic! You gave 4 praises in only one minute when you really concentrated on it. I knew you could do it. If you kept up that pace you would have 20 in five minutes, that's 10 more than you need for mastery. Well done!

An exercise such as this one provides encouragement and incentive as well as good practice for parents who are struggling with a particular skill. It is often a better strategy than continuing to provide frequent corrective feedback which can become disheartening for the parent. Other exercises that help parents to focus on particular skills include (1) asking parents to reflect everything appropriate the child says in a two-minute time period, (2) asking parents to catch every question they ask and restate it as a description or reflection, (3) asking parents to turn unlabeled praises into labeled praises, (4) asking parents to practice alternately dropping and raising the inflection of their voices to make a phrase a statement or a question, and (5) giving parents the assignment to be "extra silly" and excited for the next 3 min to promote enthusiasm.

Use Observations to Highlight Effects Often, we find that abstract discussions of how children respond positively and negatively to particular communications from parents are not sufficiently potent teaching tools. Many times, it is not until the parent actually sees it demonstrated during a coaching session that they are able to recognize and strategically alter their communication patterns to elicit desirable child responses. Therefore, in addition to coaching parental use of "do" and "avoid" skills, the therapist-coach should comment on the ways in which the child is responding to the parent. For example, if the parent praises the child for putting the red blocks together and then the child reaches for another red block, the therapist-coach may state an observation such as, "Your praise is powerful. Whatever you praise him for, he'll probably do again." Similarly, after the parent reflects the child's verbalization and the child speaks again, elaborating on the same topic, the therapist-coach may make an observation such as "You've given him positive attention for talking to you without taking his lead away, so he'll keep the conversation going." Because observations can be wordy and may interrupt the flow of the interaction, they should be used strategically. If a particular observation is lengthy or requires an extended discussion, we may choose to review our observations with the parent at the end of the coaching period.

The therapist-coach may also make observations about the child's negative responses to less desirable parental verbalizations and behaviors. For example, if a parent's "imitating" turns into the building of a far more elaborate structure than the one the child is making (despite warnings about this pitfall during the teaching session), the child may be expected to show any of several unfavorable responses: losing interest in the activity and leaving the parent to play with another toy, making negative comments about his or her own ability, or expressing frustration by damaging the parent's structure. Rather than coaching the parent early in the sequence to tone down the complexity of the building, it is sometimes more instructional to allow the parent to continue and the child to respond unfavorably and then help the parent to recognize how he or she precipitated this negative child response. In this situation, the therapist-coach might offer an observation such as "He's showing you that your building was too advanced for him and took away his chance to lead the play."

One of our goals in PCIT is to help parents improve their attitudes toward their children. One way that this can be accomplished is by pointing out to the parent good qualities about the child. During coaching, we frequently comment on the child's appearance, manners, intelligence, creativity, curiosity, sense of humor, problem-solving ability, building skills, speed, artistic prowess, and attire. Early in this book, we recounted how we often have parents tell us that they love their children, but they just do not like them anymore. When parents have given up on finding the good in their children, it is our job to train their eyes to see the positive qualities that we see. We look hard for improvements in the child's behavior and share those observations with parents. We make it a point to comment on how parents are responsible for these improvements. For example, we might say, "He's sharing much more this week. That is because you have been praising sharing." We find that if we do not show parents the direct link between their changes in parenting and their children's behavioral improvements, they often credit the child's changes to extraneous factors, such as sleeping, eating, allergies, the toys in the room, and the phase of the moon. Observations can help parents feel proud of their children and take responsibility for their children's behavioral improvements.

Make Use of Humor Although coaching and learning child-directed interaction is hard work for both the therapist-coach and the parent, it need not be an overly serious and formal process. In healthy parent-child interactions, most parents and children relax, laugh, and find humor in their activities and interactions. We find that the session is much more enjoyable for all involved if the therapist makes use of humor for reducing parental performance anxiety and helping to increase the warmth of the parent-child interaction.

Progress from More Directive to Less Directive Coaching A goal of CDI coaching is to empower parents to use the skills autonomously. This can be accomplished by gradually reducing the use of directives and corrections as parents display increased mastery of play therapy skills. For example, in the beginning of a first CDI coaching session, the therapist may need to give parents the exact words for labeled praises. As the session progresses, the therapist may only need to provide a brief prompt, such as "How about a praise?" Toward the end of the session, the parent may have developed the ability to generate his or her own praises. When this happens, the sensitive therapist-coach will step back and simply reinforce the parent's good use of praise and provide observations on its effects. Once parents near mastery of CDI skills, the therapist should rarely need to provide directives or offer suggestions for the words parents say. Toward the end of CDI, the coaching basically sounds like this: "Nice job. You're so good at this....You've got it. Just keep going.... Beautiful reflection...She's smiling!...Your praises are so warm."

Coaching Strategic Attention and Selective Ignoring To maximize the effectiveness of child-directed interaction, parents must understand the concepts of strategic attention and selective ignoring described in Chapter 4, and they must be able to implement them in tandem to shape desirable child behaviors. The therapist-coach should look for child behaviors that are pro-social, occur with low frequency, and are appropriate targets to increase through strategic attention. Often these behaviors are naturally incompatible with identified problematic behaviors. For example, a child who is bossy may have "asking politely" as a target of strategic attention. Using the double-pronged approach, bossiness in turn may be identified as a target for decrease through selective ignoring. Examples of problematic behaviors responsive to selective ignoring and their incompatible pro-social behaviors that may be increased through strategic attention are presented in Table 5.5.

When an appropriate target for selective ignoring is presented during the coaching session, the therapist-coach first identifies the problematic behavior, coaches the parent in selective ignoring until the child ceases the problematic behavior, coaches the parent to return attention to the child for positive or neutral behaviors, and coaches the parent to keep an eye out for pro-social behaviors (which are incompatible with the problem behavior) that can be responded to with strategic praise. The following example illustrates the use of selective ignoring and strategic attention in tandem.

Table 5.5 Behavioral targets for strategic attention and selective ignoring

Strategically attend to	Selectively ignore
Polite manners	Bossiness, demandingness
Playing gently with the toys	Banging toy on the table
Using a "big boy (girl)" voice	Whining
Talking softly	Yelling
Driving toy cars safely	Repeatedly wrecking cars
Being nice to toy people	Dropping people on floor
Sharing toys	Grabbing toys away
Building pro-social structures	Making toy guns
Trying even when it is hard	Giving up in frustration

Child: "Pow, pow, pow. You're all dead." (mimics shooting Lego people with a Tinkertoy gun he has made)

Therapist (to the parent): "That's aggressive. Now is a good time to begin ignoring. Drop your eyes, quickly turn away, and begin building something of your own with some Tinkertoys. Describe out loud what you are making, but speak as though you're just talking to yourself, not to him.

Parent: (turns away from child and picks up wheels) "I think I'm going to build a swamp buggy. Here's one wheel. . . ."

Child: (louder this time) "Look mom, I'm killing all of them! Pow, pow."

Therapist: "Great job of ignoring. Keep looking away. Good describing your own play. Let's see if we can get him interested in what you are doing so he stops the shooting. Be very enthusiastic about your buggy."

Parent: "I'm going to make the coolest, baddest, freshest swamp buggy in the whole world!! It's going to have red wheels. Now, I'm going to put a green seat here. I guess I'd better find a driver for my swamp buggy."

Child: "Oh, I know, this Lego-man can drive it!! Here, I'll show you."

Therapist: "Perfect! You got his attention away from the aggressive play and now he's playing appropriately with you. Let's give him your full attention now and some labeled praise."

Parent: (turns to face child) "What a great idea to have the Lego-man drive! Thanks for playing nicely with the toys so I can play with you again."

Therapist: "Nice labeled praise. You did a great job of getting him back on track."

Parent: "Now you're adding a back seat so more people can ride."

Therapist: "Good describing."

Parent: "I'm really glad you're playing swamp buggy with me. I like gentle play."

Therapist: "Excellent labeled praise."

Sometimes, during selective ignoring, parents will try to speed up the process by trying to coax children to reengage in CDI. This looks like the following: While the child is pounding aggressively on the dollhouse, the parent selectively ignores the pounding and starts talking out loud about how they like to play gently with the Tinkertoys (modeling opposite behavior). When the child does not discontinue the pounding immediately, the parent rushes the process by saying, "I sure wish that Freddie would come over here and play gently with the Tinker Toys." This verbalization breaks two of the CDI rules. First, it provides attention to Freddie for his disruptive behavior. And, second, it is an indirect command, making it hard for Freddie to lead the play. We coach parents to be patient and let the selective ignoring work. Parents can combine ignoring with distraction in which they enthusiastically describe their own play activity as though talking to themselves, rather than to the child. But, we do not want parents to use any form of distraction that involves looking at the child, addressing the child by name, or providing either direct or indirect commands.

There are times early in CDI coaching when children have extended tantrums and parents must ignore for up to 20 min. During the ignoring, parents who are not yet fully invested in treatment will give the coach nonverbal cues that they do not approve of this strategy. They roll their eyes, sigh, raise their hands in frustration, look into the observation window skeptically, and sometimes even say out loud "This isn't working people." If the therapist wants these families to return to the next session, it is important to stay confident and use motivational strategies during the extended period of ignoring the tantrum. We anticipate that the parent will have a hard time withholding attention for a prolonged period and prevent them from providing negative attention by continuously talking to them about the need to look away and enthusiastically describe their own play. We also take this opportunity to remind them that CDI is not the entire treatment program. We reassure these parents that ignoring is not the only strategy that we will be recommending for misbehavior. We remind them that an intensive discipline program is coming in which we will teach them more direct and hands-on strategies for handling tantrums. If the session ends on a negative note, we often provide a midweek call to motivate parents to hang in there with CDI.

Occasionally, we want to target a pro-social behavior that occurs so infrequently that there may be no naturally occurring opportunity to reinforce the behavior during coaching. For example, we worked with a three year old who was extremely bossy and rude, demanding that his mother do things for him (e.g., "Get me a drink," "You sit there," "Give me that!"). After three coaching sessions, we had never heard the child ask appropriately for anything. We decided to "prime the pump." Before we began CDI coaching, we showed the mother how to teach the child the skill of "asking nicely" (e.g., role-playing with the toy people). In this way, we were able to increase the chance that the child would ask nicely for something during the coaching session, and we could then coach the parent to provide labeled praise. With older children, we can prime the pump by simply telling them what we are looking for in the session. We might say, "Today, we are going to be working on using the words 'please' and 'thank you.' Your mom is going to be listening very closely for those words. If she hears you say them, I know she will get very excited, and so will I." Sometimes, after a few CDI sessions, children just need to be told directly (before CDI begins) what behavior we are hoping to see, and they will come through with it to please both the parent and the therapist. Once CDI begins, commands and reminders about the identified skill are no longer used because they take the lead away from the child.

Coaching Qualitative Aspects of the Parent-Child Interaction Although parents are instructed in a set of "do" and "avoid" skills for special playtime, these skills do not encompass all relevant aspects of parent-child interactions or the parent-child relationship. Novice PCIT therapists often focus their coaching exclusively on these "do" and "avoid" skills, neglecting other qualitative aspects of the interaction. This "tunnel vision" may result in play therapy that meets the latter but not the spirit of the mastery criteria cited earlier in this chapter and which would not be described by an objective observer as warm, nurturing, or promoting parent-child relationship enhancement. Experienced PCIT therapist-coaches integrate coaching of the core skills with coaching of more qualitative aspects of relationships, including physical closeness and touching, eye contact, vocal qualities, facial expressions, turn-taking, sharing, polite manners, developmentally sensitive teaching, task persistence, and frustration tolerance. For a DVD demonstrating advanced PCIT coaching skills with an actual client, see the American Psychological Association video by McNeil (2008).

Physical Closeness and Touching There is no "gold standard" for the optimum amount and type of physical closeness during CDI. Healthy parent-child dyads vary widely in the nature and degree of physical closeness and touching exhibited in parent-child interactions. In securely attached parent-child dyads, preschoolers will frequently move from very close physical proximity with their parents (e.g., sitting on parent's lap) to wider and wider exploration of the environment with frequent returns to the security of "home base." However, when the parent is a participant rather than observer of the child's play, such as occurs during CDI, most securely attached children will play for extended periods of time within two or three feet of their parents, and parents will intermittently touch their children in an affectionate way.

In our work with less functional parent-child dyads, we have observed anxiously attached, clinging children as well as young children who show unusually little interest in interacting closely with their parents. We have also observed parents who hover over their children, engaging in an excessive degree of controlling physical contact, as well as those who appear to be uncomfortable with physical affection (e.g., hugs, sitting on lap) expressed by their young children. Thus, depending on the needs of the particular family, the therapist may coach parents to (1) praise their children for more independent behaviors incompatible with clinging, like sitting in one's own chair; (2) combine verbal praise with physical praise such as stroking the child's hair, offering a hug, and patting the child's knee; (3) refrain from "restraining" gestures such as grabbing the child's hand to prevent a response; or (4) move closer to the child who has distanced himself or herself from the parent, praising the child for allowing the parent to join in the game.

Eye Contact, Facial Expressions, and Vocal Qualities Among US Caucasian populations, it is expected that the listener will make eye contact with the speaker during conversation, and a lack of eye contact may be interpreted as avoidance of emotional contact or poor social skills. Some of the parents we work with have significant social skills deficits or discomfort with emotional exchanges and profit from direct coaching in how to model good eye contact during special playtime. Modeling good eye contact is helpful but sometimes insufficient for encouraging young children to improve their own eye contact patterns. For young children who only occasionally make eye contact, parents are coached to praise their children strategically and enthusiastically for good eye contact. When eye contact is a very low base-rate behavior, we coach parents to shape eye contact by lifting a toy that has captured the child's attention to the parents' eye level, while they are speaking, and then strategically praising the child for good eye contact when the parent's and the child's eyes meet (e.g., "I like it when you look at me when we're talking"). This is a helpful strategy for young children with atypical development, such as those with autism spectrum disorders. Please see Chapter 12 for a full description of working with children with developmental disabilities.

Sometimes, parents master the mechanics of the praising, reflecting, imitating, and describing, but the play therapy takes on a monotonous and boring quality. These parents appear to be "going through the motions" but not to have their hearts in it. On reflection, the therapist may notice that he or she is coaching in a monotone as well. When we first notice this occurring, we exaggerate our own animation and then coach parents to play in a more animated fashion, increasing the enthusiasm in their voices, adding clapping to praises for young preschoolers, and exaggerating facial expressions. As the parents add more animation to their play, we offer observations on its effect such as: "He's looking at your face more and making better eye contact now," "Look at her face beam. Your enthusiasm means a lot to her," and "Now she can really tell you're enjoying this time with her." When a parent does not respond to this coaching by brightening his or her affect, it is sometimes an indicator of depression, substance use, or chronic fatigue. At other times, it is an indicator that the parent is resistant to treatment. When this occurs, we temporarily suspend coaching in order to have a "heart-to-heart" discussion with the parent in which we explore these issues. Sometimes adjunctive interventions for depression or substance abuse are recommended, strategies for stress reduction are presented, and sources of resistance to treatment are identified and addressed.

Turn-Taking, Sharing, and Polite Manners The "do" skills of CDI, at a basic level, represent social communication skills that people of all ages use in their interpersonal relationships. Imitation begets imitation, and when parents describe, imitate, praise, and reflect during special playtime, their young children in turn imitate these skills. Over time, young children begin spontaneously praising their parents, reflecting parental verbalizations, and describing their own and their parents' play. For many children, we believe these positive social communication skills generalize to sibling and peer interactions as well. Other valuable social skills for young children that are not listed as "do" skills for CDI may be targeted and coached, particularly turn-taking, sharing, and polite manners.

The "do" skill of imitation presents a natural opportunity to coach turn-taking. As the child performs an action, the parent may be coached to label it as the child's turn and then describe it. Then, as the parent imitates the child's action, the parent may be coached to label their own turn in play and to praise the child for allowing them to take a turn. To clarify for the parents how this sequence of interactions may be helpful to the child, the therapist may add an additional observation such as in the example below:

Child: (puts block on tower)
Therapist: "Now label his turn and describe it."
Parent: "You're taking a turn and putting a blue block on the tower."
Therapist: "Good. Now label your own turn and describe it."
Parent: (picks up another block) "Now I'll take my turn and add another blue block to the tower."

Child: "OK, go ahead mom."
Parent: "Thanks for letting me take my turn! Taking turns is fun."
Therapist: "Good labeled praise."
Child: "Yeah, and we're good at it! Now I get to go, right?"
Therapist: "You've taught him that taking turns can be fun, and if you keep praising him for it, he'll probably do it more when he plays with his sister."

Just as young children can be taught the early social skill of turn-taking during the context of CDI, they can be shaped into sharing and using polite manners. Most young children will offer the parent a toy at some point during the course of a play therapy session. We encourage parents to recognize this as sharing and reward the child with enthusiastic labeled praise followed by a parental act of sharing. Similarly, many young children will say "please" or "thank you" at least once during a CDI coaching session. Parents are coached to label these verbalizations as good manners, provide labeled praise, and be sure to say "please" and "thank you" as appropriate to the child. For young children who do not spontaneously share or use polite manners, we coach parents to periodically model these early social skills, clearly labeling their own behavior so that the likelihood of imitation by the child is enhanced.

Developmentally Sensitive Teaching Many parents choose to use CDI as a vehicle for developmental stimulation as well as parent-child relationship enhancement. Unfortunately, during our baseline observations of parent-child interactions, it may become apparent that the parent is not well-tuned into the child's developmental capabilities. With preschoolers, parents may overestimate the child's fine motor ability (e.g., building, drawing), grasp of spatial concepts, ability to remember sequentially presented information, and speed of mental processing. They may also underestimate the child's ability to persevere at a difficult task, to pick up after him- or herself, or to select the next item needed while building. This lack of accurate perception of a child's developmental level may become apparent during coaching. We have seen parents (1) command the child to perform a task that he or she is incapable of, (2) impatiently interfere in the child's problem-solving by taking over and completing a task for the child, (3) fail to recognize and praise the child for small increments of developmental advancement, and (4) model inappropriately advanced levels of play. Errors such as these may cause the child to feel bad about his or her own abilities or to lose interest in performing a play task that is too difficult. In addition, the parent's ability to effectively teach is compromised when input is pitched at either too high or too low a level.

To ensure that play therapy is conducted at the child's level of development, parents are encouraged to adhere to the overriding rule that the child is to remain in the lead. Parents are told that it is at this level that children are most interested in the play activity and most receptive to teaching from parents. The therapist should coach parents to (1) accurately perceive their child's developmental capabilities, (2) recognize the next step that is within the child's reach, and (3) teach the next step through subtle prompting, modeling, and shaping of successive approximations during special playtime. The following is an example of how a parent may be coached to work at the child's developmental level and stimulate learning:

Child: (draws a rough square on the chalkboard) "I'm drawing a doggy!"

Parent: "He needs a head, body, legs, a tail, a face, and a collar like your doggy, Mattie."

Child: (puts down chalk and studies own shoe)

Therapist: "I'm not sure I could remember to draw all of those parts! She's showing you with her long face that it's too hard for her. Let's back up and work at her developmental level. Point to her drawing and say, "You drew a wonderful doggy's head. I think I'll draw one just like it.""

Parent: "I love the doggy's head you drew. I think I'll make one too." (draws another square)

Therapist: "Good start! Let's focus just on the face now. Say something like, 'I'm trying hard to remember what doggies have on their faces.' Try to look puzzled."

Parent: "Hmmm, I wonder what doggies have on their faces?"

Child: "I know, eyes!" (hops up and draws eyes)

Parent: "What a great job of making eyes."

Therapist: "Good labeled praise and nice job of keeping her in the lead. Now, how can you help her think of the next thing to add without using a command?"

Parent: "This doggy can see us now because he has eyes. But if we gave him a bone he couldn't eat it."

Child: (giggles) "He needs a mouth! I can draw one."

Therapist: "Excellent job of giving her a hint that was within her developmental capability. Now she's drawn a dog's head with eyes and a mouth. If you keep this up, she'll draw the most detailed dog she's ever made. You've broken it down into small steps so she won't feel frustrated or overwhelmed."

Parent: "I knew you could make a doggy's face if we did just one part at a time. You're a smart girl and a good artist."

Task Persistence and Frustration Tolerance Many of the children we work with are easily frustrated during play as well as during early academic tasks at school. They may show their frustration by giving up when the activity becomes challenging, becoming destructive with materials, whining, crying, or throwing temper tantrums. Once a child has been identified as having difficulty in this area, several coaching strategies may be used to teach parents how to improve their child's frustration tolerance. It is important to note that in many cases, the parents do not have a high degree of tolerance for frustration themselves. This presents a double-edged sword. The parents may find it more difficult to teach positive coping techniques to their own child, but they may also benefit from learning new skills to cope with their own frustration, in turn modeling more appropriate coping skills for their young children.

After mastering basic CDI skills, parents can be coached to provide strategic praise for task persistence, attempting difficult tasks, and staying calm when experiencing frustration. Yet, some children require a more intensive approach. In such cases, parents are coached to demonstrate a mild degree of frustration with a play activity that is similar to one exhibited earlier by the child. The parent is coached to initially verbalize the frustration, then take a deep breath, count to five, and engage in positive coping statements and simple problem-solving strategies appropriate for the child's level of development. The parent instructs the child that this is something he or she can do too when frustrated and then prompts and rewards the child for engaging in positive coping strategies throughout special playtime. The following example illustrates how we might coach a parent to facilitate positive coping with frustration:

Child: (struggles to put stick in wheel, them slams Tinkertoy down) "Stupid thing. It never goes in. I can't do it."

Parent: "They're hard to put together. I'll give it a try too."

Therapist: "Good. Now model some mild frustration."

Parent: (struggles to fit pieces together) "This is so hard to put together."

Therapist: "Nice modeling of frustration. Now put the toy down, take a deep breath, close your eyes, and count to five out loud."

Parent: (takes a deep breath and closes eyes) "One, two, three, four, five."

Therapist: "Good relaxing yourself. Now talk about how you feel and model some positive coping statements."

Parent: "There. I took a deep breath and counted to five and now I don't feel so angry. Now I'm ready to try again. I know that if I keep trying I might get them to fit together. (tries to fit pieces together and succeeds, this time) Boy, am I proud of myself! I was mad but then I stopped, relaxed, and tried again. That's something you can do when you get mad too."

After the parent has learned how to model these steps for the child, the parent can cue the child to use positive coping in response to frustration at home, providing rewards in the form of praise or tangible reinforcers like happy-face stickers. Children can also be cued to go through this sequence of steps in response to frustration at daycare, preschool, and elementary school. However, it must be noted that very young children are rarely able to remember to initiate these coping responses at the appropriate times without direct cuing from a parent or teacher. To be most effective, the cue should come early in the child's frustration reaction, preventing the escalation of frustration to a high level that will inhibit effective coping.

Helping Parents Handle Aggressive and Destructive Child Behavior Most children are on their best behavior during special playtime and are rarely disruptive. After all, they have their parent's undivided attention, are playing with novel toys, and get to be in the lead. However, parents must have a strategy for handling disruptive behavior if it occurs during coaching sessions and during play sessions at home. As mentioned earlier, when children engage in mildly disruptive behavior (e.g., whining, talking back) during CDI in either the clinic or the home setting, parents are coached to address these problems using strategic attention and selective ignoring described earlier in this chapter. For more serious behaviors such as physical aggression and destructive behavior during home play sessions, we encourage parents to immediately end the special playtime. However, if aggressive or destructive behavior occurs during a clinic coaching session, we usually do not choose to suspend CDI because doing so will result in lost session time and inhibit treatment progress. Instead, we enter the room quickly and ask parents to exit and watch from the observation room. In a serious voice, we remind the child of the relevant rule of our playroom. So, if the child was hitting the parent, the therapist would review the "no hurting" rule. If the child was throwing heavy toys at the glass, the therapist would remind him of the safety rules of the playroom. When children calm immediately, the therapist leaves right away and the parent returns to CDI. When children engage in prolonged episodes of disruptive behavior, the therapist explains to the child that the child must be calm and safe before the parent will be able to come and play again. In rare cases, the child is so out of control that the therapist needs to do enthusiastic CDI to distract the child and interrupt tantruming behavior. Once the child regains emotional control, the CDI coaching can be resumed. On those rare occasions when a therapist must enter the room because of dangerous or destructive behavior, it is helpful to spend a couple of minutes putting the room back together (e.g., picking up overturned chairs) and removing any toys that were being misused, thrown, or broken. Please see Chapter 16 for additional strategies for coaching parents with extremely aggressive and explosive children.

Coaching Sessions with Siblings Most parents are able to extend the child-directed interaction skills to the targeted child's young siblings with little difficulty. However, when children are at different developmental levels, generalization of skills can be enhanced by having one session in which the parent is coached with the referred child and with each of his or her siblings in turn. Usually the referred child feels somewhat proprietary about special playtime in the clinic setting. For this reason, we always include some period of coaching for the referred child, even though the greater focus in this session may be on coaching the parent's use of skills with the siblings. For a more complete discussion of how to incorporate siblings into PCIT, please see Chapter 11.

End-of-Session Debriefing and Homework Assignment

We reserve the last 10 min of each coaching session for providing feedback to parents on their skills progress and discussing the upcoming week's homework. Many parents are motivated by viewing the PCIT Progress sheet. This is a record of their CDI skill acquisition and ECBI changes across sessions. They are able to view their progress from week to week, as well as monitor how close they are to reaching the mastery criteria for CDI and moving on to the discipline portion of PCIT. Feedback should begin by noting for parents areas of progress in the "do" and "avoid" skills, child responsiveness to these skills, and improvements in qualitative aspects of the parent-child interaction. It is important that constructive feedback be given as well that highlights areas needing further work. However, as with the coaching, the therapist must carefully attend to the balance of positive and corrective feedback so that parents leave the session feeling both encouraged by their progress and motivated to work hard in the upcoming week. Between CDI coaching sessions, parents are asked to complete a daily five-minute special playtime at home and to record their practice on their homework sheet.

Progression of CDI Coaching Sessions

The strategies and procedures described in this chapter apply to all CDI coaching sessions. Yet, there is a typical progression in what is emphasized in each coaching session (Table 5.6 presents the typical progression of CDI coaching sessions). In general, behavioral descriptions are focused on in the first coaching session, while there is a greater emphasis on reflections and avoiding questions in the second session. The third coaching session emphasizes labeled praise and fine tuning of PRIDE skills, and later sessions focus on specific drills for particular skills that have not been mastered. There is no fixed number of CDI sessions. CDI coaching continues until parents meet the 10-10-10 set of mastery criteria (with 3 or fewer commands + questions + negative talk). Thus, some families may be coached in CDI for only two sessions, whereas others may require six or more CDI coaching sessions.

Table 5.6 Typical progression of CDI coaching sessions

Session #1
Labeled praise for all PRIDE skills and ignoring
Provide only positive feedback. Do not point out mistakes in this session
Focus coaching primarily on behavioral description
In homework, parents are encouraged to focus on decreasing questions and increasing reflections
Session #2
Review "Parents are Models for their Children" handout and discuss anger control
Labeled praise for all PRIDE skills and ignoring
Focus coaching primarily on increasing reflections and avoiding questions
Go over CDI mastery criteria
In homework, parents are encouraged to focus on increasing labeled praise
Session #3
Review "Getting Support" handout and discuss family's social support network
Fine-tune all PRIDE skills and ignoring
Focus coaching primarily on labeled praise and qualitative aspects of the interaction
In homework, parents are encouraged to focus on skills not yet mastered
Session #4 and beyond
Review "Kids and Stress" handout
Labeled praise for all PRIDE skills and ignoring
Conduct 2–3-minute coaching drills on whatever skills are weak
If mastery criteria are met, introduce PDI, and remind them that child does not attend the next session
In homework, parents are encouraged to focus on skills not yet mastered

For handouts listed above, see Eyberg (1999) available at www.pcit.org.

What if a Caregiver Does Not Reach CDI Mastery?

We often are asked how to handle cases in which a caregiver has had numerous CDI coaching sessions (e.g., ten or more) and still has not reached mastery. The therapist should try coding this type of family more than once during a CDI session to determine whether coaching and anxiety reduction enhance performance. Sometimes a family can meet the mastery criteria at the middle of a session but not at the beginning. Unfortunately, however, these cases often involve families who do not practice CDI at home as prescribed. The first question for a therapist to consider is whether he or she has done everything to motivate the parent to buy in to CDI and to complete homework. Then, the therapist should examine the issues in failing to reach mastery. If the parent is able to follow the child's lead and is missing mastery by only a couple of questions or a few PRIDE statements, it is possible that moving forward is an appropriate step. After all, CDI coding and coaching will continue in the PDI sessions. Sometimes parents have greater CDI buy-in after PDI has begun to work. If the parent simply is "not getting CDI," the therapist should be cautious about moving forward. PDI is likely to be difficult and possibly ineffective without the relationship enhancement. Occasionally, a family may only be motivated by the consequence that treatment may be suspended or even terminated unless the caregiver is able to commit to the daily homework requirement (e.g., a family with a history of abuse that is doing only the bare minimum to regain parental rights). A similar issue that often arises is in dual-caregiver families when one parent reaches mastery faster than the other parent. Do we move forward with the caregiver who has reached mastery or hold the family until both caregivers attain mastery? With this decision, we usually consider the degree of involvement of the caregiver who has not reached mastery. If that caregiver is the primary caregiver or highly involved in the parenting of the child, we might choose to slow progression to allow that caregiver to "catch up." For us, however, the ultimate issue question is this one: "What is in the best interest of the child?" If a family is getting highly frustrated with the overabundance of CDI sessions and is at risk of dropping out of treatment, it may be in the child's best interest to move forward to PDI. Whereas PCIT will be less effective when the family does not reach mastery, it may be even more ineffective if the family terminates prematurely. As these decisions are made on a case-by-case basis using clinical experience, we recommend taking advantage of a seasoned PCIT consultant or colleagues on the PCIT list serve (sign up at www.pcit.org) when making such judgments. One of the strongest aspects of PCIT is the large change in parenting skill that occurs when enforcing the high standards of the mastery criteria. Allowing a parent to move forward without mastery should be a rare exception. By valuing and following the mastery criteria, we can ensure that each family receives its optimal "dose" of CDI.

References

Eyberg, S.M. (n.d.). *Parent-child interaction therapy: Basic coaching guidelines introduction*. A Power Point presentation retrieved 8 Apr 2008, from http://www.pcit.org

Eyberg, S.M. (1999). *Parent-child interaction therapy: Integrity checklists and session materials*. Retrieved 2 Apr 2008, from www.pcit.org

McNeil, C.B. (2008). *Parent-child interaction therapy*. A 2-hour DVD in the APA Psychotherapy Training Video Series hosted by Jon Carlson.

Reprinted by permission from Springer: McNeil, C.B., & Hembree-Kigin, T. (2010). *Parent-Child Interaction Therapy: Second Edition (Chapter 5)*. New York: Springer.

Appendix B: Understanding Your Child's Behavior: Reading Your Child's Cues from Birth to Age 2, Center on the Social and Emotional Foundations for Early Learning (CSEFEL)

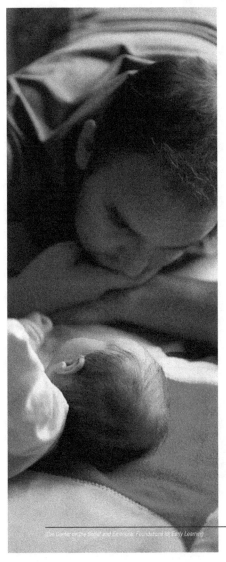

Understanding Your
Child's Behavior:

Reading Your Child's Cues from Birth to Age 2

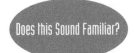

Does this Sound Familiar?

Jayden, age 9 months, has been happily putting cereal pieces into his mouth. He pauses for a moment and then uses his hands to scatter the food across his high chair tray. He catches his father's eye, gives him a big smile, and drops a piece of cereal on the floor. When his father picks it up, Jayden kicks his legs, waves his arms, and laughs. He throws another piece of cereal. His dad smiles and says, "Jayden, it looks like you are all done eating. Is that right?" He picks Jayden up and says, "How about we throw a ball instead of your food, okay?"

The Center on the Social and Emotional Foundations for Early Learning   Vanderbilt University   vanderbilt.edu/csefel

© Springer Nature Switzerland AG 2018
E. I. Girard et al., *Parent-Child Interaction Therapy with Toddlers*,
https://doi.org/10.1007/978-3-319-93251-4

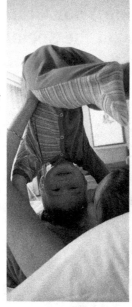

Naomi, age 30 months, is happily playing with her blocks. All of a sudden, her mother looks at the clock, gasps, and says, "Naomi, I lost track of time! We need to go meet your brother at the school bus! Let's go." She scoops Naomi up and rushes toward the kitchen door. Naomi shouts, "NO!" and tries to slide out of her mother's arms to run back to her blocks. When her mother puts on Naomi's sneakers, she kicks them off, slaps her mother's hands, and repeats, "No! I STAY! I playing blocks!" Naomi's mother sighs with frustration and buckles her into the stroller with no shoes. This sets off another round of protests: "My SHOES! Where my SHOES?" Naomi pulls at her stroller's buckle, trying to unfasten it, and kicks, screams, and cries all the way to the bus stop.

The Focus

Babies and toddlers might just be learning to talk—but they have many other ways to tell parents how they are feeling! Children can experience the same emotions that adults do, but they express those feelings differently. Jayden is giving his father many clues that he is done eating. First, he begins to play by sweeping the food across his tray. Then he drops food on the floor in an attempt to get his Dad to play the "I Drop It, You Get It" game. Jayden's father notices and responds to these "cues," by calling an end to mealtime and giving Jayden a chance to play. Naomi is also very clear about her feelings. She doesn't like having to make a transition from a fun activity (blocks) so quickly. She is giving her mother many "cues" too—her words, facial expressions, and actions are all saying, "This transition was too quick for me. I

was having fun and I can't move on so quickly."

Children's behavior has meaning— it's just that adults don't always understand what the meaning is. In the early years, before children have strong language skills, it can be especially hard to understand what a baby or toddler is trying to communicate. This resource will help you better understand your child's behavior cues and help you respond in ways that support his or her healthy social and communication development.

What to Expect: Communication Skills

Birth to 12 Months

Did you know that crying is really just a baby's way of trying to tell you something? Your baby's cry can mean many different things, including, "I'm tired," "I don't know how to settle myself," "I'm in pain or discomfort," or "I want the toy you just picked up." In the first year, babies will gradually begin to use gestures and sounds to communicate. But many parents find the first 12 months one of the most difficult times to understand the meaning of their babies' behaviors. Below are some common ways babies communicate. With time, you will figure out your baby's unique way of communicating.

Sounds: Crying is your baby's primary communication tool. You might find that your baby uses different cries for hunger, discomfort (like a wet diaper), or pain (like a tummy ache). Paying attention to the sounds of these cries helps you make a good guess about what your baby is trying to communicate.

Language: Right around the one-year mark (for some babies earlier, and for some babies later), your baby will say his or her first word. While at first your child's language skills will seem to grow slowly, right around the two-year mark they will really take off!

Facial Expressions: The meaning of a smile is easy to understand. But you will also get to know your baby's questioning or curious face, along with expressions of frustration,

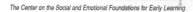

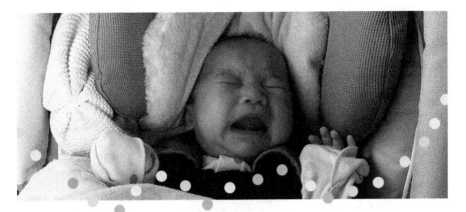

pleasure, excitement, boredom, and more. Remember, babies experience the same basic emotions we do: happiness, sadness, curiosity, anxiety, frustration, excitement, and so on.

Gaze: Look where your baby is looking and it will tell you a lot about what he or she is thinking. An overstimulated or tired baby will often break eye contact with you and look away. A baby who wants to play will have a bright gaze focused right on you or the toy she is interested in!

Gestures: Babies use their bodies in many ways to communicate. They reach for people and objects, pick objects up, sweep objects away with their hands, wave their arms and hands and kick their feet, and point (just to name a few). Babies will also turn away from sounds they don't like or arch backwards if they are upset.

Putting It Together

Babies use their whole body to communicate. So, for example, a baby might focus a bright, clear gaze on a new toy, and then look to you, then back at the toy. She might kick her legs or swing her arms excitedly. The baby might then reach for the toy while making excited "eh eh!" sounds

and smiling. While babies don't think in words yet, the message this baby is sending might be, "What is that thing? I want to see it. Can you give it to me? It looks like fun!"

Or imagine a baby who is happily playing with an older cousin. The cousin is puffing out his cheeks and then letting the air out, making a loud whooshing sound. The baby is laughing, kicking, and waving his arms. All of a sudden, though, the baby's response changes. He looks away and his expression turns to one of distress. He kicks his legs and arches his back. He starts to cry. The message this baby is sending might be, "That was fun for a while. But now it's too much. I need a break."

12 Months to 24 Months
In the second year, young toddlers are becoming more skilled at communicating their needs and desires to you. Here are more examples of how young toddlers' communication skills are growing and changing from 12 to 24 months.

Sounds and Language: Your young toddler's vocabulary is growing slowly but steadily across his or her second year of life. Pronunciation might not be perfect, like "muh" for milk, but that will

come with time. Your toddler also understands more words than ever before. In fact, he probably understands more words than he can actually say! For example, if you ask him to touch his nose, chances are, he will be able to do so.

Even as your toddler's language skills are growing, cries are still the main way to communicate strong emotions like anger, frustration, sadness, or feeling overwhelmed. You might also see your toddler squeal with laughter and scream in delighted glee when he is too excited for words!

Facial Expressions and Gaze: Toddlers make some of the best expressions ever, so keep your camera handy during this second year of life. You can see delight, curiosity, jealousy, and other feelings play across their faces. Young children also use eye contact to communicate with you. For example, you might see your toddler gazing at you to get your attention (Won't you come play with me?). You might also see your child watching you to learn something new (Now how do I press the cell phone buttons?).

Your toddler also watches your reactions to make sense of new situations (I am not sure I want Uncle Joe to hold me. I am going to check your face to see if you think he is he okay or not.) Often you will find that your child mirrors your own expressions and gestures—if you take a bite of broccoli and crinkle your nose, chances are good that your toddler will too.

Gestures: Young toddlers are more talented than ever at using their bodies to communicate. They can walk, run, point, take your hand, show you things, carry and move objects, climb, open and shut things, and more. Watching your toddler's body language and gestures will give you lots of information about what she is thinking about, what she wants, or what she is feeling.

Putting It Together

Over time, it becomes easier to understand your child's cues and messages. Young toddlers are skilled at using their bodies, expressions, and growing language skills to communicate their needs more clearly than ever before. A 14-month-old might creep over to the book basket, choose a favorite story, creep back to her uncle, and tap the book on his leg while saying, "Buh." A 20-month-old might pick up her sandals and then walk to the back door, turn to her grandmother and say, "Go park." These interactions are really an amazing developmental leap for toddlers! They are now able to hold an idea in their minds ("I want to read a book and not just any book, this book") and understand how to communicate that idea to the people who can make it happen!

Three Steps to Understanding Your Baby's or Toddler's Behavior

When you see a behavior you don't understand, think about these "clues" to try to figure out what the behavior means for your child. Remember, every child is different. The same behavior (for example, a baby who is arching her back while being held) can mean that one baby is tired and that another baby wants to be put down so she can stretch out and play. Getting to know your child's unique cues is an important way that you can show your child that you love and understand him or her.

Step 1: Observe and interpret your child's behavior:

• Notice the sounds (or words) your baby or toddler is using. Does your child sound happy, sad, frustrated, bored, or hungry? When have your heard this cry or sound before?

• What is your child's facial expression? What feelings are you seeing on your child's face? Is your baby looking at a new object with interest? Perhaps he is trying to say, "Hand that to me so I can touch it."

• Notice your child's gaze. Is your baby holding eye contact with you or has she looked away? (That is usually a sign that a baby needs a break.) Is your toddler holding your gaze? Perhaps she is trying to get your

attention or wants to see how you are reacting to a new situation.

• What gestures or movements is your child using? Is your baby rubbing her eyes and pulling on her ear when you try to hold her? She might feel sleepy and be ready for a nap. An older toddler who is on the verge of beginning potty training might start to hide behind a chair or go into a closet to have a bowel movement.

• Think about what's going on when you see a behavior you don't understand. Does this behavior happen at a certain time of day (like at child care drop-off or bedtime)? Does this behavior tend to happen in a certain place (like the brightly lit, noisy mall)? Does the behavior happen in a particular situation (like when your child must cope with many other children at one time, like at the playground)?

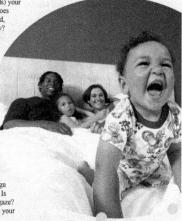

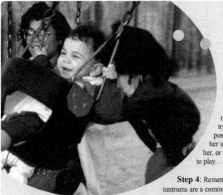

validate his feelings. If your four-month-old is crying but refuses a bottle, try changing her position—picking her up and rocking her, or putting her down to play.

Step 4: Remember that tantrums are a communication, too. A tantrum usually means that your child is not able to calm himself down. Tantrums are no fun for anyone. They feel overwhelming and even scary for young children. For adults, it is easy to get upset when you see upsetting behavior. But what frequently happens is that when you get really upset, your child's tantrum gets even bigger. Although it can be difficult, when you are able to stay calm during these intense moments, it often helps your child calm down, too.

Another strategy to try when you child is "losing it" is to re-state how your child seems to be feeling, while reflecting her strong emotions. You might say in a very excited voice, "You are telling me that you just cannot wait for the birthday party! It is just tooooo hard for you to wait! You want to go the party right now!" For some children, having you "mirror" their intense feelings lets them know that you understand them and take them seriously, which helps them calm down. Experiment to see which response works best to calm your child.

Remember: You can't always understand what your child is trying to communicate. Even in adult

Step 2: Respond to your baby or toddler based on what you think the meaning of his or her behavior is. It's okay if you are not sure if your guess is right. Just try something. Remember, you can always try again. For example, if your 11-month-old is pointing toward the window, lift him up so he can see outside. Even though you might discover he was really pointing to a spider on the wall, the very fact that you tried to understand and respond lets him know that his communications are important to you. This motivates him to keep trying to connect with you. When you respond to your child, say out loud what you think his behavior might mean. For example, you might say to the toddler you pick up, "Are you saying that you want up? I can pick you up." By using language to describe what the child is communicating, you will be teaching your child the meaning of words.

Step 3: If your first try didn't work, try again. Trying different techniques increases the chances that you will figure out the meaning of your child's behavior, understand his needs, and

relationships, we sometimes find ourselves wondering about the meaning of another person's behavior. But these moments—when your child is distressed and you can't figure out why—can be very stressful for parents. If you feel as though you really cannot handle your baby or toddler in the moment, it's okay to put him or her somewhere safe (like a crib) and take a few minutes for yourself. Taking care of you is important. You will make better parenting choices and be able to meet your child's needs more effectively if you are feeling calm and together.

Wrapping Up

Babies and toddlers experience and express thoughts and feelings. Often they communicate their strong feelings through behaviors that adults understand right away—like a baby's big toothless grin when she sees her grandma coming. Other times, very young children's behavior can be confusing or even frustrating to the adults who care for them. Being able to stay calm, make a good guess at what the behavior might mean, and then respond helps children understand that they are powerful communicators. Over the long-term, this helps children learn how to connect with others in ways that are healthy and respectful—a skill they'll use for life.

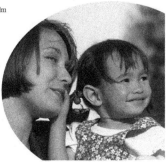

The Center on the Social and Emotional Foundations for Early Learning

Child Care Bureau

Office of Head Start

Appendix C: Sleep Needs Guide for Infants 0 to 3 Years Old, Karitane

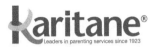

Sleep Needs Guide for Infants 0 to 3 Years
This is a guide only, variations may be needed to meet the individual child's needs

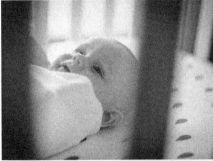

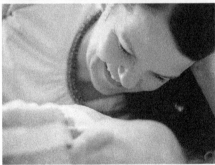

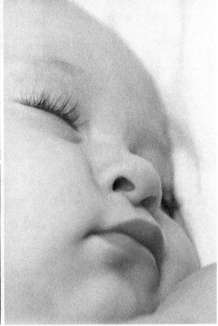

Karitane provides advice and support to families during the early years of parenting.

Karitane offers a comprehensive range of evidence-based parenting services to support families with parenting skills, including: sleep and settling, toddler behaviour, establishing routines, feeding and nutrition and perinatal mood disorders.

Our healthcare professionals guide, support and educate families to ensure a safe and nurturing environment for their children.

Parenting help is only a call away or available 24 hours on our website.

Careline: 1300 CARING (1300 227 464)
www.karitane.com.au/mybabyandme

© Springer Nature Switzerland AG 2018
E. I. Girard et al., *Parent-Child Interaction Therapy with Toddlers*,
https://doi.org/10.1007/978-3-319-93251-4

A daily guide for children 0 to 3 year

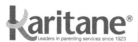

Leaders in parenting services since 1923

Our vision is for children to be safe, healthy and nurtured by confident families and communities.

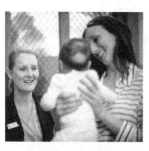

This is a guide only, variations may be needed to meet the individual child's needs.

0-6 month Guide

0-6 WEEKS

FEED
2–4 hourly

AVERAGE NUMBER OF FEEDS
6–10 feeds in 24 hours

AWAKE (FEED & PLAY)
Around 1 hour

SLEEP/REST
1.5–3 hours per sleep

AVERAGE NUMBER OF SLEEPS
5–6 sleeps in 24 hours

TYPE OF FOODS
Milk feeds

TIRED SIGNS
- Clenched fists
- Facial contortions
- Jerky movements
- Grizzling or crying
- Rubbing eyes
- Yawning
- Staring

6 WEEKS-3 MONTHS

FEED
2–4 hourly

AVERAGE NUMBER OF FEEDS
6–8 feeds in 24 hours

AWAKE (FEED & PLAY)
1 - 1.5 hours

SLEEP/REST
1.5–2.5 hours

AVERAGE NUMBER OF SLEEPS
4–5 sleeps in 24 hours

TYPE OF FOODS
Milk feeds

TIRED SIGNS
- Clenched fists
- Facial contortions
- Jerky movements
- Grizzling or crying
- Rubbing eyes
- Yawning
- Staring

3-4.5 MONTHS

FEED
3–4 hourly

AVERAGE NUMBER OF FEEDS
5–6 feeds in 24 hours

AWAKE (FEED & PLAY)
1.5 - 2 hours

SLEEP/REST
1.5–2.5 hours

AVERAGE NUMBER OF SLEEPS
3 daytime sleeps

TYPE OF FOODS
Milk feeds

TIRED SIGNS
- Clenched fists
- Facial contortions
- Jerky movements
- Grizzling or crying
- Rubbing eyes
- Yawning
- Staring

4.5-6 MONTHS

FEED
3–4 hourly

AVERAGE NUMBER OF FEEDS
4–6 feeds in 24 hours

AWAKE (FEED & PLAY)
2 – 2.5 hours

SLEEP/REST
1.5–2 hours

AVERAGE NUMBER OF SLEEPS
3 daytime sleeps

TYPE OF FOODS
Introduce solids around 6 months
Milk feeds

TIRED SIGNS
- Clenched fists
- Facial contortions
- Jerky movements
- Grizzling or crying
- Rubbing eyes
- Yawning
- Staring

rs

6 months - 3 years Guide

6-9 MONTHS

FEED
3-4 milk feeds.
Introduce solids.
Increase 3 meals + 2 snacks
per day (start with milk then solids)
AWAKE (FEED & PLAY)
2-3 hours
SLEEP/REST
1-2 hours
AVERAGE NUMBER OF SLEEPS
2 daytime sleeps
TYPE OF FOODS
Milk feeds
Solids
TIRED SIGNS
- Upset
- Irritable or whingey
- Clingy or fussy
- Unco-operative
- Short concentration span
- Lose co-ordination or clumsy
- Rub their eyes or yawn
- Bored with toys

9-12 MONTHS

FEED
3-4 milk feeds.
3 meals + 2 snacks per day
AWAKE (FEED & PLAY)
3-4 hours
SLEEP/REST
1-3 hours
AVERAGE NUMBER OF SLEEPS
1-2 hours per sleep
TYPE OF FOODS
Solids
Milk feeds
TIRED SIGNS
- Upset
- Irritable or whingey
- Clingy or fussy
- Unco-operative
- Short concentration span
- Lose co-ordination or clumsy
- Rub their eyes or yawn
- Bored with toys

12-18 MONTHS

FEED
1-1½ serves of dairy
3 meals + 2 snacks per day
AWAKE (FEED & PLAY)
4-6 hours
SLEEP/REST
1-3 hours in total
AVERAGE NUMBER OF SLEEPS
1-2 daytime sleeps
TYPE OF FOODS
Family Foods and all drinks from
a cup
TIRED SIGNS
- Upset
- Irritable or whingey
- Clingy or fussy
- Unco-operative
- Short concentration span
- Lose co-ordination or clumsy
- Rub their eyes or yawn
- Bored with toys

18 MONTHS - 3 YEARS

FEED
1½-2½ serves of dairy
3 meals + 2 snacks per day
AWAKE (FEED & PLAY)
5-7 hours
SLEEP/REST
1-2 hours
AVERAGE NUMBER OF SLEEPS
1 daytime sleeps
TYPE OF FOODS
Family Foods and all drinks from
a cup
TIRED SIGNS
- Upset
- Irritable or whingey
- Clingy or fussy
- Unco-operative
- Short concentration span
- Lose co-ordination or clumsy
- Rub their eyes or yawn
- Bored with toys

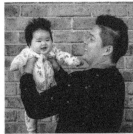
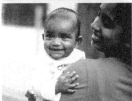
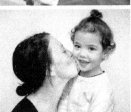
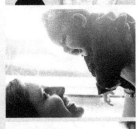
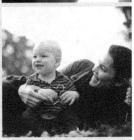

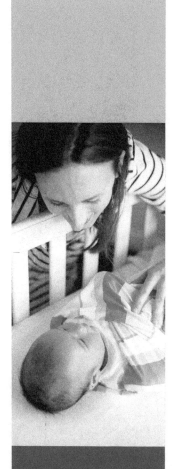

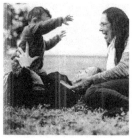

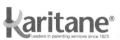
Leaders in parenting services since 1923

Contact Details

Phone	02 9794 2300
Fax	02 9794 2323
Postal	PO Box 241, Villawood NSW 2163
Email	karitane.online@sswahs.nsw.gov.au
Website	www.karitane.com.au

Karitane - Carramar
Head Office, Residential Unit, Jade House, Toddler Clinic,
Education & Research Centre, Venue Hire
126-150 The Horsley Drive, Carramar NSW 2163
(Entrance via Mitchell Street)
Phone 02 9794 2300   Fax 02 9794 2323

Karitane Camden
Residential, Perinatal Mental Health, Parenting Centre,
Toddler Clinic
Camden Hospital, Menangle Road, Camden NSW 2560
Phone 02 4654 6125   Fax 02 4654 6213

Randwick Parenting Centre
146 Avoca Street, Randwick NSW 2031
Phone 02 9399 6999   Fax 02 9399 8510

Liverpool Parenting Centre
10 Murphy Avenue, Liverpool NSW 2170
Phone 02 9821 4555   Fax 02 9821 4559

Karitane Linking Families
130 Nelson Street, Fairfield Heights NSW 2165
Phone 02 9754 2655   Fax 02 9754 2644

Connecting Carers & Talking Realities
124 The Horsley Drive, Carramar NSW 2163
Phone 02 9794 2352   Fax 02 9794 2381
www.connectingcarersnsw.com.au

Karitane Referrals and Intake
Phone 02 9794 2300   Fax 02 9794 2323
Email   karitane.referrals@sswahs.nsw.gov.au

Careline & Parenting Website
Phone   1300 CARING (1300 227 464)
Email   karitane.online@sswahs.nsw.gov.au
Website www.karitane.com.au/mybabyandme

Follow us on

ABN 25000018842   Updated May 2016 - FAM002.
References available on request. Consumer Reviewed.

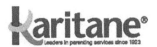

TIPS FOR SLEEP AND BEDTIME
Newborn to toddler

There are many ways you can support your child to go to sleep, and finding the strategy that best suits you and your family can be challenging. To move into sleep your child needs to feel safe, secure and relaxed plus be physically ready for sleep.

At Karitane, we use strategies which respond to your baby's cues.

If you are changing the way you settle your baby, allow a few days/weeks to adjust to the new strategy.

Remember:
• Be consistent
• If you have had enough, or your baby is becoming distressed, stop and calmly pick up your baby. Responding to your baby's cues will help them feel contained, safe and secure

It's really important that your child learns to feel safe and secure, so they can relax and move naturally into sleep.

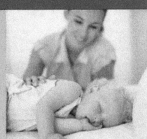

For more information, refer to our "Understanding Sleep" brochure or our parenting website www.karitane.com.au

Be patient – change takes time, don't be afraid to seek help!

| 0 mth | 3 mth | 6 mth | 9 mth | 12 mth | 15+ mth |

Settling in Arms

Hands-on Settling

Comfort Settling

Parental Presence

Gradual Withdrawal

Settling in Arms
Recommended for: 0 - 3 months and beyond

This strategy can be useful for young babies, or an older baby having difficulty settling.
• Cradle your baby in your arms, with or without gentle rocking, until your baby is calm. In the early days, you may need to hold your baby until they fall asleep.
• Gently place your baby in their cot on their back.
• If your baby stirs or becomes upset when placed in the cot, stay with your baby and offer comfort until calm
• You can combine some of the Hands-on Settling suggestions below to support your baby to move into sleep
• If your baby becomes distressed pick up your baby and return to the first step

Hands-on Settling
Recommended for: 0 - 6 months and beyond

• Following quiet time and sleep routine (e.g. wrap, story, and cuddle) place your baby in their cot on their back
• Watch and respond to the cues your baby is giving you
• If your baby remains calm, allow your baby to settle on their own. If they start to cry, try any of the following to provide comfort and reassurance:
• Gentle 'ssshhh' sounds
• Pat gently and rhythmically, e.g. thigh, shoulder, tummy or pat the mattress
• Talk quietly, using comforting tones, e.g. 'its ok', 'time for sleep'
• Gently touch or stroke your baby's head, arm, or leg
• Gently rock the cot in a slow, rhythmic movement to calm your baby.
• If at any time you feel like you've had enough, or your baby is not calming, stop and use a different strategy such as 'Settling in Arms'

Comfort Settling
Recommended for: 6 months and beyond

Comfort settling is different to 'Hands-on' setting in that it allows some space for your baby to discover their own way of going to sleep.
• Quiet time and preparation for sleep routine (e.g. bath, wrap, story, and cuddle)
• Place your baby in the cot awake on their back
• If this is a new strategy, stay in the room for a few minutes and make gentle 'shh shh' sounds
• If your baby remains calm, leave the room. If unsettled, stay and provide reassurance until calm
• When you leave the room, remain somewhere close by in case more reassurance is needed
• If your baby starts making noises, wait before you intervene. Babbling, whinging, brief cries and movement are common when a baby is trying to settle
• If your baby's cries go up and down in volume, wait a short time to see if they will go to sleep
• If the noise continues to increase, return to your baby and offer comfort while your baby is still in the cot

If this is not working, use the techniques from 'Hands-on' or 'Settling in Arms'. Try again next sleep cycle as baby learns with consistent and predictable patterns.

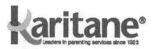

TIPS FOR SLEEP AND BEDTIME

Parental Presence

Recommended for: 6 months and beyond

This strategy is useful if your baby becomes distressed when you leave the room. It may take from 1 – 4 weeks. During the day stay in the baby's room until they are asleep and during the night sleep in the baby's room.

- Have a quiet, calm room that is dimly lit
- Have a bed or mattress in the room for you to lie on
- Stay in view, remain calm, close your eyes and breathe slowly
- If your baby wakes, make a small noise or movement to let them know that you are still there without interacting directly
- If your baby is crying and needs reassurance, offer comfort such as 'shhh' sounds or gentle soft words such as 'time for sleep now'. Move on to other forms of comfort as needed
- Aim to have your baby stay in their cot. Once your baby is calm, lie down, close your eyes and breathe slowly
- If at any time you feel like you've had enough, or your baby continues to be distressed, stop and use a different strategy such as 'Hands-on' or 'Settling in Arms'
- Once your baby has had 3 consecutive nights of relatively uninterrupted sleep, begin to leave the room before your baby is asleep and move to your own room

Gradual Withdrawal

Recommended for: 12 months and beyond

The aim of Gradual Withdrawal is for your child to learn to fall asleep without your help. This is a good strategy when moving from a cot to a bed.

Gradual Withdrawal starts with you being close to your child while they fall asleep. Over the next few days or weeks, you slowly move further away until your child is confident to settle on their own.

- Put your child in bed and start by sitting beside or on the bed. Your child may like some physical contact initially, e.g. holding hands
- Reassure your child that if they stay in bed, you will remain until they have fallen asleep (e.g. end of bed, on a chair in the room)

Reviewed February 2016 · FAM005. References available on request.

- Avoid discussions and responding to requests such as 'I want a drink' or 'another story'
- If your child continually gets out of bed, calmly take your child back to bed
- Over the following days or weeks, gradually increase the distance between you, until eventually you are outside the room
- Once outside the room, reassure your child that you are nearby. If your child leaves the bed, walk them back calmly saying "it's time for bed"

During the day, if your child does not actually go to sleep, don't be discouraged. Each attempt to settle in bed is a valuable learning experience.

Alternate Strategies to Calm your Baby

Settling in a Pram

Sometimes using a pram to settle your baby can be a short-term option, such as when you are out.

It may also work at home when your baby won't settle in the cot. We recommend that this is only done during the day and have your baby facing you.

When out and about

- It is best not to cover the pram. However if there are bright lights or other distractions, try using a hood to allow for air flow and have baby facing you
- Regularly check that your baby is not getting too hot and is settled

When at home

- Use the pram as a last resort
- Movement may help calm your baby. Try walking the pram around the house (on one level) or take your baby for a walk outside in the pram

If you are feeling overwhelmed or stressed:

S-T-O-P: Stop what you are doing - **T**ake a few breaths - **O**bserve (what is happening? how am I feeling? what is best to do next?) – **P**roceed

Here are a few suggestions you can try:

- Place your baby gently in the cot and leave the room. Your baby is safe there while you calm yourself
- Take a few deep, slow breaths. Stretch or walk outside for a moment
- Phone your Child and Family Health Centre or a friend or relative for support
- Call the Karitane Careline on 1300 227 464

Need Help?

Don't hesitate to seek help from family, friends or the Karitane Careline
1300 CARING (1300 227 464)

www.karitane.com.au
PO Box 241, Villawood NSW 2163
Tel: 02 9794 2300 Fax: 02 9794 2323
ABN 25 000 018 842 Charity No.: 12991

For Parenting information:
www.karitane.com.au/mybabyandme
Karitane.online@sswahs.nsw.gov.au
Careline 1300 CARING (1300 227 464)

Appendix D: Teaching Your Child to Become Independent with Daily Routines, Center on the Social and Emotional Foundations for Early Learning (CSEFEL)

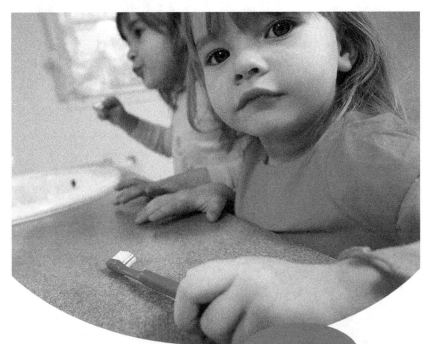

Teaching Your Child to:

Become Independent with Daily Routines

Does this Sound Familiar?

Nadine is a single mom with two young children ages 3 and 5. Her children attend preschool while she is working. When they all get home at the end of the day, Nadine is exhausted but still has household chores to complete (i.e., making dinner, doing laundry, straightening the house, etc.). In addition, she has to help the children with bathing, getting ready for bed, and brushing their teeth. She wishes that her children would start doing some of their daily self-help routines independently. The preschool teacher has said that the 5-year-old is very helpful and independent. But at home, neither of the children will get dressed and undressed independently, and they complain and whine when asked to wash their hands, brush their teeth, or help with the

The Center on the Social and Emotional Foundations for Early Learning   *Vanderbilt University*   *vanderbilt.edu/csefel*

bathtime routine. When Nadine asks the children to do one of these self-help tasks, they run around the house or whine and drop to the ground. It takes every ounce of energy Nadine has to get through the evening. Often she finds herself yelling at the children and physically helping them through the entire routine, just to get it done.

The Focus

Young children can learn how to do simple daily self-help activities—they just need to be taught what to do. When teaching a child to do self-care skills, you first need to know what you can typically expect of a young child, your child's skill level, and how to provide clear and simple instructions about how to do a task. In addition, providing children with ample encouragement that is both positive and specific will help promote their success. Children can learn, at a very young age, how to independently wash their hands, brush their teeth, and get undressed and dressed. The information below will help you understand what you can expect from your preschooler and tips for helping your child learn how to become more independent with daily routines.

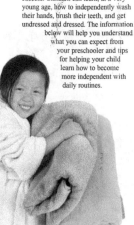

What to Expect

Children who are 8 to 18 months old often can:

- Drink from a cup, pick up finger food, and begin to use a spoon
- Help undress and dress, put foot in shoe and arm in sleeve
- Point to body parts
- Have strong feelings and begin saying "no"
- Reach for/point to choices
- Feel a sense of security with routines and expectations (e.g., at bedtime)
- Imitate sounds and movement
- Understand more than they can say

Children who are 18 to 36 months old often can do all of the above and:

- Wash hands with help
- Drink from a straw
- Put clothes in the hamper when asked
- Feed self with spoon
- Push and pull toys; fill and dump containers
- Learn to use the toilet
- Bend over without falling
- Imitate simple actions
- Become easily frustrated
- Enjoy trying to do tasks on their own (note that this is why tasks may now take more time to complete)

- Pouring, washing, dressing
- Enjoy playing dress-up
- Become fascinated with water and sand play
- Begin learning simple clear rules

Children who are 3 often can:
- Help with brushing teeth
- Understand "now," "soon," and "later"
- Put dirty clothes in the hamper independently
- Get shoes from the closet
- Put on shoes without ties
- Enjoy singing easy songs
- Listen more attentively
- At times, prefer one parent over the other
- Enjoy playing house
- Imitate
- Match like objects
- Put non-breakable dishes in the sink
- Put trash in the trash can
- Wash body with help
- Wash and dry hands, though they may need some help reaching

Children who are 4 often can:
- Use a spoon, fork, and dinner knife
- Dress without help, except with fasteners/buttons
- Learn new words quickly
- Recognize stop signs and their own name in print
- Follow two-step directions that are unrelated

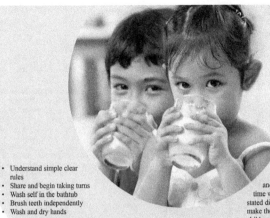

- Understand simple clear rules
- Share and begin taking turns
- Wash self in the bathtub
- Brush teeth independently
- Wash and dry hands

Children who are 5 often can:
- Follow established rules and routines (e.g., wash hands before eating, put dirty clothes in the hamper, brush teeth before going to bed)
- Independently initiate a simple routine (e.g., dress and undress, brush teeth, wash hands, eat dinner sitting at the table, take bath with adult watching)
- Understand beginning, middle, and end
- Begin to understand others' feelings
- Be independent with most self-care skills

Sometimes, children with disabilities may need special assistance to become more independent in doing daily routines. You might want to do the following:
- Expect your child to do only part of the routine, while you assist with the part that is difficult
- Provide help to your child so that he/she can complete the task
- Provide instructions in a different format, by modeling and/or using a picture or gesture so that your child understands what to do
- Allow extra time to complete the task

Teaching Your Child to Independently Complete Daily Routines

Young children like to feel independent, but sometimes they need a parent's encouragement to feel that they are capable and that adults believe that they "can" do it. Teaching independence with self-help skills like hand washing, brushing teeth, and dressing/undressing is an important step in development that can be achieved when children are taught how to do each step in each routine. Initially, it takes an adult's focused attention to teach children how to do these skills. Once the child learns how to do a skill independently, the adult can fade out of the routine completely.

When teaching your child independence in self help routines (brushing teeth, hand washing, getting dressed/undressed), try these simple, yet effective, tips:

1. Begin by getting down on your child's eye level and gaining his attention. (i.e., touch your child gently, make eye contact, physically guide, or jointly look at the same object).

2. Break down the routine into simple steps and state each step one at a time with positive and clearly stated directions. Sometimes we make the mistake of telling children what not to do or what they did wrong, such as, "Stop splashing in the water." However, it's more effective and clear to say, "All done washing, now it's time to turn off the water."

3. To clarify steps even further, you could take a photo of each step in the routine and post it where the routine takes place. For instance, with hand washing, you could post photos above the sink. As you state one step at a time, show your child the photograph to illustrate what needs to be done.

4. When teaching your child to do each step, model (i.e., demonstrate) how to do each step. After your child begins to learn the steps, you can take turns showing each other "how" to do the routine. Be prepared to provide your child with reminders about what to do. As a child first learns a skill, it's common to forget a step and need assistance. You can simply model and say, "Look, do this," and show how to do the step that is causing difficulty. If needed, you can gently physically guide your child in how to do the step so that he/she can feel successful.

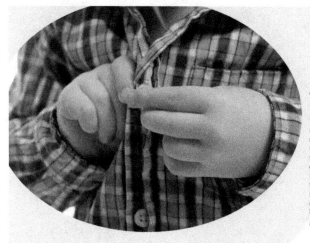

communicate that the task is too difficult. Other children might have challenging behavior because they don't want to leave a preferred activity (e.g., playing with toys) to do something that is less interesting (e.g., taking a bath). If you think you know the "message" of your child's challenging behavior, a good strategy is to validate what the behavior seems to be saying. For example, you might say, "You are telling me that you don't want to stop playing for your bath. But it's time to be all done and get in the tub."

5. For activities that might be difficult or not preferred, state the direction in a "first/then" phrase. For instance, "First wash hands, and then we can eat snack"; or "First brush your teeth, and then I can give you a minty fresh kiss"; or "First get dressed, and then you can choose milk or juice with breakfast."

6. Offering children a "choice" during routines increases the likelihood that they will do the activity. With brushing teeth, you could say, "Do you want to use the mint toothpaste or the bubble gum toothpaste?"

7. It is very important that you encourage all attempts when your child is first learning how to do a routine. If you discourage or reprimand your child because it was not done quite right, his/her attempts at trying might stop. It's important to let your child know you understand his/her feelings and then assist your child so that he/she feels successful. For example, "I know it's hard to brush your teeth. Let me help. (Singing while you help brush) Brush, brush, brush your teeth; brush the front and back . . .

brush, brush, brush your teeth, attack the germs right back." Remember that young children need a lot of practice—and your support—before they are able to do new skills independently.

8. Encourage your child as each routine is completed and celebrate when the task is done.

Why Do Children Sometimes Become Challenging When Learning to Do Self-Help Skills on Their Own?

As children grow, they are learning all kinds of new skills that will help them become more and more independent. A child might be using challenging behavior to communicate a variety of messages. For example, your child might need help with a task, and crying results in your providing that help. Or a child might have a tantrum to

What Can You Do When Children Refuse to Independently Do Daily Routines?

Remember, preschoolers are moving from the toddler stage, where much was done for them, to a new stage where they are becoming independent little people. Your child might need a bit of help or extra cueing when learning new skills that will build his/her ability to be more independent around everyday routines. Think about what your child needs and help him/her be successful...success builds independence! For instance, your child:

- Might want your attention because inappropriate behavior got attention in the past. Your child might refuse to listen or cooperate to gain your attention because this has worked before.
  - Remember to ignore the challenging behavior and teach calmly and clearly while guiding him/her through the task.

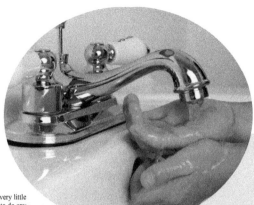

- Praise every little attempt to do any step. Attention to your child's use of a new skill will strengthen that skill.
• Might not understand what you are trying to get him/her to do.
  - Restate your expectation in positive terms and show him/her how, with either photo cues and/or modeling.
• Could need a warning a few minutes prior to the routine.
  - Let him/her know there are only a few more minutes of "play time" and then it's time to ____ (i.e., wash hands, eat dinner, undress/dress, brush teeth, etc.).
• Might not have heard what you asked him/her to do.
  - Gain attention and calmly and clearly restate the direction.
  - Try pairing the verbal direction with a gesture or model.
• Might feel rushed and confused.
  - As children learn new tasks, we need to slow down the routine and expect that it might take extra time to complete.
  - If you are feeling frustrated with your child and think your child is reacting to your

frustration, you might take a few deep breaths to feel calmer. First, take a deep breath in through your nose and out through your mouth several times, and then proceed with clearly stating your expectation to your child.
• Might find the routine too difficult and need some modeling or partial help.
  - First, model how to do the first step and then say, "Now you show me." Show one step at a time, allowing time for your child to process the information and imitate what you did before moving to the next step.
  - If needed, assist your child by gently guiding him/her through the steps.
  - Praise every attempt.

• Might need encouragement and to be validated.
  - You could say, "I see you are sad. This is hard. You can do it. Let me show you how."

It is important to try to understand your child's point of view and feelings. This will help you respond with the most appropriate cue. Encouragement and supporting your child's attempts will build confidence.

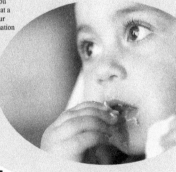

The Center on the Social and Emotional Foundations for Early Learning

Child Care Bureau

Office of Head Start

Appendix E: Responding to Your Child's Bite, Center on the Social and Emotional Foundations for Early Learning (CSEFEL)

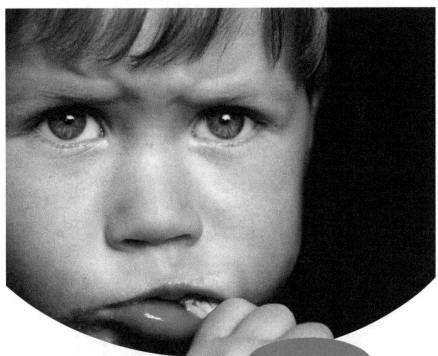

Does this Sound Familiar?

Responding to Your Child's Bite

Marc is preparing dinner and his two children—Jack (3 years) and Jalen (1½ years)—are playing with cars on the kitchen floor. Suddenly, Marc hears a bloodcurdling scream coming from Jack that quickly turns into sobs. Between sobs, Jack shows his dad his arm and slowly says, "He bit me." Jalen has bitten Jack. Marc is frustrated. He doesn't know what to do. Jalen bites often. He bites his brother, other children on the playground, and children in his childcare class. Marc is not sure how to respond. He wonders if he should use "time out" as a consequence, but thinks that Jalen is just too young to understand the relationship between biting and a "time out."

The Center on the Social and Emotional Foundations for Early Learning   Vanderbilt University   vanderbilt.edu/csefel

The Focus

Many toddlers and young children bite. Developmentally, most toddlers don't have enough words to express how they are feeling. They primarily rely on sounds and actions to communicate what they are thinking and feeling. . Biting is one of the ways toddlers express their needs, desires, or feelings. While biting might be very frustrating, your child is not biting purposefully annoy you or hurt anyone. Your child might be biting to say, "I'm scared," "People are crowding me," or, "I'm frustrated." Naturally, parents and caregivers worry that biting might seriously injure another child. And they worry about the negative impact for the biter as well, such as being avoided by other children. The good news is that there are many ways to reduce and to stop a child's biting.

Why Do Children Bite?

Young children bite for many different reasons. Understanding why your toddler might be biting is the first step in reducing or stopping the behavior. The following are some of the reasons young children bite.

- **Communicating frustration**—Many young children bite out of frustration. They often do not know other ways to express their strong feelings. Biting might communicate messages such as, "I don't like that" or "I want that toy" or "You are in my space."

- **Challenges in playing with others**—Some young children can become overwhelmed when playing near or with others. They might not know how to share, take turns, or communicate their wishes or interests.

- **Cause and effect**—Toddlers might bite to see the effect it has on others. They learn quickly that it gets a BIG reaction and has a major impact from both the children they bite and the adults who witness it.

- **Exploration and learning**—One of the most important ways toddlers learn about their world is through their senses. Biting might be a way to find out what an object, or person, feels like. In other words, their biting might be trying to communicate, "You seem interesting. I wonder what you feel and taste like?"

- **Oral stimulation**—Some children bite because they enjoy and seek out the physical sensation of biting or chewing.

- **Teething**—Many children experience pain when they are teething. Biting or chewing on something can help ease the pain of teething.

- **Monkey see, monkey do**—Toddlers love to imitate or copy the behaviors of others. They learn so much by practicing behaviors they observe. For example, if Jalen sees Sara bite and sees that Sara receives quite a bit of attention for biting (even if it is negative attention), Jalen might want to try out that biting behavior to see how the various adults in his life react.

- **Coping with uncomfortable feelings**—When children are hungry, sleepy, bored, or anxious, they are less able to cope with life's ups and downs (for example, a toy being taken, not getting that second cookie after lunch) and might resort to biting instead of finding other ways to express their needs or feelings.

Normal but Unacceptable

While biting is a typical behavior for young children, that doesn't mean it is acceptable. Biting can cause discomfort, angry feelings, and on occasion serious injury. Other children may begin to make negative comments about (e.g., "he's mean") or avoid playing with children who frequently bite. Social reactions such as these can be very harmful to a child's relationships with other children and his feelings about himself.

What Can You Do?

Children can be taught more appropriate ways to express their needs and feelings.

Observe

Observe your child to attempt to understand more about why he/she bites. Identify any patterns, such as what happens before your child bites. Notice when, where, and who your child bites. Does he/she bite when crowded in a small space with other children, or when he/she is hungry or sleepy? Does he/she bite when there are a number of children present or when the noise level is high?

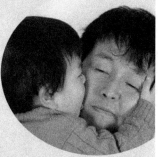

Try to prevent biting

Once you understand why and when your child is likely to bite, you can try to change situations in order to prevent it. The following are just a few ways you can use your observations to this end:

- **If your child seems to bite when frustrated:**
  You can say, "You are so frustrated. You want that toy." Teach your child simple words such as "mine" or "no." Teach some basic sign language or gestures for things like "help" or "stop."

- **If your child seems to bite because he/she is overwhelmed by playing near or with others:** Join your child in play by sitting on the floor and coaching him/her in play. Your child might need help to understand other children's ideas. He/she might also need guidance to learn and practice how to join play, take turns, share, communicate with other children, and get help if he/she needs it. For example, if another child tries to take your child's doll, you might say, "Molly thinks your doll looks fun. She wants to play too. Can we show Molly where the other dolls are?"

- **If you think your child is biting to see what happens when he/she bites:** Clearly and calmly let your child know that biting hurts. Keep your reaction neutral, non-emotional, short, and as uninteresting as possible to avoid teaching that biting has a big effect on the adult. An adult's big reaction can be very rewarding and reinforcing. Encourage your child to experiment with cause and effect in other ways. For example, you might want to show him/her how to wave "bye bye" so that others will wave back, or let your child tickle you and then give him/her a big laughing reaction.

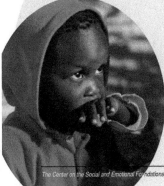

- **If you think your child might be biting for oral stimulation:** Offer crunchy healthy foods such as crackers, rice cakes, or pretzels at snack intervals throughout the day. Or, provide appropriate and interesting items for your child to chew on (e.g., teething toys).

- **If your child is biting because he/she is teething:** Give him/her a teething ring or cloth to chew on. Chilled teethers can also soothe sore gums.

- **If your child tends to bite when he/she is tired:** Provide increased opportunities for your child to rest. Gradually move naps or bedtime up in 10- to 15-minute intervals to earlier times. Ask your child's other caregivers to watch and stay close when he/she seems tired. Minimize stressful or stimulating activities when your child is tired.

- **If you believe your child might be biting when he/she is hungry:** Try to offer more frequent healthy snacks. Show your child what he/she can bite—food.

- **If you believe your child might bite when he/she is bored:** Provide novel, interesting activities and toys to explore and play with. Change the environment as needed (when you see your child becoming bored or unfocused) by rotating toys or going outdoors or into different play spaces.

- **If you believe your child might bite when he/she is anxious:** Talk about any changes he/she might be experiencing. Help your child put words or signs to his/her feelings. Attempt to keep confusion and uncertainty at a minimum by talking about transitions, schedules, plans, etc.

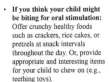

What Can You Do in the Moment When Your Child Bites?

1. Quickly yet calmly remove your child from the person he has bitten. Calmly (e.g., without yelling or scolding), clearly, and firmly say, "Stop. No biting. Biting hurts." Show and explain the effect of the bite on the other child. For example, you might say, "Jack is crying and sad because the bite hurts him."

2. Focus most of your attention on the child who was bitten. Understandably, adults often react strongly to the child who bit as they try to correct the biting behavior. However, even negative attention can encourage the biting. Helping to soothe the child who was bitten teaches empathy and helps the child who bit to understand the power of his actions. It might be helpful to say to the child who was bitten, "I'm so sorry this happened. I know biting really hurts," as a way to model apologies and empathy. Avoid trying to get your child to apologize. While it is important for your child to develop empathy, trying to get your child to apologize typically results in paying more attention to the biter and not the child who was bit.

3. Acknowledge your child's feelings. You might say something like, "You are frustrated. Let's find another way. Touch gently or ask for the toy. You can say, 'Can I have that?'"

4. When your child is calm (not in the heat of the moment), teach him/her other ways to express his/her needs and desires. For example, you might say to your child, "Biting hurts. Next time, if Sienna is grabbing your toy you can say stop or ask a grownup for help." It might be helpful to role play scenarios where your child can practice saying "stop" or "help."

The Center on the Social and Emotional Foundations for Early Learning   Vanderbilt University   vanderbilt.edu/csefel

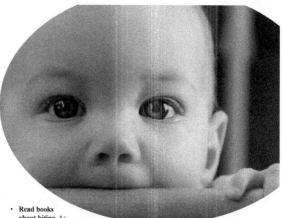

What to Do When Biting Continues

- **Be patient.** It can take time to learn a new way to cope with difficult feelings. Continue to observe and try to understand as best you can the purpose of the biting, the need it is meeting. Stay calm when it happens and focus on teaching your child alternative ways to get needs met. Continue to help put words to your child's experience: "You don't like it when Jalen bites. You can say 'stop.'"

- **Shadow or stay within arm's distance of your child during playtime** with other children and/or at times when you believe your child might be more likely to bite. Staying close gives your child a sense of security and makes it easier to intervene before your child bites.

- **Talk to others who care for your child.** Share with your child's daycare provider or other caregivers the strategies you use when your child bites. Share the observations you have made about when your child seems to be more prone to biting. Ask your childcare provider for help and suggestions for preventing and responding to biting. Try to have all caregivers approach the biting in the same way.

- **Provide your child with education about teeth and what teeth are for.** Teeth are for chewing foods, not people. Offer your child appropriate things to chew.

- **Read books about biting.** As you read, ask your child how the different characters might be feeling. If you have an older toddler, you can ask him/her to "read" the book to you by telling you what is happening based on the pictures. Some recommended titles include

  - *Teeth Are Not for Biting* by Elizabeth Verdick
  - *No Biting* by Karen Katz
  - *No Biting,* Louise by Margie Palatini

What Not to Do

- **Don't bite back.** Biting a child back to show what it feels like creates confusion and fear. Young children often cannot make the connection between why you bit them and their own biting. And it teaches that biting is an acceptable problem-solving method. Biting hurts and can be considered a form of child abuse.

- **Don't use harsh punishment.** Yelling, scolding, lecturing, or using any form of physical punishment has not been demonstrated to reduce biting. Harsh reactions such as these might increase your child's level of anxiety or fear and might cause more biting. They also do not teach children a new skill to use instead of biting.

When to Seek Professional Help

If your child's biting does not decrease over time, you might want to consider seeking guidance from your pediatrician or the nurse in your doctor's office or medical clinic. If your child is enrolled in an early childhood or Head Start program, ask if there is somewhere there who might be able to address the biting or refer you to another professional. A child therapist or a child development professional can help you to sort out potential reasons for your child's biting and to devise a plan to address it.

Portions adapted with permission from "ZERO TO THREE. (n.d.). Chew on This: Responding to Toddlers Who Bite." Retrieved June 5, 2008, from http://www.zerotothree.org/site/PageServer?pagename=ter_key_social_biting&JSevSessionIdr009=4rzxepxog4.app2a

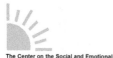

The Center on the Social and Emotional Foundations for Early Learning

Child Care Bureau

Office of Head Start

Appendix F: Making the Most of Playtime, Center on the Social and Emotional Foundations for Early Learning (CSEFEL)

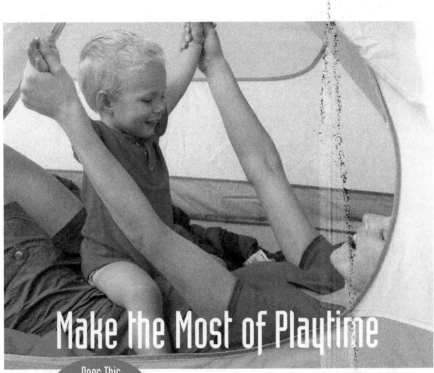

Make the Most of Playtime

Does This Sound Familiar?

Eight-month-old Jamia loves the game of peek-a-boo she and her father play. Jamia's father, Tomas, hides his face behind the couch then pops up and with a big smile says, "Here's Daddy!" Tomas and Jamia repeat the interaction over and over. Each time Tomas pops up from behind the couch, Jamia expresses sheer glee. After a number of repetitions, Tomas becomes tired of the game and is ready to move on to things he needs to do. Once Tomas stops playing and starts to fold laundry, Jamia screams and shrieks, stretching and waving her arms out to her dad as if to say, "Don't stop!" or "More! More!"

Jackson (age 14 months) throws his sippy cup in the trash. His mother, Danette, gently picks it out, washes it off, and hands it back to him. Only seconds later, Jackson throws his sippy cup in the trash again, giving his mother a wide smile. Danette, a bit distracted and frustrated, takes the sippy cup out again, washes it off, and gives it back to him. This time, she scolds Jackson. She tells him the sippy cup doesn't go in the trash and to stop playing in the trash. Before Danette can distract Jackson with another game or remove the trash can to another location, he throws the sippy cup in the trash again. He looks to his mother with another wide smile, appearing proud and eager for her reaction.

The Focus

Babies and toddlers love to play. As a parent, it can feel overwhelming at times. You might feel like your young child thinks everything is a game. Often young children want to repeat their games over and over. They also want to test the boundaries to learn what is appropriate and what is not. For busy parents, this can test your patience. Sometimes it might seem as though your child wants to "play" exactly at the time when you have other things that must be done.

© Springer Nature Switzerland AG 2018

E. I. Girard et al., *Parent-Child Interaction Therapy with Toddlers*,

https://doi.org/10.1007/978-3-319-93251-4

Development of Play Skills for Infants and Toddlers

Babies Birth to 4 Months	• Smile (usually around 6 weeks of age) and begin to coo (make sounds like "oooooo" or "aaaaaa") (usually around 4 months) • Prefer human faces over objects or toys • Turn toward familiar voices and faces • Follow objects with their eyes and recognize familiar faces and objects • Begin to explore their hands by bringing them to their face or putting them in their mouth
Babies 4-7 Months	• Enjoy social games with a caregiver such as peek-a-boo and patty cake • Bring toys to their mouth • Can use their fingers and thumb to pick up objects • Enjoy looking at themselves in a baby-safe mirror • Laugh and babble (saying things like "ba-ba-ba-ba") • Distinguish feelings by listening to the tone of your voice and the voices of other loved ones. (Babies can tell when you are sad, upset, or happy just by the tone of your voice.)
Babies 8-12 Months	• Might begin to make recognizable sounds (like "Ma" or "Da") and repeat or copy sounds/word they hear you say, like "Hi!" or "Bye bye!" • Communicate nonverbally by pointing, gesturing, pulling up, or crawling • Play games such as peek-a-boo and patty cake • Use some objects correctly to imitate actions, like holding a toy phone to their ear or holding a cup to their mouth • Explore objects by shaking or banging them • Might become shy around strangers • Might cry when Mom or Dad or a primary caregiver leaves
Toddlers 13-24 Months	• Enjoy playing with objects such as wooden spoons, cardboard boxes, and empty plastic food containers. Toddlers also enjoy toys like board books, balls, stackable cups or blocks, dolls, simple puzzles, etc. • Have fun filling containers up with water, sand, or toys and then dumping them out • Enjoy watching other children play. Your child might carefully look on or smile as other children play, but might not want to join the group • Usually plays alone or next to other children • Might offer toys to caregivers or other children, but might want them right back • Might choose to play close to other children using the same kind of toy or materials, but not necessarily interact with them • Will struggle with sharing and turn taking
Toddlers 25-36 Months	• Might play with other children but in an occasional, brief, or limited way. For example, a child might play "monsters" or run around chasing other children for a brief period • Older toddlers might begin to cooperate with other toddlers in a shared play activity. For example, children might work together to build a block tower. Or, they might work together to paint a picture together, complete a puzzle, or take on roles and act out a story. One child might pretend to be the "baby," while another is a "mom." • Begin to use their imaginations in their play. For example, toddlers might pretend to give a doll a bottle, pretend to do household chores like cooking or cleaning, or pretend that the shoebox is a garage for toy cars. • Still play alone frequently. • Will struggle with sharing and turn taking.

The Center on the Social and Emotional Foundations for Early Learning   Vanderbilt University   vanderbilt.edu/csefel

Playing with your child in the first three years of life helps the two of you build a warm and loving relationship. Playing together also supports the development of essential social skills (like sharing and turn taking), language skills (like labeling objects, making requests, commenting), and thinking skills (like problem-solving).

For babies and toddlers, play is their "work." It is through play and repetition that babies and toddlers try out and master new skills. Through play, they learn what can happen as a result of an action, explore their imagination and creativity, learn to communicate, and learn about relationships with other people. Any activity can be playful to young children, whether it's a game of peek-a-boo or helping you wipe the table with a sponge. And all types of play help children learn and practice new skills.

As a parent, you are your child's very first and favorite playmate. From the very beginning of his/her life, he/she is playing with you, whether watching your face at meal time or listening to your voice as you sing during a diaper change. Your baby needs you to help him/her learn to play and develop social skills to connect and build friendships with others. As your child grows, he/she will use the skills learned with you and other caregivers to have fun, enjoy, and play with other children. Your child will also learn what is appropriate to play with and what is not. For example, he/she might learn that it is okay to play with a sippy cup but it is not okay to put it in the trash.

Playtime is special. Playing together with your child is not only fun, but a critical time to support your baby or toddler's healthy development. Making time to play with your child each day is not always easy. However, setting aside a brief period every day to play together goes a long way in building a loving relationship between you and your child. Making time for play, especially active play, can also help in reducing your child's challenging behavior.

So what can you do to make the most of your child's playtime? Check out the tips below.

Follow Your Child's Lead

Provide an object, toy, or activity for your baby or toddler and then see what he/she does with it. When your child plays, it's okay if it's not the "right" way...let him/her show you a "new way." For example, when you hand your child a plastic cup, instead of pretending to drink from it, he/she might put it on his/her head as a "party hat". Support your child's creativity and join in the birthday play.

Go Slowly

It's great to show your child how a toy works, but try to hold off on "doing it for him/her" every time. You can begin something, such as stacking one block on another, and then encourage your child to give it a try. Providing just enough help to keep frustration at bay motivates your child to learn new skills.

Read Your Child's Signals

Your little one might not be able to tell you with words when he/she's had enough or when he/she's frustrated. But your child has other ways—like using sounds, facial expressions, and gestures. Reading these signals can also tell you what activities your child prefers. Reading the signals that come before a tantrum help you know when to jump in or change to a new activity.

Look at Your Play Space

Is the area where you play child-friendly and child-safe? Is there too much noise or other distractions? Is the area safe to explore? Is this a good place for the activity you've chosen, such as running, throwing balls, or painting? Checking out your space beforehand can prevent a tantrum, an accident, or a broken lamp.

Play It Again, Sam

While doing things over and over again is not necessarily thrilling for Mom and Dad, it is for young children. They are practicing in order to master a challenge. And when your child can do it "all by myself!" he/she is rewarded with a powerful sense of his/her own skills and abilities—the confidence that he/she is a smart and successful being. The more children have a chance to practice and master new skills, the more likely they are to take on new challenges and learn new things. So when you're tempted to hide that toy because you don't think you can stand playing with it one more time, remember how important repetition is to your child's development.

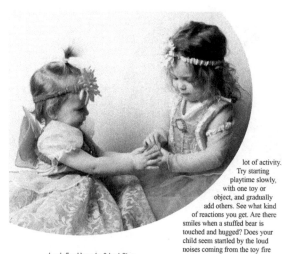

Ideas for How to Play With Your Child

Sometimes it is difficult to figure out how to play with a very young child, especially if he/she is too young to play with toys or other children. Remember that your smile and attention are your baby's favorite "toys." Watch for your child's cues that he/she is ready to play. Play when he/she is calm, alert and content. Let him/her cuddle and rest when he/she is tired, fussy, or hungry. Below are just a few ideas to spark your own playtime adventures.

For Babies Under 6 Months

- Imitate the sounds your baby makes and try to have a "conversation" with your baby as you coo or babble back and forth to each other.
- Sing your favorite songs or lullabies to your baby.
- Talk to your baby about what you are doing. You might say, "I'm starting to cook dinner. First I wash my hands, etc." or "I'm going to change your diaper now. First we take off your pants."
- Talk to your baby about his/her surroundings, for example, "Look at your brother—he is laughing and having so much fun!" or "Look at those bright lights."
- Read to your baby. Point out bright colored pictures with contrasting bright colors.
- Let your baby touch objects with different textures. Hold a toy within reach so he/she can swat it with his/her hands or feet.

Look For Ways to Adapt Play Activities to Meet Your Child's Needs

All children learn through play, and any play activity can be adapted to meet a child's unique needs. The suggestions below can help parents of children with special needs as well as other parents think about how to make playtime enjoyable and appropriate to their child's skills, preferences, and abilities.

- **Think about the environment.** How do variables like sound or light affect your child? What is the background noise like in your play area? Is there a television or radio on? Are there many other kids around? If your child seems distressed during playtime, and you've tried everything else, move to a quieter, less stimulating area to play.
- **How does your child respond to new things?** Some infants and toddlers, particularly if they have a special need, are easily overstimulated, while others enjoy a lot of activity. Try starting playtime slowly, with one toy or object, and gradually add others. See what kind of reactions you get. Are there smiles when a stuffed bear is touched and hugged? Does your child seem startled by the loud noises coming from the toy fire engine?
- **How does your child react to different textures, smells, and tastes?** For example, some objects might be particularly enjoyable for your little one to touch and hold. Others might "feel funny" to them. Read your child's signals and change the materials you are using accordingly.
- **Involve peers.** It is important for children to establish relationships with other children their age. Encourage siblings to play together. Arrange times to play with other children or family members. Check out opportunities to play with other kids at the park or during free public library story hours. Having fun with peers is an important way for children to learn social skills like sharing, problem solving, and understanding others' feelings—and also helps prepare children for the school setting later on.

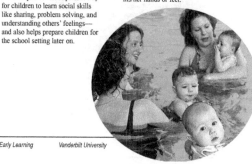

For Babies 6 to 12 Months

- Start a bedtime routine that includes time to interact with your baby and read or describe pictures from books.
- Use bath time as a time to gently splash, pour, and explore the water.
- Play peek-a-boo by covering your face and then removing your hands while you say, "Surprise!" or "Peek-a-boo!" and make a surprised facial expression.
- Hide your child's favorite toy under a blanket and ask him/her where the toy went. Encourage your child to look for it and/or help him/her find it. You can ask, "Where did your bear go? Is it on the couch? Is it behind the pillow? Oh, here it is under the blanket!"
- Play hide and seek. "Hide" yourself (leave lots of you showing!), and if your child is crawling, encourage him/her to come and find you.

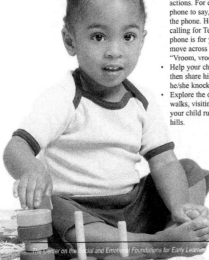

- Imitate your child's sounds. Encourage a dialogue by taking turns listening and copying each other's sounds.
- Use containers to fill with objects like toys or sand, and dump them out. You might use a shoebox with soft foam blocks or other baby-safe small toys.

For Toddlers 12-24 Months

- Sing special songs while changing a diaper or getting ready for bed.
- Keep reading and talking together. When looking at a book, ask your child questions about the pictures like, "Where is the doggy?" Show your excitement by acknowledging when your child points to the object: "Yes, you know where the doggy is!"
- Hide behind a door, the couch, or the high chair, then pop up and say, "Surprise!" If your child enjoys this game, change the location where you pop up. For example, if you usually pop up from under the high chair, try popping up from under the table. This switch will delight him/her!
- Use play objects to act out pretend actions. For example, use a toy phone to say, "Ring ring ring. It's the phone. Hello. Oh, you are calling for Teddy. Teddy, the phone is for you." Use a toy car to move across the floor saying, "Vroom, vroom, go car go!"
- Help your child stack blocks and then share his/her excitement when he/she knocks it down.
- Explore the outdoors by taking walks, visiting a park, or helping your child run up or down grassy hills.

For Toddlers 24-36 Months

- Continue to read and talk often to your child. When looking at books together, give your child time to look at the pictures before reading the words. Begin to ask questions about the book such as, "Why did he do that?", "What happens next?", and "Where did she go?"
- Dance and jump around to music and encourage your child to join you.
- Support your child's imagination by providing dress-up clothes like scarves, hats, pocketbooks, or your old shoes; and props such as plastic kitchen bowls and plates, or toy musical instruments.
- Encourage your child's creativity by playing with crayons, markers, play dough, finger paint, paints, etc.
- Use play objects that look like the "real" thing: child-sized brooms and dust pans, pots and pans, toy cash registers, etc.

What can you do when your child's play is inappropriate or dangerous (e.g., throwing the sippy cup in the trash, pulling at the lamp, etc.)?

- Try to give your child an acceptable way to meet his/her goal. For example, show him/her how to throw the ball into a laundry basket instead of into the trash.
- Use words to validate your child's desires: "You want to pull that lamp. You want to see what will happen. You are playing a game. You want me to come close and play with you."
- Show your child what he/she can do: "You can put it in this basket"; "You can put the socks in the hamper"; "You can push this block tower down."
- Distract or redirect your child to another toy or game with you: "Look at this toy." "Do you see how this toy moves?"

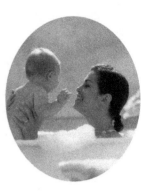

- When you tell your child, "No" or "No touch, it is dangerous," direct him/her to what he/she can do: "No touch, look with your eyes."
- Remove the object, if possible, to make the play area more child-friendly.
- Remove the child from the area or activity: "Let's play over here instead."
- Use humor and join the game: "You just want me to come chase you. Now I'm going to tickle you."

What happens when my baby or toddler has difficulty moving on from play time? What if, like Jamia, she doesn't want to stop?

- Tell your child when a transition is coming: "one more time," "last time."
- Give your child a visual reminder of the transition. Set a kitchen timer or egg timer for "two more minutes" or "five more minutes."
- Explain what is happening: "I have to stop playing now. I have to make dinner."

- Provide an alternative activity: "I can't play anymore, but you can sit at the table while I cook and color with crayons."
- Provide a choice: "You can do a puzzle or play with cars."
- Use words to validate your child's feelings: "You want to play longer." "Again? You want to do it again." "You feel sad that it is time to leave the park."
- If your child becomes upset, validate his/her feelings and try to provide words of comfort: "I know you are mad because I have to change your diaper now. You want to keep playing. We'll play again after your diaper change."

Adapted with permission from: "ZERO TO THREE. (n.d.) Make the most of play time." Retrieved May 22, 2008, from www.zerotothree.org/site/PageServer ?pagename=ter_key_play_tips&Add Interest=1154

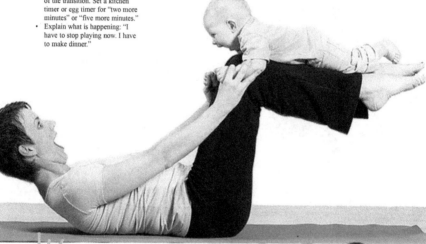

The Center on the Social and Emotional Foundations for Early Learning

Child Care
Bureau

Office of
Head Start

Appendix G: Toddler Book Suggestions, Parents Magazine

Toddler Book Suggestions

Source: Parents Magazine

http://www.parents.com/fun/entertainment/books/best-toddler-books/?slideId=39592

Book Title	Author
The Very Hungry Caterpillar	Eric Carle
We're going on a Bear Hunt	Michael Rosen & Helen Oxenbury
Freight Train	Donald Crews
The Napping House	Audrey Wood
The Happy Egg	Ruth Krauss
Fast Food	Saxton Freymann
Yummy Yucky	Leslie Patricelli
Where's My Teddy	Jez Alborough
Counting Kisses	Karen Katz
Sheep in the Jeep	Nancy Shaw
Baby Happy, Baby Sad	Leslie Patricelli
Green Eggs and Ham	Dr. Seuss
Corduroy	Don Freeman
How I became a Pirate	Melinda Long
The Family Book	Todd Parr
Are You My Mother?	P.D. Eastman
Diary of a Worm	Doreen Cronin
Walter the Farting Dog	William Kotzwinkle & Glen Murray
Cookie Count: A Tasty Pop-Up	Robert Sabuda
I Hope You Dance	Mark D. Sanders & Tia Sillers
The Big Shiny Sparkly First Words Book	Willabel Tong
I Know a Rhino	Charles Fuge
Baby Beluga	Raffi
Brown Bear, Brown Bear, What Do You See?	Bill Martin Jr.
A Pocket for Corduroy	Don Freeman

© Springer Nature Switzerland AG 2018
E. I. Girard et al., *Parent-Child Interaction Therapy with Toddlers*,
https://doi.org/10.1007/978-3-319-93251-4

Appendix H: Developmental Tip of the Day Cards

The developmental tip cards presented are derived from the incredible work produced by the University of Minnesota in their reference material entitled, "Positive Discipline: A Guide for Parents." This complete work can be found at https://www.extension.umn.edu/family/school-success/professionals/tools/positive-discipline/docs/positive-discipline-guide-english.pdf.

Toddler Tip of the Day!

Most toddlers will not understand how to share. Parents can demonstrate sharing and praise their children when they do. Be sure to have lots of items around so sharing is not always necessary.

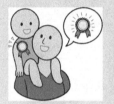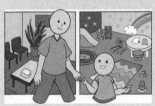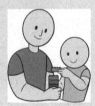

Toddler Tip of the Day!

Talk and read to toddlers often. Their vocabularies are still growing. The more words they learn early on, the more words they will be able to understand as they grow.

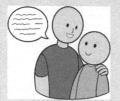 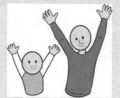 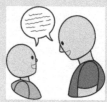

Toddler Tip of the Day!

Toddlers are always on the move. Be sure to pack extra activities or food to keep toddlers busy when you need them to be still and calm. Try singing songs or playing games to help them wait.

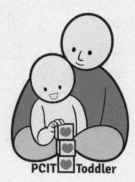

PCIT♥Toddler

Toddler Tip of the Day!

Toddlers are still learning how to control their emotions. When they are hungry, sleepy, have a dirty diaper, or need attention, they may tantrum. Think about and try to satisfy their need in the moment to help them calm down.

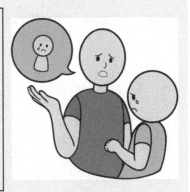

Toddler Tip of the Day!

Children often begin to toilet train around the age of 2. Never reprimand a child for having an accident. Accidents are an expected part of the toilet training process.

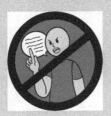 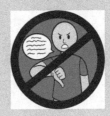

Toddler Tip of the Day!

Toddlers thrive on routine. Try to structure aspects of each day (nap time, bath time) similarly so your child knows what to expect.

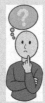 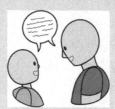 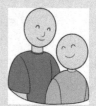

Toddler Tip of the Day!

It is a toddler's job to explore. Sometimes this can result in a mess. Be sure your child is safe at all times. Keep items that are not safe away from toddlers.

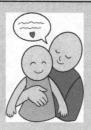 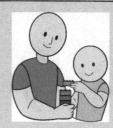

Toddler Tip of the Day!

Parenting can be very tiring. Be sure to give yourself a break to relax when others are available to care for your toddler.

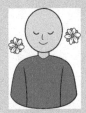 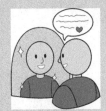

Toddler Tip of the Day!

Toddlers learn by copying what they see and hear around them. Behave how you want your child to behave.

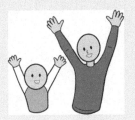 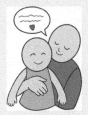

Appendix I: Additional Resources

Useful websites with parent handouts related to a variety of child behaviors, emotions, and daily tasks include video modules and examples:

- Center on the Social and Emotional Foundations for Early Learning: http://csefel. vanderbilt.edu/resources/family.html
- Child Development Video (University of Minnesota Institute of Child Development):
  - Part One: https://www.youtube.com/watch?v=SpqLzFew9bs
  - Part Two: https://www.youtube.com/watch?v=u0_Y7jSGnp8
  - Part Three: https://www.youtube.com/watch?v=kivv2BJhzbA
  - Part Four: https://www.youtube.com/watch?v=20DdwzhMTTA
- Positive Discipline:
  - https://www.extension.umn.edu/family/school-success/professionals/tools/ positive-discipline/docs/positive-discipline-guide-english.pdf
- Helping Children to Regulate Emotions:
  - https://www.zerotothree.org/espanol/challenging-behaviors

References

Center on the Social and Emotional Foundations for Early Learning. *Make the most of playtime*. Retrieved from http://csefel.vanderbilt.edu/documents/make_the_ most_of_playtime2.pdf

Center on the Social and Emotional Foundations for Early Learning. *Responding to your child's bite*. Retrieved from http://csefel.vanderbilt.edu/documents/biting-parenting_tool.pdf

© Springer Nature Switzerland AG 2018   359

E. I. Girard et al., *Parent-Child Interaction Therapy with Toddlers*,

https://doi.org/10.1007/978-3-319-93251-4

Center on the Social and Emotional Foundations for Early Learning. *Teaching your child to become independent with daily routines.* Retrieved from http://csefel.vanderbilt.edu/documents/teaching_routines.pdf

Center on the Social and Emotional Foundations for Early Learning. *Understanding your child's behavior: Reading your child's cues from birth to age 2.* Retrieved from http://csefel.vanderbilt.edu/documents/reading_cues.pdf

Karitane. (2018). *Resources.* Retrieved from https://karitane.com.au/page/our-services/resources

Parents.com. *The all-time best books for toddlers.* Retrieved from https://www.parents.com/fun/entertainment/books/best-toddler-books/?slideId=39592

Index

E. I. Girard et al., *Parent-Child Interaction Therapy with Toddlers*,
https://doi.org/10.1007/978-3-319-93251-4